Opportunistic Pathogens

Edited by
James E. Prier and Herman Friedman

UNIVERSITY PARK PRESS
Baltimore · London · Tokyo

UNIVERSITY PARK PRESS
International Publishers in Science and Medicine
Chamber of Commerce Building
Baltimore, Maryland 21202

Copyright © 1974 by University Park Press
ISBN 0-8391-0710-2

Printed in the United States of America by the Maple Press Company

Second printing, June 1976

All rights, including that of translation into other languages, reserved. Photomechanical reproduction (photocopy, microcopy) of this book or parts thereof without special permission of the publisher is prohibited.

Library of Congress Cataloging in Publication Data

American Society for Microbiology. Eastern
 Pennsylvania Branch.
 Opportunistic pathogens.

  "Fourth Annual symposium of the Eastern Pennsylvania Branch of the American Society for Microbiology, held in Philadelphia on November 2–3, 1972."
  1. Medical microbiology—Technique—Congresses. 2. Micro organisms, Pathogenic—Identification—Congresses. I. Prier, James E., ed. II. Friedman, Herman S., ed. III. Title. DNLM: 1. Cross infection—Congresses. 2. Infection—Congresses.   3. Microbiology—Congresses.   QW 4 S9890 1972
QR46.A49   616.01   73-6708

Contents

Participants ix

Introduction xiii

1. **Superinfection: A Partial Overview** · *Donald B. Louria*   1
   - I. Superinfection in patients whose lives are prolonged by therapy
   - II. The influence of antibiotic therapy on the incidence of superinfection
   - III. Adrenal hormones
   - IV. Needles and catheters
   - V. Antitumor agents
   - VI. Transplantation
   - VII. Superinfection arising in a geographically non-endemic area
   - VIII. Unnecessary environmental exposure
   - IX. The problem of dual superinfection
   - X. Use of hypertonic media to detect superinfection
   - XI. The necessity for a close liaison between the laboratory and the clinicians

2. **Culture and Identification of Commonly Encountered Gram-negative Bacilli:** *Pseudomonas, Klebsiella-Enterobacter, Serratia, Proteus,* **and** *Providencia* · *Robert B. Lindberg*   19

Contents

3. **Opportunistic Pathogens: Immunological Aspects** · *Erwin Neter*   37

4. **Bacteriocin Typing of** *Pseudomonas, Proteus,* **and** *Klebsiella-Enterobacter-Serratia* · *J. J. Farmer, III*   49
   - I. Bacteriocin production–scrape and streak method
   - II. Bacteriocin production–growth in broth method
   - III. Bacteriocin sensitivity
   - IV. Reporting bacteriocin production or bacteriocin sensitivity patterns
   - V. Automated application of bacteriocins
   - VI. Computer selection of bacteriocin indicators or producers
   - VII. Application of bacteriocin typing–investigating the known outbreak
   - VIII. Application of bacteriocin typing–determining cause of cross-infection
   - IX. Bacteriocin typing of *P. aeruginosa*
   - X. Typing *Proteus* by bacteriocin production
   - XI. Typing *Klebsiella-Enterobacter-Serratia* by bacteriocin production or sensitivity

5. **Miscellaneous Facultatively Anaerobic Bacilli in Opportunistic Infections** · *Alexander von Graevenitz*   65
   - I. Nonfastidious, Gram-negative opportunists
   - II. Fastidious opportunists

6. **Anaerobic Bacteria: Culture and Identification** · *Earle H. Spaulding, Valerie Vargo, Thomas C. Michaelson, Myroslawa Korzeniowski, and Robert M. Swenson*   87
   - I. Methods used by the Anaerobe Laboratory
   - II. Methods used by the Diagnostic Laboratory
   - III. Results of comparative study
   - IV. Summary of results

Contents

7. **Antibiotic Susceptibility Testing of Anaerobic Bacteria** · *Tracy D. Wilkins*   105
   I. Antibiotics used
   II. Methods for antibiotic susceptibility testing
   III. Summary of current status

8. **In Vitro Susceptibility Tests of Opportunistic Pathogens: A Clinical Appraisal** · *Robert M. Swenson*   119
   I. Methods of susceptibility testing
   II. Technical considerations of disc diffusion tests
   III. Interpretation of zone size–MIC values
   IV. Correlation of microbial susceptibility and clinical response

9. **Identification and Ecology of Yeasts of Medical Importance** · *Donald G. Ahearn*   129
   I. Introduction
   II. Methods
   III. Ecology of principal pathogens
   IV. Classification

10. **Serodiagnosis of Opportunistic Mycoses** · *Morris A. Gordon*   147
    I. Introduction
    II. Cryptococcosis
    III. Candidiasis
    IV. Torulopsosis
    V. Aspergillosis
    VI. Mucormycosis
    VII. Immunoelectroosmophoresis

11. **Opportunistic Phycomycetes and Aspergilli in the Compromised Host** · *Roger Denio Baker*   163
    I. Mucormycosis
    II. Aspergillosis
    III. Mechanisms of opportunism

12. *Nocardia* Species as Opportunists and Current Methods for Their Identification · *Lucille K. Georg*   177

    I. *Nocardia* species as opportunists
    II. Current methods for the isolation and identification of *Nocardia* species from clinical materials
    III. Appendix

13. Toxoplasmosis and Pneumocystosis: Clinical and Laboratory Aspects in Immunocompetent and Compromised Hosts · *J. K. Frenkel*   203

    I. Introduction
    II. Toxoplasmosis
    III. Pneumocystosis

14. Cytomegalovirus, A Model for Herpesvirus Opportunism · *John L. Randall and Stanley A. Plotkin*   261

    I. Clinical manifestations of herpes agents
    II. Epidemiology and biology
    III. Pathology, classification, and morphology
    IV. Cytomegalovirus

15. Control of Opportunistic Infections in Hospitals—A Position Paper · *N. Joel Ehrenkranz, George W. Counts, J. Leilani Kicklighter, and Phineas J. Hyams*   281

    I. Introduction
    II. Organization of the Infection Control Service
    III. Responsibilities of the Infection Control Service
    IV. Summary

Index   295

Opportunistic Pathogens

Fourth Annual Symposium of the Eastern Pennsylvania Branch of the American Society for Microbiology, held in Philadelphia

PROGRAM CHAIRMAN: Earle H. Spaulding

CONFERENCE COORDINATOR: Josephine Bartola

SYMPOSIUM CHAIRMAN: Jay E. Satz, Ph.D.

SYMPOSIUM SPONSORS:
Bureau of Laboratories, Pennsylvania Department of Health, Philadelphia
Department of Microbiology, Hahnemann Medical College and Hospital, Philadelphia
Flow Laboratories, Rockville, Maryland

CONTRIBUTORS:
Cooke Laboratory Products, Alexandria, Virginia
Hotpack Corporation, Philadelphia

Participants

AHEARN, DONALD G., Ph.D.
Department of Biology
Georgia State University
Atlanta, Georgia

BAKER, ROGER DENIO, M.D.
College of Medicine and Dentistry of New Jersey
Rutgers Medical School
Piscataway, New Jersey

BARTOLA, JOSEPHINE, M. A.
Bureau of Laboratories
Pennsylvania Department of Health
Philadelphia, Pennsylvania

COUNTS, GEORGE W., M.D.
Assistant Professor of Pathology and Medicine
University of Miami School of Medicine, and
Director of Infectious Control Department
Jackson Memorial Hospital
Miami, Florida

EHRENKRANZ, N. JOEL, M.D.
Professor and Chief of Medicine
Cedars of Lebanon Hospital
University of Miami School of Medicine
Miami, Florida

Participants

FARMER, JOHN J., III, Ph.D.
Bacteriophage-Bacteriocin Laboratory
Enteric Unit
Center for Disease Control
Atlanta, Georgia

FRENKEL, JACOB K., M.D., Ph.D.
Department of Pathology and Oncology
University of Kansas Medical Center
Kansas City, Kansas

FRIEDMAN, HERMAN, Ph.D.
Head, Department of Microbiology
Albert Einstein Medical Center, and
Associate Professor
Temple University School of Medicine
Philadelphia, Pennsylvania

GEORG, LUCILLE K., Ph.D.
Mycology Branch
Center for Disease Control
Atlanta, Georgia

GORDON, MORRIS A., Ph.D.
Division of Laboratories and Research
New York State Department of Health
Albany, New York

HYAMS, PHINEAS J., M.D.
Assistant Professor of Medicine
University of Miami School of Medicine, and
Hospital Epidemiologist
Jackson Memorial Hospital
Miami, Florida

KICKLIGHTER, J. LEILANI, R.N.
Infectious Control Coordinator
Cedars of Lebanon Hospital
Miami, Florida

Participants

KORZENIOWSKI, MYROSLAWA, B.S.
Anaerobe Laboratory
Department of Microbiology
Temple University Health Sciences Center
Philadelphia, Pennsylvania

LINDBERG, ROBERT B., Ph.D.
Chief, Microbiology Department
U. S. Army Institute of Surgical Research
Fort Sam Houston, Texas

LOURIA, DONALD B., M.D.
Professor and Chairman
Department of Preventive Medicine and Community Health
New Jersey Medical School
Newark, New Jersey

MICHAELSON, THOMAS C., M.D.
Anaerobe Laboratory
Department of Microbiology
Temple University Health Sciences Center
Philadelphia, Pennsylvania

NETER, ERWIN, M.D.
Professor of Microbiology
State University of New York at Buffalo
Buffalo, New York

PLOTKIN, STANLEY, M.D.
Associate Professor of Pediatrics
University of Pennsylvania, and
Director of Infectious Diseases
Children's Hospital of Philadelphia, and
Associate Member
Wistar Institute
Philadelphia, Pennsylvania

PRIER, JAMES E., D.V.M., Ph.D.
Director, Bureau of Laboratories
Pennsylvania Department of Health, and
Adjunct Professor of Microbiology
Temple University School of Medicine
Philadelphia, Pennsylvania

Participants

RANDALL, JOHN L., M.D.
Attending Physician, Pediatrics
Philadelphia General Hospital, and
Department of Infectious Diseases
Children's Hospital of Philadelphia
Philadelphia, Pennsylvania

SPAULDING, EARLE H., Ph.D.
Anaerobe Laboratory
Department of Microbiology
Temple University Health Sciences Center
Philadelphia, Pennsylvania

SWENSON, ROBERT M., M.D.
Assistant Professor of Medicine and Microbiology, and
Head, Section of Infectious Diseases
Temple University Health Sciences Center
Philadelphia, Pennsylvania

VARGO, VALERIE, M.S.
Anaerobe Laboratory
Department of Microbiology
Temple University Health Sciences Center
Philadelphia, Pennsylvania

VON GRAEVENITZ, ALEXANDER, M.D.
Departments of Laboratory Medicine and Microbiology
Yale University School of Medicine
New Haven, Connecticut

WILKINS, TRACY D., Ph.D.
Anaerobe Laboratory
Division of Basic Sciences
College of Agriculture
Virginia Polytechnic Institute and State University
Blacksburg, Virginia

Introduction

Earle H. Spaulding

Opportunistic infections, particularly in hospitalized individuals, have become major infectious disease problems in recent years. Furthermore, this problem is likely to continue because of the increasing use of instrumentation, antibiotics, and drugs which either bypass or reduce the level of natural resistance and/or the specific immune mechanisms of the host. Thus, microorganisms previously considered as innocuous commensals or contaminants now are able to multiply extensively in the tissue and cause disease which often may be severe.

The emergence of one opportunistic pathogen after another has also created problems for many clinical laboratory microbiologists, who frequently have not been able to keep up with the literature and do not know when to look for opportunists, how to recognize them, or what pitfalls there are in laboratory methods. The primary objective of this conference, therefore, was to review the present state of knowledge, especially from the point of view of the laboratory.

The second objective was to provide practical information which we can put to use in our laboratories. The panel of speakers was selected with this objective in mind, for all of them have acquired the expertise which comes from practical experience with the opportunists they will discuss.

The third objective of this symposium was to make it both a rewarding, educational experience and a pleasant one as well. The large attendance was evidence that the subject is of far-reaching interest.

This will not be the last symposium on opportunistic pathogens. A repeated theme throughout this one is the changing etiology and nature of infectious disease because of the emergence of new pathogens. I cite the frequency of reference to medically exotic genera such as *Erwinia, Yersinia, Herbicola-Lathyri* group, *Aeromonas, Pneumocystis, Torulopsis, Rhizopus,* cytomegalic virus, and so on.

The etiology and nature of opportunistic infections will continue to change, and the incidence is likely to rise even more as advances in the technology of medicine succeed in prolonging lives of individuals but at the same time compromise their abilities to resist and overcome infectious disease. Today, these compromising agents are instrumentation, such as with catheters or inhalation therapy machines, and administration of antibiotics, steroids, or immunosuppressants; tomorrow, there may be other attempts to abrogate the laws of immunology.

There probably is no other component of the biological world so resilient and so adaptable to environmental change as the microbial one. Microbes often exist as enormous populations which spin off, faster than do other forms of life, low-frequency mutants with selective advantage when there is environmental change. Thus, they often have the capacity as a population to develop resistance to antibiotics. The capacity of opportunists to do so is even greater than that of most bacteria, for they are generally hardy, saprophytic types with a higher innate resistance to such agents. Furthermore, they are able to multiply rapidly in the nutritionally rich tissues of the human host, especially in one whose defense mechanisms are jeopardized.

As a result, we in the laboratory are faced with the prospect of encountering a continuum of uncommon, and sometimes bizarre, species. Thus, we must maintain the "prepared mind" and learn to ask ourselves whether the diptheroid "contaminant" in a blood culture could really be a *Listeria*, whether the mold "contaminant" from a wound actually may have been in the specimen, whether the yeast-like organism from sputum may in fact represent an aberrant *Cryptococcus*.

One of the contributions of this symposium, at least for me, is to point up certain developments in technology which promise to be valuable additions to our laboratory methodology. I suggest

Introduction

you watch the literature during the ensuing months for progress in the development of bacteriocin typing (Farmer), the use of hypertonic media (Louria) and fluorescent antibody for the identification of anaerobes (Dowell), as well as increasing application of the approach described by Neter in which the patient's own blood is examined for passive hemagglutination for antibody response to antigens of opportunistic pathogens.

It is clear that the clinical laboratories will be adopting more sophisticated methods in the future to keep pace with advancing knowledge and technology. I predict that gas-liquid chromatography will become standard procedure for the identification of some types of microorganisms, including opportunists. There will be increasing use of paper chromatography too. In immunoserology laboratories, application of counter-immunoelectrophoresis will become relatively commonplace (Gordon).

I see also an increasingly more responsible role for clinical microbiologists in the hospital setting. Both Drs. Louria and Swenson, as clinicians, emphasized their dependency on the laboratory and therefore the importance to them of good-quality laboratory work. The complexities of the host-parasite relationships being produced by iatrogenic measures are making clinical understanding of the infectious process very difficult indeed, and thus clinicians are being forced into even greater dependency on the laboratory.

Hospitals, in general, have only begun to establish meaningful programs of infection control, and the microbiology laboratory should play a central role in these procedures (Ehrenkranz). In order to function effectively in these areas, we must try to keep abreast of advancing knowledge and new techniques. One way to do this, of course, is to read the literature diligently. Another way is to attend symposia such as this one. Today's research methods become tomorrow's diagnostic tools. The discussions presented here surely will bring about some improvement in the level of performance in the considerable number of laboratories represented at this symposium. Since these laboratories are, for the most part, involved directly in support of physicians, this symposium has made a contribution toward fulfillment of our collective professional obligation to society, i.e., improvement in the delivery of health care.

1

Superinfection: A Partial Overview

Donald B. Louria

Superinfection is clearly an increasing problem in the United States. In part, the increase is apparent because of our ability to better define underlying abnormalities. Thus, for example, a decade ago, we would not have considered *Serratia* bacteremia in a child as a form of superinfection; rather, it would have been thought of as a strange and unusual occurrence in an otherwise apparently normal individual. Now, the occurrence of this type of infection prompts an immediate search for a leukocyte defect, such as the inability to generate hydrogen peroxide, as in chronic granulomatous disease of childhood. Similarly, chronic severe mucocutaneous candidiasis was considered to be a disease of those who were otherwise healthy. However, we now know that some of those apparently healthy individuals suffer from serious defects in delayed immune mechanisms. Patients suffering from bacteremia because of chronic granulomatous disease of childhood or acquiring candidiasis because of defects in delayed immune mechanisms are now considered as examples of superinfection. Thus, some of the increased prevalence of superinfection is, in reality, merely recognition of specific, infection-promoting, underlying diseases.

Nevertheless, there also appears to have been a definite increase in the incidence of superinfection because of prolongation of life in persons with severe underlying diseases, use of antibiotics and adrenal steroids, administration of antitumor agents, and immunosuppressive therapy during transplantation.

I. Superinfection in Patients Whose Lives Are Prolonged by Therapy

The best example in this category is acute leukemia. Most patients dying of acute leukemia suffer from bacterial infections. Additionally, they have a substantial incidence of fungal superinfection, especially that attributable to species of *Candida*, *Mucor*, and *Aspergillus*. The increase in *Candida* infection has been particularly emphasized by Bodey (1). He found that, during the 1954–1958 period, 7% of patients dying with acute leukemia had severe *Candida* infection. During the next five-year period, the prevalence of serious candidiasis increased to 20%.

A similar striking increase has been reported in the incidence of mucormycosis and aspergillosis in leukemia patients (2, 3). With both fungi, there is a striking proclivity for vascular invasion. Currently, however, the greatest problem for the acute leukemic is still overwhelming bacterial sepsis. Recent studies suggest that not only have Gram-negative organisms replaced staphylococci as the most frequent invader, but, in addition, one among the Gram-negatives, *Pseudomonas*, shows increasing predominance. It was thought that the propensity to bacterial superinfection was related almost exclusively to the profound leukopenia and lack of mature polymorphonuclear leukocytes capable of performing phagocytosis, but studies from the Memorial Hospital in New York City now suggest that, in addition to polymorphonuclear leukocyte defects, there is a deficiency in heat-stable opsonins that predisposes to severe infections with species of both *Pseudomonas* and *Aeromonas* (4, 5).

Those suffering from acute leukemia and under treatment are also inordinately susceptible to infections with cytomegaloviruses and *Pneumocystis carinii*.

The unanswered question is "how much of the increased infection is due to longer life in the leukemia patient and how much is due to the multiple agents administered to these patients?" Thus far, no prospective study has been carried out that might answer the question; indeed, even a prospective study might not separate the influences of leukemia and its therapies. The prevailing opinion is that most of the infections, particularly those due to fungi, *Pneumocystis*, and cytomegaloviruses, result from treatment. Even the bacterial superinfections may be treatment induced; for example, the defect in heat-stable opsonins associated with *Pseudomonas* infections most probably occurs as a consequence of antileukemia therapy.

Lymphoma presents a strikingly different picture. It is clear that in this group of reticuloendothelial malignancies, especially in the Hodgkin's variety, the patient is prone to certain superinfections even if no treatment is given. Such patients, unlike the acute leukemic, have no defects in polymorphonuclear leukocyte function, and in most cases there is no defect in immunoglobulins. On the other hand, characteristically, delayed immune mechanisms are impaired. The resulting infections are the following: *Mycobacterium tuberculosis, Cryptococcus neoformans, Toxoplasma gondii, Listeria monocytogenes, Nocardia asteroides*, and occasionally either *Histoplasma capsulatum* or *Coccidioides immitis*.

It is clearly important to keep the differences in susceptibility in mind. We have made unnecessary errors in presumptive diagnoses merely because we ignored the setting in which superinfection occurred. Thus, in a patient with lymphoma who is not leukopenic or hypogammaglobulinemic, there is little likelihood of *Aspergillus, Candida,* or *Pseudomonas* infection, but there is a considerable possibility of cryptococcal or nocardial superinfection.

II. The Influence of Antibiotic Therapy on the Incidence of Superinfection

For the last decade, we have been interested in the incidence of superinfection following various antibiotic regimens. In an attempt to introduce quantitative data, we homogenized sputum, serially diluted the homogenate, and plated the various dilutions on various aerobic media. The results of several studies are summarized in Table 1. In these studies, bacteriological superinfection was defined as the appearance of new organisms (Gram-negatives and/or staphylococci) in the sputum in a five-day period, in a titer of at least 10^5 per ml in pure culture, or, if in higher titer in mixed culture, the Gram-negative organism or *Staphylococcus* had to be in clear numerical predominance to be considered as superinfection. If only small numbers of new organisms were found or if the newly found organisms were not in numerical predominance, this was called "acquisition" as contrasted to "superinfection." There has always been the question of interpretation of the quantitative results in regard to differentiating superinfection from so-called "supercontamination." We find that approximately one in three persons bacteriologically superinfected develop clinical disease.

In patients who had acute pneumonia or acute exacerbations of chronic bronchitis and who were producing sputum, material was analyzed before treatment and at least twice during the subsequent five days. We have examined only a small number of agents and combinations; in general, these can be divided into three groups: those with a limited likelihood of superinfection (maximum 5%), those with a moderate chance (6-20%), and those with a considerable likelihood of superinfection (greater than 20%). Most of the single antibiotics given in conventional dosage caused bacteriological superinfection in 5% of cases or less (see Table 1). The broad spectrum agent, tetracycline, although long accused of having considerable superinfection potential, did not demonstrate this effect. In fact, it was in the lowest category, as was chloramphenicol. Gentamicin, when given as therapy for Gram-negative pneumonia, did not carry a substantial superinfection risk, nor did clindamycin, which was used for anaerobic pneumonia. Hetacillin, closely related to ampicillin, did result in a moderate degree of superinfection, as did the combination of penicillin and streptomycin, each given in conventional dosage.

The most interesting data related to oral phenethicillin and injectable penicillin. When oral phenethicillin was given in dosages of 250 mg every 6 hr, the bacteriological superinfection rate was about 3%. Merely increasing the dosage to 500 mg every 6 hr increased the superinfection rate some seven-fold. Similarly, penicillin (1.2 million units daily) resulted in no superinfection at all;

Table 1. Bacteriological sputum superinfection rate on different antibiotic regimens

Rate		
Low (< 5%)	Moderate (6–20%)	High (> 20%)
Penicillin, 2.4 million units/day	Penicillin, 2.4 million units/day and streptomycin, 1–2 g/day	Phenethicillin, 500 mg q.i.d.
Tetracycline, 2.0 g/day		Penicillin IV, 10 million units daily
Chloramphenicol, 2.0–3.0 g/day	Hetacillin, 2.0 g/day	Penicillin, 2.4 million units/day and tetracycline, 2.0 g/day
	Cephaloridine, 1.0–6.0 g/day	
Gentamicin, 3 mg/kg/day		Penicillin, 2.4 million units/day and chloramphenicol
Clindamycin, 150–300 mg/day		Cloxacillin or nafcillin, 3.0 g/day (for staphylococcal pneumonia) IM

increase in the dosage to 10–20 million units each day for treatment of pneumonia of similar severity resulted in a superinfection rate of over 25%.

Our studies clearly show that the best approach to administration of antibiotics to the patient with pneumonia is to give the smallest amount of a single agent that will suppress or eradicate an invading microorganism. Increasing the dosage of a single agent or using multiple antibiotics will increase the likelihood of superinfection.

Our studies suggested that the mechanism of superinfection was suppression of the normal flora. Even though the patient continued to bring up sputum, aerobic cultures obtained after two days of therapy often showed no growth at all, a finding which permitted a reasonably confident prediction that superinfection would supervene during the next few days. Other studies suggested that broad spectrum antibiotics interfere with phagocytosis (6). These older studies have not been adequately confirmed, but recently, investigations by Martin et al. (7) suggest that tetracycline may interfere with leukocyte mobilization. Thus, superinfection consequent to antibiotic usage may result both from a direct effect on the microbial flora and, in some instances, from an impairment of host defense mechanisms.

When our studies were first published, there was considerable controversy about the data indicating that multiple antimicrobials given concurrently or large amounts of a single agent produced a very considerable risk of superinfection. Even if there is some disagreement about the precise risk of superinfection and the likelihood of clinical manifestations supervening, there is currently no quarrel with the general thesis. However, there continues to be substantial debate about the uses of the quantitative sputum analysis technique. It is our opinion that there are three major uses for quantitative sputum analysis. First, in a sick patient with a putative, hospital-acquired lung infection, quantitative analysis can help to separate acquisition of a small number of organisms from true superinfection. We have not observed hospital-acquired Gram-negative or staphylococcal pneumonia unless the organism was present in high titer either in pure culture or in clear, numerical predominance. Second, if there are two superinfecting organisms, quantitative sputum analysis may show a very substantial difference in numbers of the two organisms, thus permitting a rational approach to therapy, directing treatment primarily against the numerically predominant organism. Serial quantitative studies will then permit an effective monitoring of the dual superinfection; in some cases, as the concentrations of the predominant organism remain stationary or diminish, the secondary organism may become numerically dominant. Failure to change therapy at this time may be catastrophic.

Third, if a patient does develop clinical evidence of superinfection, quantitative sputum analysis may be a very valuable method of following the efficacy of antibiotics directed against the superinfecting organism. For the most part, such quantitative analyses are used only to monitor new antimicrobial agents. In most cases, a combination of careful clinical observations and routine sputum cultures will suffice to determine antibiotic efficacy.

The above three situations currently provide the only reasons for doing quantitative analysis. Certainly, the technique is not recommended for the general clinical laboratory. Some patients will show large numbers of Gram-negative organisms in sputum cultures in nearly pure culture, yet have negative cultures when the specimen is obtained by transtracheal puncture. An increasing number of clinicians are calling for the use of transtracheal puncture as the preferred way of establishing a definitive diagnosis in patients suffering from pneumonia. It seems to me that this is highly undesirable. A transtracheal puncture carries a certain risk and should be reserved for a small number of cases in which an intelligent therapeutic decision cannot be made otherwise. For the most part, smelling the expectorated sputum, carefully reviewing the clinical situation, doing a Gram stain, and examining the results of sputum cultures will permit institution of a sensible antibiotic regimen. Transtracheal puncture then can be reserved for the few patients who remain a clinical and microbiological enigma.

Antibiotic administration also promotes systemic yeast infections, particularly those attributable to species of *Candida*. At least 90% of those developing the renal-myocardial type of systemic candidiasis have been treated with one or more antibiotics, usually for a period of at least seven days. The data suggest that the sequence of pathogenesis is 1) suppression of normal bacterial flora, 2) colonization with *Candida*, and then, in many cases, 3) invasion through holes in the skin created by indwelling needles or catheters. There is no convincing evidence that the antibiotics directly promote growth of the yeast.

III. Adrenal Hormones

Virtually any experimental infection can be augmented by pretreatment of the animal with adrenal steroids. Even if infection and steroid therapy are initiated simultaneously, enhancement of infection is likely. If, on the other hand, host defenses are allowed to react to the invading organism for one to three days, the enhancing capacity of the steroids is markedly reduced. At least 25% of patients developing systemic candidiasis have been treated with adrenal hormones prior to the onset of the yeast infection. In other disseminated mycotic infections, the percentage is even greater; thus, the majority of those infected with species of *Aspergillus* or *Mucor* have been so treated.

The relationship is not nearly so clear for most bacterial superinfections, nor is the mechanism of enhancement fully established. Studies by Hirsch and Church (8) showed that phagocytosis and intracellular killing were not affected in vitro. Their data, among those of others, suggested that the major effect of steroids was to delay the mobilization of polymorphonuclear leukocytes into parasitized areas. More recent experiments by Sidransky and his colleagues (9) with mice infected with *Aspergillus* by the aerosol route showed that, in steroid-treated animals, lysozomes within macrophages were stabilized. As a result of failure of lysozomal degranulation, ingested spores survive and, in addition, there is reduced mobilization of polymorphonuclear leukocytes.

IV. Needles and Catheters

In patients acquiring systemic candidiasis, half have no evidence of invasion from the esophagus or stomach (10). Presumably, in these cases, the organism gains direct access to the bloodstream through needles or catheters. It has been assumed that the risk of infection is greater with the large-bore catheters in comparison to small-bore needles, and there are some data which support this supposition. Crossley and Matsen (11) carried out a prospective study of complications from use of scalp vein needles; they found that pathogens were recovered from 4.2% of needle tips, but there were no instances of bacteremia. On the other hand, the bacteremia incidence following use of intravenous catheters ranges from 0.4–5.6%; consequently, the scalp vein needle appears to be substantially safer.

The most impressive relationship between vascular catheters and infection occurs in patients receiving hyperalimentation. Curry and Quie (12) observed 33 cases of yeast fungemia in a 20-month period in a university hospital setting. Of the 33 cases, 22 occurred in patients being treated with intravenous hyperalimentation. In 19 of the 22, *Candida* species were involved (*C. albicans* in 17 cases, *C. parakrusei* in two cases). Curry and Quie then carried out a prospective study of 49 patients who received hyperalimentation for at least 48 hr. Bloodstream infection supervened in 13 of the 49 (27%); in 8 of the 13 cases, the organisms isolated were yeasts. Williams, Chandler, and Orloff (13) observed 27 cases of *Candida* fungemia; 18 of the 27 were receiving parenteral hyperalimentation. It is not entirely clear why hyperalimentation is followed by such a high incidence of infection. It may be that a combination of large-bore catheters and the concomitant administration of antibiotics, suppressing the endogenous flora, results in a propensity to acquire yeast fungemia. An alternate possibility is that the hyperalimentation fluid supports *Candida* growth to an unusual degree. We have not found any supporting in vitro evidence, however; 24-hr growth in hyperalimentation fluid is identical to that found in conventional fluids.

V. Antitumor Agents

It is clear that antitumor agents increase the likelihood of superinfection because of adverse side effects such as leukopenia or hypogammaglobulinemia. Perhaps the best example of the enhancing effects of antitumor agents is infection with *P. carinii*.

The first major outbreak in the United States was described at the St. Jude Children's Research Hospital in Memphis, Tennessee, where 19 cases of clinically apparent *Pneumocystis* infection occurred in a two-year period (14). Review of 301 autopsies showed 40 cases of inapparent *Pneumocystis* infection, 39 of which occurred in patients with underlying malignancies, primarily of the hematopoetic system. The data suggested that the inapparent cases had been occurring with regularity for years, but the clinically apparent *Pneumocystis* infection was associated with the utilization of vigorous treatment regimens, including steroids and vincristine. Presumably, the endogenous infection was activated by a combination of antitumor drugs and adrenal glucocorticoids.

Antitumor agents also increase the prevalence of infection attributable to exogenously acquired superinfecting agents. Thus, for example, at the Memorial Hospital in New York City, Dr. Donald Armstrong and his colleagues have described an increasing incidence of *Aspergillus* and *Mucor* infections in patients suffering from leukemia. As in the St. Jude experience, their evidence suggests that antitumor agents played a major role in the increasing frequency of those frequently lethal fungal superinfections (2, 3).

VI. Transplantation

Patients being treated with immunosuppressive agents and steroids related to renal transplantation have a tendency to acquire bacterial, fungal, viral, and protozoan infections. This has been well recorded by Rifkind (15) and by Remington and his colleagues (16, 17). In many cases, patients are infected with more than one agent.

Among patients receiving renal transplants, early deaths were, in the majority of cases, due to sepsis, whereas among those dying after the first few postoperative weeks, only about one-third were due to infections. The most important infecting organisms were *Pseudomonas*, other Gram-negative microbes, *N. asteroides*, and species of *Aspergillus* and *Candida*. Additionally, there were a substantial number of cases due to cytomegaloviruses and *P. carinii*.

In one extraordinary case, reported by Hood et al. (18), superinfection was not due to any particular therapeutic regimen, but rather to the fact that the transplanted kidney was infected with *H. capsulatum*. The recipient then developed systemic histoplasmosis and subsequently died. Recent studies also suggest that papovaviruses can be activated in some patients after renal transplantation. In some cases, this takes the form of warts, but, in rare cases, multifocal leukoencephalopathy supervenes, this being a progressive, lethal disease of the central nervous system, apparently attributable to papovaviruses (19). Gurwith and his colleagues (17) observed that approximately 25% of patients dying following cardiac transplantation had evidence of significant infection with species of *Aspergillus*.

VII. Superinfection Arising in a Geographically Nonendemic Area

We have seen patients with leukemia or lymphoma who traveled through areas endemic for histoplasmosis or coccidioidomycosis and who have then manifested the superinfection only weeks or months after leaving that area. Under these circumstances, the diagnosis often is delayed an inordinate amount of time. The following case illustrates the difficulties that may arise when the disease occurs outside the endemic area.

A man in his early 40's was hospitalized for severe pneumonia involving the midportion of the right lung. Because he was an alcoholic and routine sputum cultures were unrevealing, a presumptive diagnosis of aspiration pneumonia was made. For the next four weeks, the patient became progressively sicker, despite presumably appropriate antibiotic and supportive treatment. Gradually, the entire right lung field became massively involved with a dense infiltrate. Concomitantly, the rectal temperature persisted at 104–105°F daily, and the breathing rate increased to between 40 and 60 per min. Review of the patient's history revealed that he had left North Carolina eight years previously and then had resided for four years in Connecticut and four years in New York City, never returning to North Carolina. Indeed, during that eight-year period, he had not traveled even transiently outside the southeastern Connecticut and New York City metropolitan areas.

Two bronchoscopic examinations were performed, but these were not helpful diagnostically. Material obtained from the right mainstem bronchus on the second bronchoscopy showed, after incubation on Sabouraud's agar, a fungus thought to be *Blastomyces dermatitides* by a laboratory technician. However, the morphology of the isolate was not clear-cut, and the infectious disease consultant, who was considered authoritative in mycotic infections, dismissed the possibility because the patient had not been in the endemic area for eight years. A third bronchoscopy was then performed; in the aspirated material sent to pathology for cytology studies, an astute pathologist thought he saw typical yeast phase *B. dermatitides*. A further examination of the morphology of the isolate from the second bronchoscopy now showed mycelial growth entirely consistent with *B. dermatitides*. The expectorated sputum was then restudied with sodium hydroxide preparations. These had initially been called negative by a house staff member who was inexperienced in mycology, but in fact, when the sputum was examined by an experienced technician, many typical *Blastomyces* forms were found in each low-power microscopic field. With the diagnosis finally established after five weeks of confusion, the now-moribund patient was treated with Amphotericin B; thereafter, he showed a prompt clinical response, eventually recovering completely. In this case, the diagnosis was missed because the patient had not resided recently in an area known to be endemic for blastomycosis. In retrospect, it seems clear that the patient had a quiescent blastomycotic focus in the right lung which was activated by the aspiration of gastric contents. The obvious lesson is that clinical disease can become apparent long after the patient has left the endemic area.

VIII. Unnecessary Environmental Exposure

Patients with certain underlying diseases have a propensity to acquire specific superinfections; in a few instances, the likelihood of such infection can be reduced by avoiding unnecessary environmental exposure. For example, several years ago, a 26-year-old man who suffered from Hodgkin's disease was hospitalized with occipital headache and stupor. Lumbar puncture revealed many cryptococci on India ink preparation of spinal fluid. Despite vigorous intravenous and intrathecal treatment with Amphotericin B, the meningitis progressed inexorably, and the patient died two weeks later. Investigations into possible environmental exposure revealed that the patient kept his own pigeon cotes and had continued this avocation despite a diagnosis of Hodgkin's disease five years prior to the onset of the cryptococcal meningitis. This, of course, is inexcusable. Since the careful mycological observations of Chester Emmons (20), it has been well known that pigeon excreta are perhaps the most important environmental reservoir for *C. neoformans.* Consequently, it is foolish to permit any patient with known or strongly suspected lymphatic malignancy to be inordinately exposed to an organism known to attack patients with lymphomas.

Similarly, patients with Hodgkin's disease should be warned about excessive contact with old chicken coops, in view of Dr. Emmons' studies that indicated that *H. capsulatum* multiplies luxuriantly in chicken droppings (21).

We have also observed patients with Hodgkin's disease who had not been warned to forego their spelunking adventures despite the data showing that cave bats and bat droppings are an important reservoir for *H. capsulatum.*

Some superinfection can be avoided merely by using some common sense. Thus, for example, patients with acute leukemia should be warned to assiduously avoid contact with children who have overt varicella. This would appear to be perfectly obvious, but we have seen patients with florid herpes zoster in beds adjacent to persons suffering from known leukemia.

Even if we cannot reduce the incidence of superinfection, we can prevent it from becoming more severe in certain cases by appropriate immunization procedures. A prime example of this is virus influenza. Observations made in the pandemic of 1958 suggested that a disproportionate number of deaths occurred in those who suffered from rheumatic valvular disease or chronic lung disease and in those who were pregnant (22). Clearly, during periods in which influenza is epidemic in a given geographic area, those who are more likely to develop potentially lethal influenza virus pneumonia (or combined influenza virus-bacterial pulmonary disease) should be protected by immunization with the appropriate vaccine.

IX. The Problem of Dual Superinfection

There are an increasing number of cases of superinfection with two or more organisms. This is especially true of patients with acute leukemia under treatment and among those undergoing organ transplantation. Those who have defective delayed immune mechanisms may also be superinfected by more than one organism simultaneously. We have observed cases of concomitant tuberculosis and cryptococcosis, cryptococcosis and nocardiosis, and listeriosis and cryptococcosis in patients suffering from Hodgkin's disease.

Dual superinfection is also frequent among heroin addicts who use unsterile materials. We have recently observed one young woman who entered the hospital with multiple pulmonary emboli, suggesting a diagnosis of tricuspid endocarditis. Sputum and blood cultures showed *Staphylococcus aureus*, confirming that suspicion. However, in addition, blood cultures repeatedly showed a nonpigmented strain of *Serratia*. Since the patient had aortic valvular disease, the assumption was made that she had concurrent right-sided staphylococcal and left-sided serratia endocarditis. Since the patient recovered after intensive antibiotic treatment, this presumptive anatomical diagnosis could not be confirmed. In other cases, *Candida* and a Gram-negative organism have been present in the bloodstream simultaneously. Indeed, in about 5% of cases of endocarditis superimposed upon addiction, two organisms have been cultivated from the bloodstream.

X. Use of Hypertonic Media to Detect Superinfection

On relatively infrequent occasions, a patient with apparent superinfection has negative cultures with routine media. In these cases, it is sometimes helpful to place the specimen in hypertonic media under both aerobic and anaerobic conditions. We use a battery of such media, including 10% sucrose, 77 broth (a hypertonic sodium chloride medium), 30% sucrose, and a cooked meat-sucrose anaerobic medium. For aerobic organisms, the hypertonic sucrose has proved better than any other medium we have used.

For example, we reported the case of a man who developed chills, fever, and splenomegaly after cardiac valvular surgery (23). Routine cultures were negative repeatedly, and the clinical illness persisted despite massive doses of a variety of antibiotics, all of whose pharmacological actions were directed against microbial cell walls. Blood specimens placed in hypertonic media then showed aberrant organisms that reverted to corynebacteria when subcultured onto solid agar. Following these findings, the patient was given erythromycin for six weeks and recovered uneventfully. Serological studies on the patient's sera showed that he had precipitins against his own organism. Thus, the data clearly pointed to a significant role for this organism in the patient's postoperative illness.

Recently, we have seen a patient who was an intravenous user of heroin and who developed an indolent meningitis characterized by a spinal fluid lymphocytic pleocytosis and depressed glucose concentrations. A presumptive diagnosis of cryptococcal meningitis was made, but cultures of the cerebrospinal fluid were repeatedly negative, and no cryptococcal antigen or antibody was found in either spinal fluid or blood. Because the patient was a drug user, the serum was tested for anti-*Candida* precipitins; these were found in high titer, and because of this, the spinal fluid was cultivated in hypertonic media. *C. albicans* was readily recovered from the 10% sucrose medium.

It is important to stress that about half the organisms isolated exclusively in hypertonic media are never seen in aberrant or wall-defective form. Whether they were present in vivo in wall-defective form or whether they grew in hypertonic media because such broths are so highly enriched is not at all clear. But it is clear that, on occasion, the use of hypertonic media can be enormously helpful in making a definitive diagnosis of microbial superinfection.

Donald B. Louria

XI. The Necessity for a Close Liaison between the Laboratory and the Clinicians

We continue to see mistakes made because there is inadequate communication between the laboratory and bedside personnel. Two examples will suffice to emphasize this point.

A patient who suffered from renal failure was hospitalized with mental deterioration. Cultures of spinal fluid were reported as showing no pathogens. Weeks later, a posterior fossa exploration showed an *Aspergillus* brain abscess. It was only then that it was discovered that the first spinal tap showed a colony of *Aspergillus* on culture but that the laboratory personnel decided it was likely to be a contaminant. Clearly, this decision was not their prerogative to make. In fact, this patient was under treatment with antibiotics and adrenal steroids, so that he had every right to have an *Aspergillus* superinfection. The judgment as to the significance of the *Aspergillus* isolate should not have been made unilaterally by the laboratory; rather, it should have been a joint interpretation by the clinicians and the laboratory personnel.

Recently, a very good infectious disease clinician admitted to his hospital service an addict with overt hepatitis. Blood cultures were obtained because the patient was febrile. The initial two cultures were reported as showing a "nonpathogenic" species of *Candida*. This report misled the physician into delaying a diagnosis of *Candida* endocarditis for about two weeks. The fact of the matter is that there are no nonpathogenic species of *Candida* as far as human infection is concerned. Any species can cause disease. Indeed, at least one-third of cases of *Candida* endocarditis in the addict are due to so-called "nonpathogenic" species. Furthermore, in the compromised host during treatment with antibiotics and/or steroids, any species can cause the myocardial-renal form of systemic infection.

Superinfection surely will be an increasing problem as the pool of compromised hosts increases. It is therefore crucial to 1) try to match a given patient's disease pattern and therapeutic program to the likely superinfecting microorganisms; 2) establish better laboratory-clinician liaison; and 3) utilize all the serological and cultural techniques at our disposal in order to make a prompt and correct diagnosis so that a potentially effective treatment regimen can be initiated.

Literature Cited

1. Bodey, G. P. Fungal infections complicating acute leukemia. J. Chronic Dis. 19: 667, 1966.
2. Meyer, R. D., P. Rosen, and D. Armstrong. Phycomycosis complicating leukemia and lymphoma. Ann. Intern. Med. 77: 871, 1972.
3. Meyer, R. D., L. S. Young, and D. Armstrong. Aspergillosis complicating neoplastic disease. Amer. J. Med. 54: 6, 1973.
4. Young, L. S., and D. Armstrong. *Pseudomonas aeruginosa* infections. Crit. Rev. Clin. Lab. Sci. 3: 291, 1972.
5. Ketover, B. P., L. S. Young, and D. Armstrong. *Aeromonas hydrophila* septicemia: Clinical and immunologic aspects. Presented at the 12th Interscience Conference on Antimicrobial Agents and Chemotherapy, September 26–29, Atlantic City, N. J., 1972.
6. Munoz, J., and R. Geister. Inhibition of phagocytosis by aureomycin. Proc. Exp. Biol. Med. 75: 367, 1950.
7. Martin R., G. Warr, H. Yeager, R. Couch, and V. Knight. Effects of tetracycline on leukotaxis. Presented at the 12th Interscience Conference on Antimicrobial Agents and Chemotherapy, September 26–29, Atlantic City, N. J., 1972.
8. Hirsch, J. G., and A. B. Church. Adrenal steroids and infection: The effect of cortisone administration on polymorphonuclear leukocytic functions and serum opsonins and bactericidins. J. Clin. Invest. 40: 794, 1961.
9. Merkow, L., M. Pardo, S. M. Epstein, E. Verney, and H. Sidransky. Lysozomal stability during phagocytosis of *Aspergillus flavus* spores by alveolar macrophages of cortisone-treated mice. Science 160: 79, 1968.
10. Louria, D. B., D. P. Stiff, and B. Bennett. Disseminated moniliasis in the adult. Medicine 41: 307, 1962.
11. Crossley, K., and J. M. Matsen. The scalp vein needle. JAMA 220: 985, 1972.
12. Curry, C. R., and P. G. Quie. Fungal septicemia in patients receiving parenteral hyperalimentation. New Engl. J. Med. 285: 1221, 1971.
13. Williams, R. J., J. G. Chandler, and M. J. Orloff. *Candida* septicemia. Arch. Surg. 103: 8, 1971.
14. Perera, D. R., K. A. Western, H. D. Johnson, W. W. Johnson, M. G. Schultz, and P. V. Akers. *Pneumocystis carinii* pneumonia in a hospital for children. JAMA 214: 1074, 1970.

15. Rifkind, D., T. L. Marchioro, W. R. Waddell, and T. E. Starzl. Infectious diseases associated with renal homotransplantation. I. Incidence, types and predisposing factors. JAMA 189: 397, 1964.
16. Remington, J. S. The problem of infections in transplantation patients. *In* Changing Patterns of Bacterial Infections and Antibiotic Therapy Neu. HC. Ed. Excerpta Med. 1971.
17. Gurwith, M. J., E. B. Stinson, and J. S. Remington. *Aspergillus* infection complicating cardiac transplantation. Arch. Intern. Med. 128: 541, 1971.
18. Hood, A. B., F. G. Inglis, L. Lowenstein, J. B. Dossetor, and L. D. MacLean. Histoplasmosis and thrombocytopenic purpura: Transmission by renal homotransplantation. Can. Med. Assoc. J. 93: 587, 1965.
19. Papovaviruses and human disease. Brit. Med. J. ii: 540, 1972.
20. Emmons, C. W. Saprophytic sources of *Cryptococcus neoformans* associated with pigeon (*Columba livia*). Amer. J. Hyg. 62: 227, 1955.
21. Emmons, C. W. Histoplasmosis. Bull. N. Y. Acad. Med. 31: 627, 1955.
22. Louria, D. B., H. L. Blumenfeld, J. T. Ellis, E. D. Kilbourne, and D. E. Rogers. Studies on influenza in the pandemic of 1957-58. II. Pulmonary complications of influenza. J. Clin. Invest. 38: 213, 1959.
23. Louria, D. B., T. Kaminski, M. Grieco, and J. Singer. Aberrant forms of bacteria and fungi found in blood or cerebrospinal fluid. Arch. Intern. Med. 124: 39, 1969.

2

Culture and Identification of Commonly Encountered Gram-negative Bacilli: *Pseudomonas, Klebsiella-Enterobacter, Serratia, Proteus,* and *Providencia*

Robert B. Lindberg

It is a common observation that a major change in the etiology of infectious disease has occurred in the past two decades. Formerly, specific infections were the greater problem. As examples, streptococcal diseases, pneumococcal pneumonia, and enteric infections were of major concern. These diseases have not disappeared, but opportunistic infections attributable to organisms formerly regarded as innocuous have become a far more serious problem than was formerly the case. Nosocomial infection is a continuing and a growing problem in hospital populations. We are confronted today with a greatly enlarged need for control of infecting organisms which, until recently regarded as part of the normal human flora, now behave as active and frequent pathogens. Their prompt recognition has become a necessity in every hospital laboratory. As would be expected, their pathogenic role is often equivocal. The presence of fecal flora in the respiratory tract is now a common occurrence, but the species involved are not necessarily the cause of pneumonia. Similarly, a severe burn wound will, in most instances, harbor an extensive enteric flora, but not all of the species present play a part in invasive wound infection. Sepsis involving these organisms, however, has become increasingly common. Their prompt recognition can be a vital matter in diagnosis and treatment of an opportunistic invader.

Table 1 summarizes, as an illustration of Gram-negative colonization, the flora found on burn patients at our Institute over a period of five years. The proportion of enteric organisms present has increased with the passage of time. Gram-negative enteric flora are now a major part of the microbial flora in such patients. *Pseudomonas, Klebsiella-Enterobacter, Proteus*, and, more recently, *Providencia* are of major concern. This colonization has continued despite the use of topical therapy designed to control invasive infection.

That these species are not merely surface contaminants is shown in Table 2, in which species recovered from the bloodstream of burn patients are summarized.

Bacteremia, attributable to *Pseudomonas* and various species of Enterobacteriaceae, has become a major concern in management

Table 1. Gram-negative bacterial species on burns: Proportion of total wound isolates, 1963–1968

Species	Per cent of total burn isolates		
	1963	1966	1968
Pseudomonas	24	17	26
Klebsiella-Enterobacter	15	14	22
Proteus mirabilis	6.5	14	30
Providencia stuartii	1.2	8	22
Escherichia coli	5	5	13

of trauma. Severe sepsis is typical in such bacteremia, and endotoxic shock is a major problem, with a high mortality rate. Such findings emphasize the pathogenic importance of these organisms and add urgency to the need for prompt, effective recognition of this class of pathogens.

The genus *Pseudomonas* contains a large number of species, most of which are not of medical importance. Of the clinically significant species, *P. aeruginosa* is by far the most common and the most important. Other species which may be recovered from patient material include: *P. fluorescens*, *P. maltophila*, *P. putida*, *P. acidovorans*, *P. stutzeri*, and *P. multivorans* (synonymous with *P. cepacia*). *P. pseudomallei* recently created a furor as a pathogen of potential future significance when it was recovered from cases of melioidosis in soldiers who had been exposed to infection in Vietnam. The end of active campaigning in endemic areas has, it is hoped, removed the hazard of exposure.

Pseudomonas may be found in wounds, sputum, pus, exudate, blood, urine, stool, and in biopsy and autopsy tissue samples. In many of these, mixed flora are commonly present, and a selective as well as a nonselective medium should be used in primary culture (1–3). Since contamination with swarming *Proteus* strains is com-

Table 2. Gram-negative bacilli recovered from blood culture in burn patients, 1963–1969

Species	Per cent of positive blood cultures			
	1963	1966	1968	1969
Pseudomonas	31	14	26	24
Klebsiella-Enterobacter	18	21	18	20
Proteus mirabilis	6	21	28	15
Providencia stuartii	0	4	6	28
Escherichia coli	5	12	16	8

mon in wounds after several days, a *Proteus*-inhibitor plate should be included in the primary culture set. Blood agar, phenylethyl alcohol blood agar, and eosin methylene blue agar have served well in our laboratory. Many laboratories include cetrimide agar as a selective medium. Cetrimide (cetyltrimethylammonium bromide, a quaternary ammonium compound) inhibits many Gram-negative bacilli and enhances fluorescence, which may be an aid in recognizing the presence of *P. aeruginosa*. A modification of cetrimide agar, in which the cetrimide content is reduced from 0.03% to 0.02% and to which 15 µg of nalidixic acid is added per ml, has been described as recovering more *P. aeruginosa* colonies and fewer enteric forms (1).

Presumptive identification of *P. aeruginosa* can be made from blood agar plates when pyocyanin-producing strains are present. When more than a few isolated colonies are present, the unmistakable odor of trimethylamine in the Petri dish is a valuable aid. However, nonpigmented colonies, which are relatively common, require more detailed study. Cultural characteristics of the species of *Pseudomonas* of clinical importance are shown in Table 3.

Flagella numbers and location are of major importance in classification of this genus, but it is regrettably true that many laboratories lack the skill or patience to prepare effective flagellar stains. Many workers find recognition of fluorescence under a Wood's lamp a useful test. The usefulness of nitrate reduction and of gelatin liquefaction is controversial with reference to the principal species, *P. aeruginosa*. In our hands, these reactions have been reliable; nitrate is reduced and gelatin is liquefied. Starch hydrolysis is not a needed reaction unless *P. stutzeri* is suspected. Oxidase production is a common characteristic, but is lacking in *P. maltophila*. Arginine dihydrolase aids in recognition of *multivorans*, *maltophila*, or *stutzeri*.

Flow charts aid in distinguishing reactions for species. Figure 1 is an abbreviated structure for this purpose. This schema starts with the alkaline triple sugar slant. Oxidase-negative strains, forming lysine decarboxylase, are recognized as *P. maltophila*. Oxidase-positive strains include the lysine-positive *multivorans* and the lysine-negative strains. Fluorescent strains include *aeruginosa*, *fluorescens*, and *putida*; the last two do not form nitrogen gas.

Table 3. Diagnostic characteristics for species of *Pseudomonas*

Culture	P. aeruginosa	P. fluorescens	P. putida	P. multivorans	P. maltophila	P. stutzeri
Flagella	1	>1	>1	>1	>1	1
Fluorescence	+	+	+	−	−	−
No. 3 red		Varies	−	−	−	+
Gelatin lysed	+	+	−	+	+	+
Starch split	−	−	−	−	−	+
Oxidase	+	+	+	+	−	+
Arginine dihydrolase	+	+	+	−	−	−

From Ref. 2.

```
                    Triple sugar iron agar alkaline
                    ───────────────────────────────
                         +       Oxidase        −
                       ┌───────────────┐    ┌──────────┐
                       + Lysine −          + Lysine −
                    ┌──────┐                ┌──────┐
                 P. multivorans          P. maltophila
                   Lactose +
                       │
                    + Fluorescence −
                  ┌──────────────┐
                  + Gas −       + Gas −
               ┌────────┐    ┌──────────┐
            P. aeruginosa    P. acidovorans
                              Fructose +
              P. Fluorescens
              P. putida
                       │
                    + Lactose −
                 ┌──────────────┐
                + Motility    + Starch −
              ┌─────┐       ┌──────────┐
           P. pseudomallei  P. stutzeri   P. aeruginosa
                            Fructose +
```

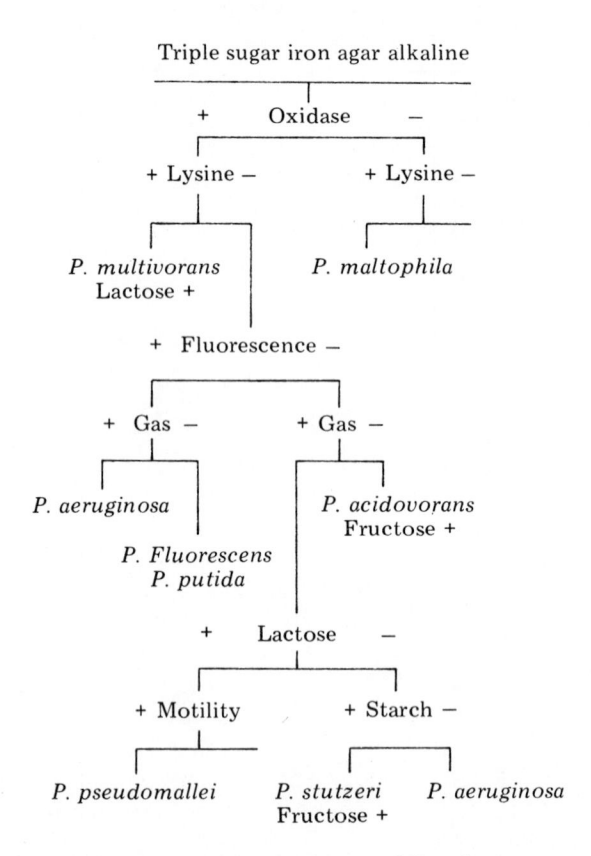

Figure 1. Presumptive speciation of *Pseudomonas*.

Nonfluorescent *P. aeruginosa* strains are differentiated from *P. acidovorans* and *P. stutzeri* by their failure to split lactose or starch and to oxidize fructose.

A widely used substrate for differentiating oxidative Gram-negative rods is the Hugh and Leifson OF medium. Table 4 summarizes the oxidative as opposed to fermentative capability of *P. aeruginosa* in Seller's agar, which is useful in characterizing nonfermentative bacilli. In our laboratory, we have not found this somewhat intricate substrate essential to use, but it is a valid multiple-reaction medium and has received wide acceptance.

Table 4. Reactions in Seller's medium

	Pseudomonas aeruginosa
Slant	
Fluorescence	+
Blue color	−
Yellow band	
Glucose oxidized	−
Butt	
Alkaline	+
Anaerobic growth	+
Nitrogen	
Gas produced	+

From Ref. 3.

Although the incidence of melioidosis attributed to *P. pseudomallei* in patients who had served in Vietnam has fallen sharply in the past two years, this organism, which is a natural inhabitant of moist soil in Southeast Asia and northern Australia, retains a potential for causing disease for some time after initial exposure. The organism would be confused readily with *P. stutzeri* if one were not aware of its potential presence. In our laboratory, the key differentiating attribute for prompt presumptive recognition has been the distinctive umbonate colony, i.e., with a raised central papilla and a raised rim, followed by appearance of radial striae. These changes at room temperature are seen on primary isolates within 72 hr. The musty, earthy odor of the colony is also unique. Addition of polymyxin B (100 units per ml) and penicillin (10 units per ml) furnishes a selective substrate for its recovery from mixed cultures. A wrinkled surface pellicle forms on broth in 24–36 hr. Motility is best demonstrated in hanging drop preparations. Its failure to form pigment and to grow in 4% NaCl or in the presence of sodium azide or cetrimide aids in its differentiation. It is described as oxidase positive; however, in our study of 45 strains recovered from 13 patients with melioidosis in our Institute, we were unable to demonstrate cytochrome oxidase, despite repeated attempts and use of a variety of techniques (4).

The recognition of *Pseudomonas* species other than *P. aeruginosa* is to be borne in mind, but at present the total involvement of clinical specimens with such organisms is not great. In our laboratory, where we recover several hundred pseudomonads annually, the majority of strains are recognized on primary isolation. All isolates are phage typed, and further scrutiny of pigment-forming strains is made only on nontypable forms. *P. maltophila* and *P. stutzeri* are the other species which we have encountered. In the past 14 months, *P. maltophila* was the predominant organism in two burn autopsies.

Turning to the Enterobacteriaceae, it is gratifying to note that, after generations of microbiologists had struggled with the biochemical differentiations of species in the poorly defined *Klebsiella-Aerobacter* group, the contribution of Moeller (5) in describing amino acid decarboxylation and the exhaustive and definitive studies of Edwards and Ewing (6) have placed the topic on reasonably firm ground in characterizing and differentiating these forms. Such differentiation may be of slight value in stool cultures, but when clinical disease is produced in the urinary tract, in the lung, and in Gram-negative sepsis in wounds, precise speciation becomes important.

Isolation of *Klebsiella* and *Enterobacter* species is readily achieved; the organisms are not fastidious and, in clinical laboratories, are recovered from primary isolation substrates. Blood agar, eosin methylene blue, and MacConkey's agar are effective recovery media. Triple sugar agar or Kligler's agar slants offer a useful start for differentiation, and these mixed sugar media are almost universally used.

Table 5 summarizes pertinent reactions of the *Klebsiella-Enterobacter* group. The organisms are H_2S-negative, mainly indole-negative, methyl red-negative, and Voges-Proskauer-positive. There are methyl red-positive, Voges-Proskauer-negative strains of *Klebsiella*, and some may be citrate-negative, but they are still included in the genus. The species most often encountered is *Klebsiella pneumoniae*. *K. ozaenae* and *K. rhinoscleromatis* are distinguished by differences in citrate utilization, lactose fermentation, and urease and by a cluster of less definitive differential reactions. Routine procedures do not often include this differentiation, since these species are relatively rare. Gelatin is not

Table 5. Biochemical reactions of *Klebsiella-Enterobacter* organisms

Reaction	Klebsiella pneumoniae	Enterobacter cloacae	aerogenes	hafniae	liquefaciens 37°C	liquefaciens 22°C
Indole	−(+)	−	−	−	−	−
H₂S	−	−	−	−	−	−
Methyl red	−	−	−	−(+)	+(−)	−(+)
Voges-Proskauer	+	+	+	+(−)	−(+)	+(−)
Citrate	+	+(−)	+	−(+)	+	+
Urease	+	−	−	−	−	−
Motility	−	−(+)	−(+)	+	+(−)	+
Gelatin	−	−	+	−	+(−)	+
Lysine	+	−	+	+	−	+
Arginine	−	+	−	+	+	+
Ornithine	−	+	+	+	−	−
Phenylalanine	−	−	−	−	−	−
ONPG	+	+	+	−(+)	−	−
Inositol	+	−(+)	+	+	+	+

(+): late or uncommon.

liquefied by most *Klebsiella* strains; gelatin-liquefying strains may be designated as the "oxytocic" biotype of *K. pneumoniae*.

The most useful differentiating reactions for *Klebsiella* and *Enterobacter* are motility, the decarboxylases, arginine dihydrolase, and phenylalanine, which is not split.

Differentiation of *Enterobacter* species involves primarily *E. cloacae* and *E. aerogenes*. *E. hafniae* and *E. liquefaciens* are species which require differential temperature observations for complete characterization, but this is not necessary in most clinical laboratories. Rhamnose is not fermented by *E. liquefaciens*, and neither sorbitol nor raffinose are split by *E. hafniae;* these reactions serve to distinguish these species when such differentiation is needed.

Decarboxylation and dihydrolase reactions are summarized in Table 6. These reactions serve to distinguish *E. cloacae*, *E. aerogenes*, and *Klebsiella*. It is apparent, of course, that without special attention, the *hafniae* and *liquefaciens* strains would be included with *E. aerogenes*.

The recognition of *K. pneumoniae* involves acceptance of the presumption that the vast majority of strains of *Klebsiella* are consistent in their decarboxylase reactions. The behavior of 705 strains of *K. pneumoniae* is summarized in Table 7. Routine screening procedures would detect 96% of the strains; the occasional exception will require special study.

Serratia species comprise, in clinical material, essentially only *S. marcescens*. Pigment formation, when it occurs, makes the species

Table 6. *Enterobacter* spp.: Decarboxylation and dihydrolase reactions at 37°C

Species	Lysine	Arginine	Ornithine
E. cloacae	−	+	+
E. aerogenes	+	−	+
E. hafniae	+	−	+
E. liquefaciens	+(−)	−	+
Klebsiella sp.	+	−	−

From Ewing, 1965.

Culture and Identification of Gram-negative Bacilli

easily recognizable, but in clinical microbiology, the majority of strains encountered are nonpigmented. Differentiating reactions are summarized in Table 8. In actual practice, gas formation from glucose is the most useful, prompt differentiating criterion to distinguish *Serratia* from *Klebsiella* and *Enterobacter*. Gas is either absent or present with *Serratia* only in a small amount (less than 10% in the Durham's tube). Decarboxylation reactions correspond to those of *E. aerogenes*, so that this differentiation is not of value. Gelatin liquefaction is prompt and is an aid in recognition of *Serratia*. Failure to ferment arabinose constitutes a definitive

Table 7. Decarboxylation reactions of *K. pneumoniae*

No. of strains	Lysine	Arginine	Ornithine
683	+	−	−
2	+	+	−
4	−	+	−
16	−	−	−

From Ewing, 1965.

Table 8. *Serratia marcescens:* Differentiating reactions (24 hr)

Reaction	*Serratia*	*Klebsiella pneumoniae*	*Enterobacter* (*cloacae* and *aerogenes*)
H_2S	−	−	−
Urase	+ or −	+	− or +
Indole	−	− or +	−
Methyl red	−(+)	−	−
Voges-Proskauer	+	+	+
Motility	+	−	+
Gelatin liquefaction	+	−	+ or −
Ornithine	+	−	+
Gas from glucose	−*	+	+
Arabinose	−	+	+

* Gas, when formed (Durham's tube), is in small volume (< 10%).

difference between *Serratia* and *Klebsiella-Enterobacter* species and precisely differentiates *S. marcescens*.

The remaining major group with which this chapter is concerned is the genus *Proteus*, comprised of four species. *P. mirabilis* is by far the most commonly encountered species, but the others are found in clinical specimens and must be recognized. Differentiation of *Proteus* species is summarized in Table 9.

A conspicuous attribute of *P. mirabilis* and *P. vulgaris* is swarming. This phenomenon, when present, makes recognition of these two species possible only with the indole reaction, since the other two species do not exhibit swarming. Species differentiation among nonswarming strains is readily accomplished with the indole, ornithine decarboxylase, hydrogen sulfide, and inositol reactions, as shown (7). Although other reactions also differentiate these species, they are not needed in the great majority of cases.

Atypical strains of *P. mirabilis*, which swarm actively but which form indole, have been described (8). Although they are not commonly encountered, their existence must be borne in mind, since the swarming indole-negative strains are assumed to be *P. mirabilis*. To exclude this error, the ornithine decarboxylase reaction is required.

The genus *Providencia* includes two species (formerly designated *Providencia* "*A*" and "*B*"). These organisms do not form hydrogen sulfide, which distinguishes them from *P. vulgaris* and *P. mirabilis*, nor do they split urea. This latter reaction is the critical

Table 9. Differentiating reactions of *Proteus* sp.

Species	Indole	Ornithine	H_2S	Inositol
P. vulgaris	+	–	+	–
P. mirabilis	–	+	+	–
P. morganii	+	+	–	–
P. rettgeri	+	–	–	+
P. mirabilis atypical	+	–	+	–

characteristic which separates *Providencia* from the urease-positive *Proteus* species. Their pathogenic role has been equivocal; in our Institute they are now a common cause of pneumonia and of sepsis in severely burned patients. Since we find them on patients at the time of admission, they are not a phenomenon confined to our installation. *Providencia stuartii* has been described as less commonly encountered than *Providencia alcalifaciens*, although in our population the incidence has been almost entirely *P. stuartii*. *P. alcalifaciens* does not ferment inositol and is thus distinguished from the inositol-fermenting *P. stuartii*.

Two flow sheets, abbreviated to include the genera discussed here, are set down as potentially useful algorithmic classification systems. Figure 2 presents the reactions of strains showing as lactose-positive on MacConkey's agar. This selective substrate will, of course, exhibit lactose fermentation for some strains of *Kleb-*

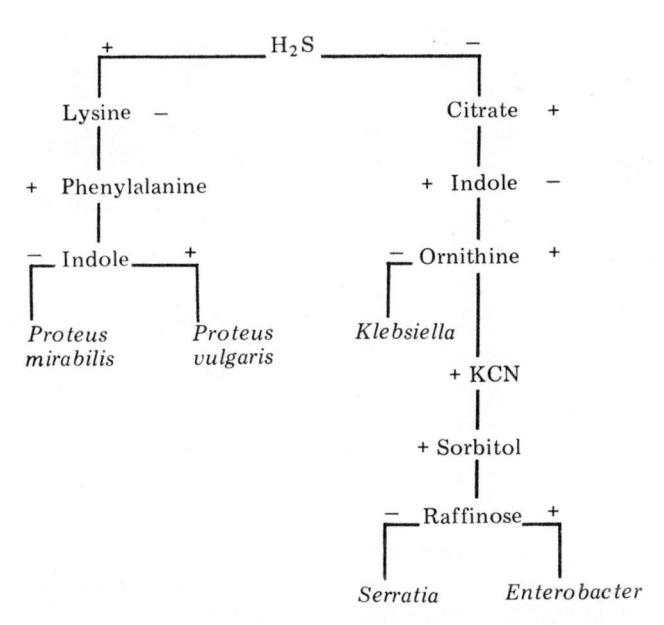

Figure 2. Lactose-positive Gram-negative rods: *Klebsiella*, *Enterobacter*, *Serratia*, and *Proteus*.

siella, Enterobacter, Serratia, Proteus, and *Providencia.* Such lactose negatives are set down in Figure 3. The lactose-positive *Klebsiella-Enterobacter-Serratia* strains are subdivided in this schema with the KCN-tolerance test, but this reaction is not essential for making these generic distinctions.

Identification of lactose-negative, Gram-negative bacilli by using the same criterion of lactose fermentation on MacConkey's agar is summarized in Figure 3. Here, the pseudomonads are included,

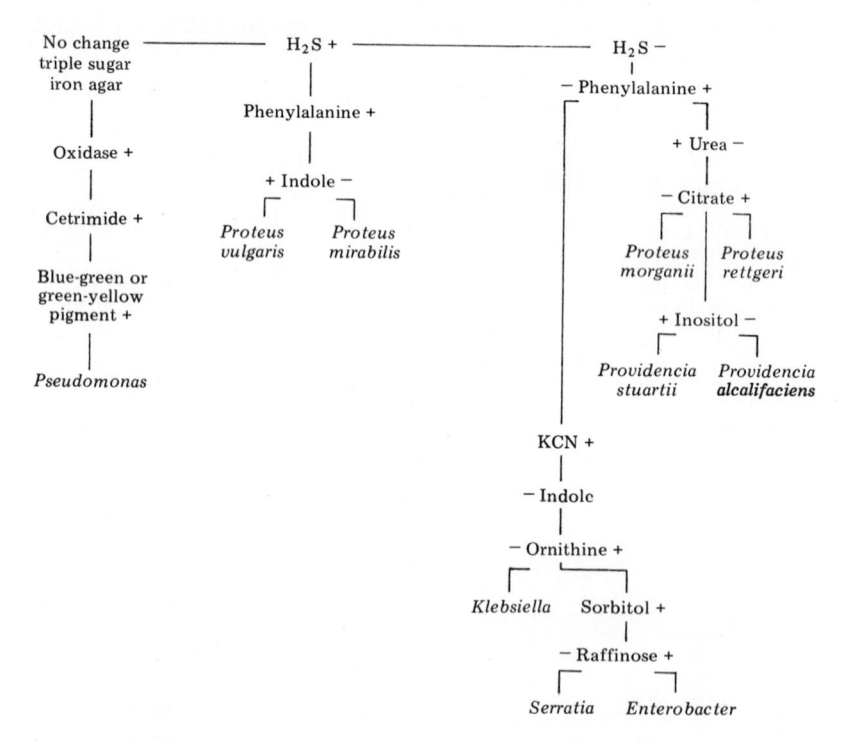

```
No change ──────── H₂S + ─────────────────── H₂S −
triple sugar                │                      │
iron agar                   │                  − Phenylalanine +
    │                 Phenylalanine +          ┌──────────┐
Oxidase +                   │                         + Urea −
    │                   + Indole −                      │
Cetrimide +             ┌────────┐                − Citrate +
    │                Proteus   Proteus          ┌──────────┐
Blue-green or        vulgaris  mirabilis      Proteus │ Proteus
green-yellow                                  morganii│ rettgeri
pigment +                                              │
    │                                            + Inositol −
Pseudomonas                                   ┌──────────┐
                                            Providencia  Providencia
                                             stuartii    alcalifaciens

                              KCN +
                                │
                             − Indole
                                │
                            − Ornithine +
                          ┌──────────┐
                       Klebsiella   Sorbitol +
                                        │
                                   − Raffinose +
                                  ┌──────────┐
                               Serratia   Enterobacter
```

Figure 3. Lactose-negative Gram-negative rods, including *Pseudomonas, Klebsiella, Enterobacter, Serratia, Proteus,* and *Providencia.*

with the interpretation that the reaction on the triple sugar iron agar slant is negative, since no H_2S is formed. *Proteus* species are delineated by the H_2S differential, and the *Klebsiella, Enterobacter, Serratia, Proteus,* and *Providencia* strains, all of which can show nonlactose fermentation on MacConkey's agar, are delineated by H_2S, phenylaline, indole, urea, decarboxylase, and specific sugar reactions.

This brief summary of characterization of several genera of commonly encountered Enterobacteriaceae has, in each case, described an approach that requires subculture of the primary isolate and the carrying out of further identification procedures. Taxonomic criteria require that definitive tests be performed, but in the hospital laboratory, a presumptive overnight identification can be of great value to clinicians treating a seriously ill patient. In our laboratory, we have directed a specific effort toward prompt presumptive identification of an isolate, based on morphology of the colony on blood agar and on EMB. The colonies are observed microscopically by oblique and transmitted light, and the organism is assigned to a presumptive genus, if possible. The colony is then subcultured, and a definitive identification is made and reported as soon as possible on the follow-up report. The techni-

Table 10. Presumptive recognition of *Pseudomonas, Providencia,* and *Enterobacter* spp. on EMB and blood agar plates

Genus	Presumptive identification	Confirmed	Erroneous
Pseudomonas	201	200	1 (*Providencia*)
Providencia	117	111	6 (*Serratia:* 1) (*Proteus:* 1) (*Enterobacter:* 4)
Enterobacter	134	91	43 (*Serratia:* 14) (*Providencia:* 13) (*Mima:* 10) (*Klebsiella:* 5) (*Pseudomonas:* 1)

cian is enjoined always to correct, if necessary, the presumptive generic finding. The degree of accuracy that has been attained by this approach is summarized in Table 10.

Three commonly encountered genera are shown here as examples of the degree of correctness that can be attained by colony inspection alone. *Klebsiella* are recognized correctly somewhat more often than *Enterobacter*. *Serratia* are most often classed presumptively with *Enterobacter*. *Proteus*, which is not listed here, is usually correctly classified, since few nonswarming species are seen. *Mima-Herellea* group organisms are recognized with moderate effectiveness. This group is not encountered with great frequency.

In 35 of 43 erroneous identifications of *Enterobacter*, the least effectively distinguished genus, the organism was correctly identified as one of Enterobacteriaceae. To this extent, the clinician was not misled, and the preliminary report states that this is a tentative identification based on colony morphology. There is a constant, positive encouragement to study colony morphology carefully, since the technicians take pride in their ability to recognize genera, and, of course, rapid definitive identification is facilitated by correct presumptive grouping.

This brief summary of cultivation and recognition of *Pseudomonas* and of several of the common genera of Enterobacteriaceae has, of course, omitted many details that must be considered if correct identifications of these organisms are to be made in all instances. However, with the major part of isolates, the criteria presented will serve to achieve identification. At the reference laboratory level, more complete schemata can be employed, but in even a small clinical laboratory, correct identification can be achieved in most instances without an unacceptable level of expense and effort. The long-standing practice of lumping coliform bacteria into an ill-defined category of "paracolon" organisms is now less excusable than ever. The long history of taxonomic study of enteric bacilli has given us tools with which to achieve correct identifications.

Literature Cited

1. Lilly, H. A., and E. J. L. Lowbury. Cetrimide-nalidixic acid agar as a selective medium for *Pseudomonas aeruginosa*. J. Med. Microbiol. 5: 151, 1972.
2. Stanier, R. Y., N. J. Palleroni, and M. Doudoroff. The aerobic pseudomonads: A taxonomic study. J. Gen. Microbiol. 43: 159, 1966.
3. Sellers, W. Medium for differentiating the Gram-negative bacilli of medical interest. J. Bacteriol. 87: 47, 1964.
4. Kovacs, N. Identification of *Pseudomonas pyocyanea* by the oxidase reaction. Nature 178: 703, 1956.
5. Moeller, V. Activity determination of amino acid decarboxylases in Enterobacteriaceae. Acta Pathol. Microbiol. Scand. 34: 102, 1954.
6. Edwards, P. R., and W. Ewing (eds). Identification of Enterobacteriaceae. 3rd Ed. Burgess Publishing Co., Minneapolis, 1972.
7. Ewing, W. H. "Biochemical Reactions Given by Enterobacteriaceae in Commonly Used Tests." Center for Disease Control, Atlanta, 1969.
8. Matsen, J. M., D. J. Blazeric, J. A. Ryan, and W. H. Ewing. Characterization of indole-positive *Proteus mirabilis*. Appl. Microbiol. 23: 592, 1972.

3

Opportunistic Pathogens: Immunological Aspects

Erwin Neter

Since the golden days of microbiology in the latter quarter of the past century, numerous infections have been etiologically clarified. The responsible microorganisms include bacteria, fungi, protozoa, and viruses, and Henle-Koch's postulates have been fulfilled for many of these pathogens. Many microorganisms are found on the skin and mucous membranes that do not cause discernible ill-effects, and our environment contains many additional microorganisms which are not pathogenic for man, animals, or plants. With the use of an ever-increasing number of drugs, the availability of more complex surgical procedures, and the prolonged survival of patients with serious diseases, a host population has arisen in whom microorganisms of low virulence or otherwise avirulent strains are causing clinical infection and sometimes even fatal disease. It is these opportunistic pathogens that are the subject of this conference. Since their presence in given specimens from patients does not unequivocally prove their etiological role in disease, our laboratories have studied the immune response of these patients to these suspected pathogens. It is the premise of this investigation that documentation of the production of anti-

---

Supported by U. S. Public Health Service Grant No. AI00658 from the National Institute of Allergy and Infectious Diseases.

bodies that are specific for these microorganisms supports the assumption of their clinical significance. The studies reported here follow previous investigations dealing with the immune response of patients with salmonellosis (1), various enterobacterial (2) or urinary tract infections (3), and other types of infection as well (4).

Opportunistic infection is concerned with the pathogenicity of certain microorganisms that are usually nonvirulent or of limited virulence, rather than with the colonization by such microorganisms in the absence of disease. Pathogenicity or virulence can be defined adequately only by reference to both microorganism and host, and the same considerations apply to opportunistic infections. These latter infections may arise from the flora of the host or may be introduced from outside, endogenous or exogenous infection. It is particularly the changes in host resistance, rather than changes in microbial factors of pathogenicity, that account for these infections. Although opportunistic infections have become increasingly important during the last decade, such infections had been recognized for many decades. For example, subacute bacterial endocarditis caused by *Streptococcus mitis* (*Streptococcus viridans*) represents such a long-known opportunistic infection, developing in patients with either rheumatic heart disease or congenital heart anomalies. Among the reasons for the increasing frequency of these opportunistic infections are the prolonged survival of patients with underlying diseases and the wider use of many drugs and surgical procedures.

The studies reported here were done on patients at Children's Hospital in Buffalo with suspected or established infection caused by Gram-negative bacteria. Conventional methods were used to isolate and identify the microorganisms. To quantitate the immune response, antibody titers, usually in serial blood specimens, were determined by the passive hemagglutination method, as described previously (2, 5, and 6). In addition to antigen(s) prepared from the patient's own organism(s), control antigens were used, comprising five O groups of enteropathogenic *Escherichia coli*, five O groups of *Salmonella* (B, C_1, C_2, D, and E), and five serogroups of *Shigella*. In accordance with the observations of Strohm, Knothe, and Sietzen (7), the use of five antigens in this polyvalent hemagglutination test does not result in decreased sensitivity of the procedure.

Opportunistic infections may be categorized under two headings, one related to the particular microorganisms and the other related to the abnormally susceptible hosts. For these reasons, data are given first on the immune response of patients to a few selected opportunistic pathogens, followed by observations on special groups of patients who represent unusually susceptible subjects.

Many species of microorganisms usually are considered to be nonpathogenic for man. However, their role in human infection is emerging from careful studies of these potential pathogens. A few representative examples are presented here.

Erwinia was isolated from the bloodstream of a two-week-old infant with hydronephrosis of the right kidney and absent left kidney (patient number 459-761). Obviously, contamination of blood cannot be excluded with certainty, particularly because only a single blood culture was available. For these reasons, documentation of a specific antibody response, as shown in Table 1, supports the assumption of true infection, rather than contamination. It should be pointed out that the more than eight-fold increase in antibody titer within a period of less than two weeks is all the more remarkable because the subject was only two weeks of age.

Present-day biochemical characterization makes it possible to identify certain species within genera of Enterobacteriaceae that were not adequately characterized previously in many diagnostic laboratories. *Enterobacter cloacae* belongs to this group of micro-

Table 1. Antibody response to *Erwinia* sp. of two-week-old infant with right hydronephrosis and absent left kidney

Dates of blood specimens	*Erwinia* sp. Hemagglutinin titers (reciprocal)
May 29	< 4
June 10	32

organisms. The antibody response of a patient (patient number 477-281) to this microorganism is summarized in Table 2. It should be mentioned that control antigens were employed in all these studies, and a parallel increase in the titers of antibodies to these 15 O antigens of Enterobacteriaceae did not take place.

A similar antibody response to *E. cloacae* could be demonstrated in a child with cystic fibrosis who harbored this microorganism in the respiratory tract. As shown in Table 3, a greater than eight-fold increase in the antibody titer was demonstrated within an eight-day period. It may be seen, too, that a rise in antibody titers against 15 other antigens did not take place.

Both pigmented and nonpigmented strains of *Serratia* are encountered with increasing frequency. The antibody response of a child (patient number 015-072) to a pigmented strain is shown in Table 4. This patient had jejunal atresia and volvulus. Parts of the small bowel were resected. Subsequently, the patient developed diarrhea. *Serratia* was isolated from the feces, the conjunctiva, and the catheter used for hyperalimentation. It may be seen that the

Table 2. Antibody response to *Enterobacter cloacae* of patient with bacteremia

Dates of blood specimens	E. cloacae
	Hemagglutinin titers (recriprocal)
December 24	80
December 28	1280
January 5	1280

Table 3. Antibody response to *Enterobacter cloacae* of patient with cystic fibrosis

Dates of blood specimens	E. cloacae	15 other O antigens
	Hemagglutinin titers (reciprocal)	
December 21	< 20	< 20
December 29	160	< 20

Immunological Aspects

antibody titer to the patient's isolate increased at least eight-fold, whereas the titers against five O groups of *E. coli* remained at the same level of 1:8. Thus, *Serratia* probably contributed to the patient's illness.

The approach of utilization of the immune response as an aid to characterization of the potential pathogenicity of a poorly described microorganism is provided by the following observation. An organism that was identified as "HB1," according to the Center for Disease Control in Atlanta, Ga., and whose identity was confirmed by the Division of Laboratories and Research of the New York State Department of Health in Albany, N.Y., was isolated from the peritoneal fluid of a patient (patient number 02-29-29) with peritonitis, which had developed upon rupture of the appendix. Antibody studies revealed the data shown in Table 5. It may be seen that the antibody titer to the patient's organism rose from less than 5 to 20 within three days, thus providing

Table 4. Antibody response to pigmented *Serratia* of two-month-old infant with postoperative diarrhea

Dates of blood specimens	*Serratia*	Enteropathogenic *E. coli* (5 serotypes)
	Hemagglutinin titers (reciprocal)	
January 3	< 4	8
January 17	< 4	8
February 21	16	8

Table 5. Antibody response to HB1 of patient with peritonitis

Dates of blood specimens	HB1
	Hemagglutinin titers (reciprocal)
June 19	< 5
June 22	20
June 26	20

evidence strongly suggesting the potential pathogenicity of this microorganism.

It is well known that numerous microorganisms live on skin and mucous membranes in symbiosis with human subjects without causing any discernible ill-effects and, in fact, may contribute to resistance to infection by pathogens. It is equally clear that these same microorganisms may cause significant infection elsewhere in the body and in subjects with reduced resistance. Thus, perforation of the intestine leads to peritonitis; organisms present in the upper respiratory tract following aspiration may cause pneumonia; intestinal organisms, when introduced into the urinary tract with either anatomical or physiological obstruction, give rise to infection. Conversely, the premature infant is more susceptible to infection than the older child; the male newborn is more susceptible than the female newborn; children with leukemia are more susceptible than nonleukemic children of similar age; and diabetic patients are more susceptible than nondiabetic subjects. Such examples could be multiplied almost ad infinitum.

Cystic fibrosis presents an unusually instructive example of lowered susceptibility to infection of the respiratory tract and normal resistance against systemic disease (including sepsis, meningitis, osteomyelitis, etc.). It has long been recognized that coagulase-positive staphylococci and *Pseudomonas aeruginosa* are frequently present in the upper respiratory tract of these patients. The antibody response to the latter microorganism has been studied by Diaz, Mosovich, and Neter (8) and compared to that of patients with neoplastic diseases (9). That other Enterobacteriaceae may play a role as well is illustrated by recent unpublished observations made in collaboration with Dr. Luis L. Mosovich and Mr. Edward J. Seidmon. In these studies, antigens were prepared from all isolates of Enterobacteriaceae present in the sputum of subjects with cystic fibrosis. A striking antibody response of one such patient to a nontypable strain of *E. coli* is recorded in Table 6. Since the antibody titer increased in parallel against a strain of *P. aeruginosa* that was present in the same sputum sample, absorption tests were carried out to differentiate between cross-reactivity and two specific antibody responses. The data shown in Table 6 clearly indicate that antibodies of different specificity were present in the second blood sample. It is likely, therefore, that *E. coli*

Table 6. Antibody response to both *Pseudomonas aeruginosa* and *E. coli* NT* of patient with cystic fibrosis

Dates of blood specimens	P. aeruginosa	E. coli NT
	Hemagglutinin titers (reciprocal)	
August 23	< 20	< 20
August 26	640	320
Absorbed		
E. coli NT	640	< 40
P. aeruginosa	< 40	320

* NT, nontypable strain.

Table 7. Antibody response to *E. coli* O18 and O50 of patient with cystic fibrosis

Dates of blood specimens	E. coli O18	O50
	Hemagglutinin titers (reciprocal)	
Unabsorbed	320	320
Absorbed		
O18	< 20	320
O50	160	< 20

played a role in the infection of the subject. Similar data on another patient with cystic fibrosis, who harbored two different serogroups of *E. coli* in the respiratory tract, are summarized in Table 7. It may be seen that antibodies to the two microorganisms differed in specificity, since only the homologous microorganism absorbed its own antibodies.

Patients with leukemia present a particularly susceptible group of subjects. The study of the immune response may be complicated because of impairment of the immune apparatus by the disease and/or by cancer therapy. The data of the antibody response to *Klebsiella*, isolated from the throat of such a patient, are recorded in Table 8. It is evident that a four-fold increase in antibody titer took place, although the absolute levels were relatively low. Significantly, there was no parallel increase in the titers of antibodies against control organisms. Even under these unfavorable conditions, production of antibodies against an opportunistic pathogen could be documented.

Organisms considered to be of limited pathogenicity may cause infection in patients with burns. Their presence in the lesion, however, does not necessarily indicate their etiological role. A triple antibody response to three different isolates from the infected burn of a representative patient is shown in Table 9.

Patients with indwelling catheters and other foreign bodies all too often are subject to opportunistic infection. Observations of one such patient undergoing peritoneal dialysis because of renal insufficiency are recorded in Table 10. *Enterobacter aerogenes* was isolated from the dialysis fluid on two occasions. It may be seen

Table 8. *Klebsiella* infection in child with leukemia

Dates of blood specimens	*Klebsiella* (throat)
	Hemagglutinin titers (reciprocal)
July 4	10
July 18	40
August 30	40

Table 9. Triple antibody response of patient with infected burn

Dates of blood specimens	*E. coli* NT (July 22, 1972)	*Klebsiella* (July 22, 1972)	*E. coli* O16 (July 24, 1972)
	Hemagglutinin titers (reciprocal)		
July 18	20	< 20	< 20
August 4	320	80	80
August 19	320	160	80

that the antibody titer to this microorganism increased from 1:40 to 1:5120 within a 10-day period.

Opportunistic infections in patients with the nephrotic syndrome have been known for many years, and pneumococcal peritonitis is the best-known example. In a patient with this syndrome, *E. coli* O6 was isolated from a single blood culture, and a definitive antibody response to this microorganism could be demonstrated, as shown in Table 11. It is particularly significant that the increase in titer took place within a five-day period.

Patients with renal transplants, too, may become subject to opportunistic infection, particularly when immunosuppressive therapy has to be employed. The data of the antibody response of such a patient are recorded in Table 12. Although infection was recognized clinically only on March 27, 1971, the immunological findings clearly indicate that the infection must have existed for at least 10 days, since the titer of antibodies had risen from 1:320 to

Table 10. Hemagglutinin response of patient with renal failure caused by absent left kidney and hypoplastic right kidney treated with peritoneal dialysis

Dates of blood specimens	*E. aerogenes* from dialysis fluid	
	April 7, 1970	April 11, 1970
	Hemagglutinin titers (reciprocal)	
February 13	40	40
April 6	40	40
April 16	5120	5120

Table 11. Antibody response to *E. coli* O6 of patient with nephrotic syndrome and *E. coli* bacteremia

Dates of blood specimens	*E. coli* O6
	Hemagglutinin titers (reciprocal)
January 9	20
January 14	160

Table 12. Hemagglutinin response to *E. coli* O18 of patient with acute infection (clinical onset March 27, 1971) and 6 months after renal transplant because of chronic glomerulonephritis

Dates of blood specimens	*E. coli* O18 Hemagglutinin titers (reciprocal)
September 25, 1968	160
December 23, 1970	320
January 13, 1970	320
February 3, 1971	320
March 17, 1971	2560
March 29, 1971	2560

1:2560 between February 3 and March 17, 1971. Thus, immunological investigation may shed light also on onset of infection.

Patients with surgical bypasses of the excretory urinary system also may develop opportunistic infection. In one such patient, infection took place in the ileal loop, and the findings on the titers of antibodies to two isolates, obtained at various times, are recorded in Table 13. It may be seen that the titer of antibodies to one isolate was already high (1:320) and that a significant increase in the titers of antibodies to the other isolate took place during the two ensuing months.

Opportunistic infection may also develop in patients with colon transplanted for correction of esophageal stricture. Findings on one such patient are recorded in Table 14 and clearly indicate that, within a seven-day period, the antibody titer to the isolate *(Bethesda* of the genus *Citrobacter)* rose from 1:20 to 1:640. In contrast, no change was observed in the titers of antibodies to other enteric pathogens.

Documentation of the immune response to microorganisms usually considered of limited virulence has supported the assumption of their etiological role as opportunistic pathogens. These organisms include *Erwinia* sp., *E. cloacae*, pigmented *Serratia*, and

Immunological Aspects

Table 13. Hemagglutinin response to *Klebsiella* and *Enterobacter* of patient with ileal loop for correction of extrophy of bladder

Dates of blood specimens	*Klebsiella* (May 25)	*Enterobacter* (July 5)
	Hemagglutinin titers (reciprocal)	
May 25	320	40
July 5	320	640

Table 14. Antibody response to *Bethesda (Citrobacter)* of patient with esophageal stricture and necrosis of transplanted colon

Dates of blood specimens	*Bethesda*	*Shigella*	*Salmonella*	Enteropathogenic *E. coli*
	Hemagglutinin titers (reciprocal)			
August 8	20	20	40	80
August 15	640	20	40	80

HB1. In addition, rises in titers of antibodies directed against various species of bacteria have been demonstrated in patients with opportunistic infections attributable to the presence of underlying diseases or preconditioning entities, including cystic fibrosis, burns, leukemia, nephrotic syndrome, and renal and other transplants. It is concluded that the demonstration and titration of antibodies directed against suspected opportunistic pathogens provide significant information for a better understanding of the source, etiology, pathogenesis, and onset of these bacterial infections.

Literature Cited

1. Neter, E., A. M. Drislane, A. H. Harris, and G. T. Jansen. Diagnosis of clinical and subclinical salmonellosis by means of a serologic hemagglutination test. New Engl. J. Med. 261: 1162, 1959.
2. Neter, E., A. H. Harris, and A. M. Drislane. The detection of enterobacterial infection in institutionalized children by means of the hemagglutination test. Amer. J. Pub. Health 55: 1164, 1965.

3. Neter, E., O. R. Oberkircher, M. I. Rubin, J. M. Steinhart, and I. Krzeska. Patterns of antibody response of children with infections of the urinary tract. Pediat. Res. 4: 500, 1970.
4. Neter, E. The immune response of the host: An aid to etiology, pathogenesis, diagnosis, and epidemiology of bacterial infections. Yale J. Biol. Med. 44: 241, 1971.
5. Neter, E., E. A. Gorzynski, R. M. Gino, O. Westphal, and O. Luderitz. The enterobacterial hemagglutination test and its diagnostic potentialities. Can. J. Microbiol. 2: 232, 1956.
6. Neter, E., A. H. Harris, and A. M. Drislane. Comparative study of hemagglutination and agglutination tests for the determination of the antibody response of patients with *S. sonnei* dysentery. Amer. J. Clin. Pathol. 37: 239, 1962.
7. Strohm, W. D., H. Knothe, and W. Sietzen. Hämagglutinationstest mit Kaninchenimmunseren und polyvalenten *E. coli*-Antigenen. Med. Microbiol. Immunol. 157: 251, 1972.
8. Diaz, F., L. L. Mosovich, and E. Neter. Serogroups of *Pseudomonas aeruginosa* and the immune response of patients with cystic fibrosis. J. Infect. Dis. 121: 269, 1970.
9. Diaz, F., and E. Neter. *Pseudomonas aeruginosa:* Serogroups and antibody response in patients with neoplastic diseases. Amer. J. Med. Sci. 259: 340, 1970.

4

Bacteriocin Typing of *Pseudomonas, Proteus,* and *Klebsiella-Enterobacter-Serratia*

J. J. Farmer, III

Three groups of opportunistic bacteria, *Pseudomonas, Proteus,* and *Klebsiella-Enterobacter-Serratia,* often cause infections in hospital patients. The ecology and epidemiology of these organisms still are not completely known, so that new investigators continue to discover the mechanism by which they cause infections. Several epidemiological typing methods have been used to place markers, or "epidemiological fingerprints," on these bacteria: serological typing, bacteriophage susceptibility, antibiotic susceptibility, the Dienes reaction (1), and bacteriocin production or sensitivity. The purpose of any of these methods is to answer the epidemiological question, "Is this isolate the same strain (in a genetic and epidemiological sense) as that isolate?" If this question can be answered satisfactorily, then the relationships among the patient and environmental strains can be determined, and the epidemiology of the pathogen can be defined. If the typing method does not answer this question satisfactorily, then it is not doing its job, and another method should be sought. Bacteriocin typing almost always answers the pertinent epidemiological questions.

This research was supported by Research Grant No. CC 00592 from the Center for Disease Control, Atlanta, Ga. 30333.

Bacteriocins are proteins that many bacteria produce during the exponential growth phase (2-4). They are bactericidal for strains of the same species or closely related species and are detected by the zones of inhibition they produce against a suitable indicator strain (see Figs. 1, 2, and 3).

Bacteriocin typing can be done in two ways: determining the bacteriocin production pattern of a strain against a set of standard indicators or determining the bacteriocin sensitivity pattern of the strain against a set of bacteriocins which are applied to it. Each method has been used in epidemiology and will be discussed below. To determine if two isolates from different sources are the same strain, one compares their bacteriocin production or sensitivity patterns. If the isolates are the same strain, the patterns will be identical. By comparing the patterns of all isolates from an outbreak or hospital, one can determine the epidemiology of the infections.

Bacteriocin typing is a technique for use primarily in epidemiological studies. If there are five cases of *Pseudomonas aeruginosa* sepsis in the nursery and *P. aeruginosa* is isolated from the formula bottles, then the question to be asked is, "Is the formula bottle isolate the same strain as the one from the infants?" For a typing method to be reliable, it must be sensitive enough to answer this kind of question, and bacteriocin typing almost always does when it is performed correctly.

Table 1. Bacteriocin production—scrape and streak method

1. Inoculate test strains in a band about 2 cm wide on an agar surface (Fig. 1,*A*)
2. Grow at optimum temperature; typically 24 hr at 32 or 37°C
3. Scrape the growth from the plate (Fig. 1,*B*)
4. Expose the surface to chloroform vapors for 30 min
5. Evaporate traces of chloroform
6. Streak the bacteriocin indicator strains perpendicular to original growth
7. Incubate at 37°C for 24 hr
8. Read and record the bacteriocin production pattern of the test strain against the bacteriocin indicators (Fig. 1,*C* and *D* shows the bacteriocin production patterns of two different strains)

I. Bacteriocin Production—Scrape and Streak Method

This method has been used to type *Shigella sonnei* (5), *Proteus* (6), *P. aeruginosa* (7), and other organisms. The method is outlined in Table 1. The advantage of the scrape and streak method is that it is simple to perform and can be done in most clinical laboratories, because no special equipment is required,

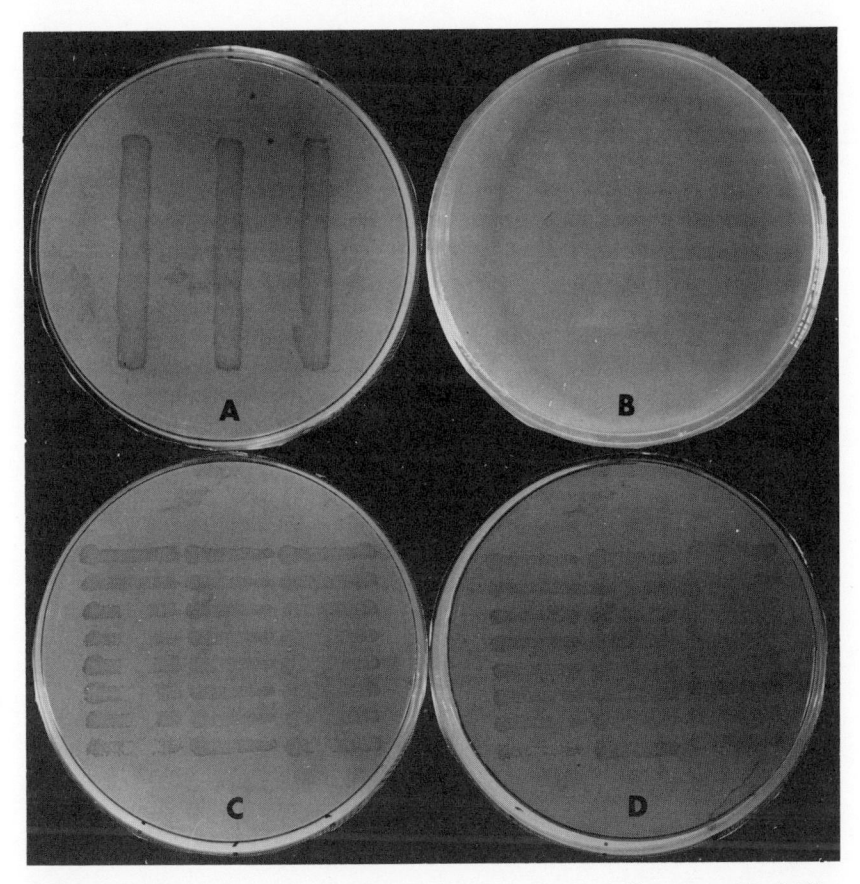

Figure 1. Bacteriocin typing of *Proteus* by the Cradock-Watson method. The isolates on plates C and D have different bacteriocin production patterns and would be considered different strains.

only a set of bacteriocin-indicator strains. The disadvantages are the lack of reproducibility and the large number of untypable strains which often are found, since it is difficult to stimulate bacteriocin production. The scrape and streak typing of *Proteus* is illustrated in Figure 1.

II. Bacteriocin Production—Growth in Broth Method

This method has become popular recently and is an alternative to the scrape and streak method (8–10). The steps are outlined in Table 2. The advantages are that a large number of strains can be tested, standardization is easy to obtain, and bacteriocin production can be stimulated with mitomycin C or ultraviolet rays (11). The disadvantage of the growth in broth method is that it requires more sophistication than does the scrape and streak method, thus making it more difficult for the small laboratory, but it is the method of choice for those who have the resources to attempt bacteriocin typing. Figure 2 illustrates typical results obtained by this method. Bacteriocins were prepared from 11 isolates of *Serratia marcescens* and were added to lawns of indicator strains 1, 2, and 3. The bacteriocin production pattern of the

Table 2. Bacteriocin production in broth
---
1. Inoculate the test strains into a rich peptone broth, such as Trypticase soy broth; grow 24 hr (usually at 32 or 37°C)
2. Start the culture back into the experimental growth phase by adding 1 ml of 24-hr culture to 8 ml of fresh broth
2a. After 1 hr, add 1 ml of 10 µg per ml mitomycin C to stimulate bacteriocin production (This step is optional and depends on the particular typing system)
3. Incubate for 24 hr
4. Add 1 ml of chloroform and shake vigorously on orbital mixer for 10 sec
5. Loosen cap and evaporate chloroform for 1 hr
6. Remove top 1 ml of fluid into tuberculin syringe or mechanical applicator and add to each bacteriocin indicator strain
7. Incubate for 24 hr
8. Read and record bacteriocin production pattern of test strain against indicators

Bacteriocin Typing of Enterics

11 isolates against these three and another 15 indicator strains were then recorded and compared.

III. Bacteriocin Sensitivity

Typing by bacteriocin sensitivity is different from typing by bacteriocin production. To determine the bacteriocin sensitivity of a bacterium, one must obtain a set of standard bacteriocin pro-

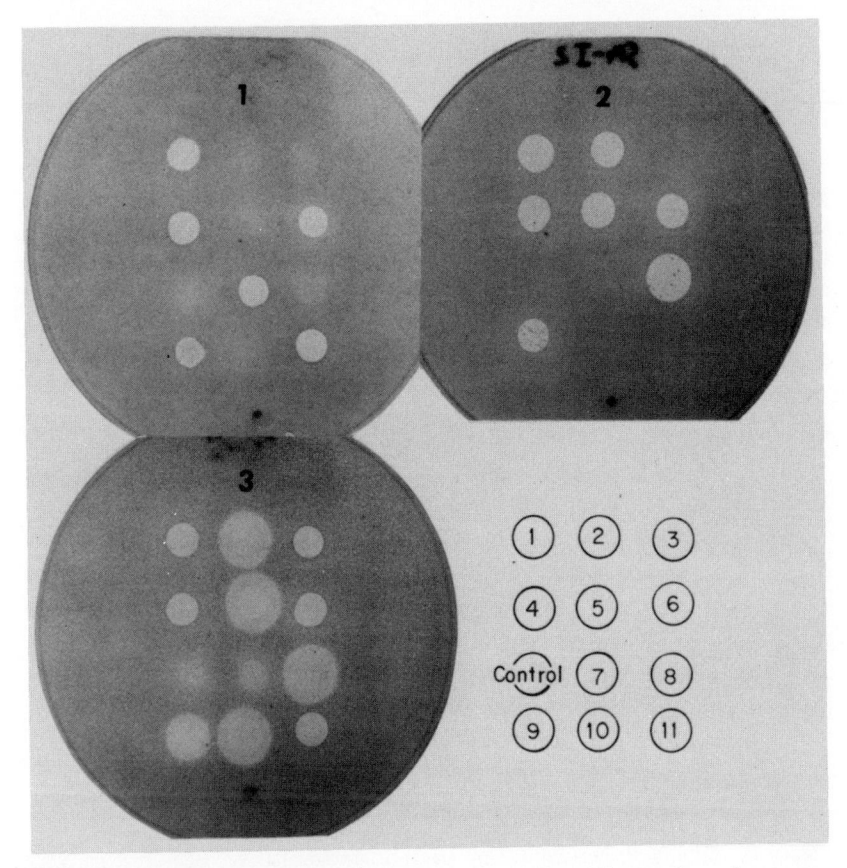

Figure 2. Bacteriocin typing of *S. marcescens*. Bacteriocins have been prepared from 11 isolates and added to indicator strains 1, 2, and 3.

ducers and grow them under standard conditions, during which they produce bacteriocins. The viable cells are killed with chloroform, and the bacteriocins then are added to the strains which are being compared. Typing by bacteriocin sensitivity is similar to typing by bacteriophage susceptibility and has been used to type *Shigella* (5), *P. aeruginosa* (11), *Klebsiella-Enterobacter-Serratia* (9, 10), and other bacteria. Figure 3 shows that isolates A and B, even though they are from different sources, have identical bacteriocin sensitivity patterns and are the same strains.

IV. Reporting Bacteriocin Production or Bacteriocin Sensitivity Patterns

This has been the subject of much confusion and has been very complicated in the past. Most authors simply assigned an arbitrary designation to each new pattern as it was encountered, and with different authors making arbitrary assignments, great confusion resulted. A set of rules was recently proposed (12) which has overcome this difficulty. With these rules, each pattern is assigned a unique number in a systematic fashion. The simplified

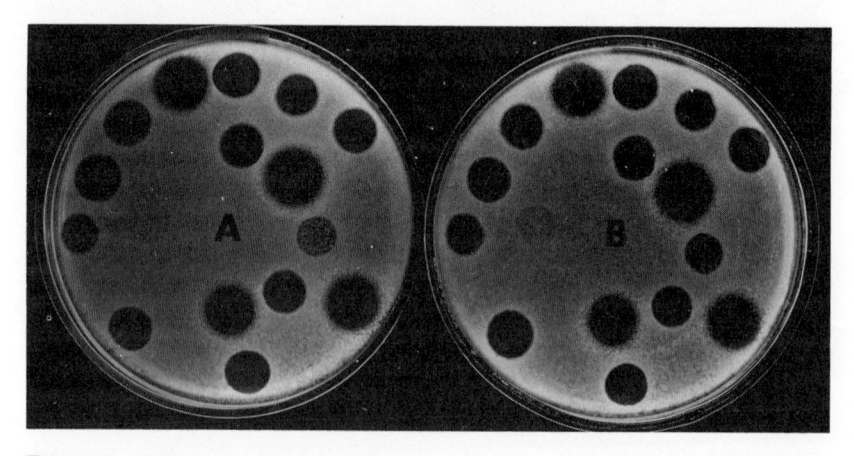

Figure 3. Typing *P. aeruginosa* by bacteriocin sensitivity. Bacteriocins were prepared from 24 standard strains and added to isolates A and B, which are really the same strains.

notation is shown in Table 3. If N is the number of bacteriocin reactions, then each of the 2^N possible patterns is assigned the correct designation according to these rules.

V. Automated Application of Bacteriocins

The ACCU-DROP bacteriophage-bacteriocin applicator is commercially available (Sylvana Corp., Milburn, N. J.) and applies 24 standardized drops in a single operation (12). We have modified it slightly so that it can apply 57 drops to a 150- × 15-mm dish

Table 3. Simplified method for reporting bacteriocin and bacteriophage patterns[a]

Reaction[b]	Notation
+ + +	1
+ + −	2
+ − +	3
− + +	4
+ − −	5
− + −	6
− − +	7
− − −	8

[a]If the number of tests is not evenly divisible by 3, a second (+ + = A, + − = B, − + = C, and − − = D) or third (+ = E, − = F) notation is required for the remaining tests.

[b] + − +   − − +   − − −   + − +
   3   7   8   3
− + = 378 3C
C

(details will be furnished on request). Bacteriocin typing is greatly facilitated with this device. Also, for the scrape and streak method of bacteriocin typing, there are a number of streakers which apply the bacteriocin indicators simultaneously.

VI. Computer Selection of Bacteriocin Indicators or Producers

Until recently, the main difficulty with bacteriocin typing has been its lack of epidemiological sensitivity. This has been due to poor choices of indicator strains. When typing is done against a limited number of indicators, the results are confusing, and, much of the time, the question, "Is isolate A the same strain as isolate B?" cannot be answered. The probability is too great against two strains' having the same bacteriocin pattern by chance alone. However, when impartial computer analysis is used to choose the indicators, the resulting typing method is more sensitive, and definitive epidemiological conclusions can be made with no additional work. We have written a computer program which reads in bacteriocin production or sensitivity patterns and prints out the set of bacteriocin indicators (or producers) which are best suited for routine typing.

These new methods are applicable to other organisms for which typing methods are not available, and work is now in progress to formulate systems for other pathogens of interest.

VII. Application of Bacteriocin Typing—Investigating the Known Outbreak

Table 4 shows that during months 4 and 5 there was a significant increase in isolates from infants in the nursery. During this type of situation there is little doubt that an outbreak is occurring, but the more important question is, "What is the source(s) of the strain(s) causing infections?" Table 5 shows how bacteriocin (pyocin) typing was used to reveal the epidemiology of this nursery outbreak. The strain with bacteriocin production

Table 4. *P. aeruginosa* isolates from an intensive care unit and nursery

Month	Isolates of *P. aeruginosa* in	
	Intensive care	Nursery
1	2	0
2	3	0
3	5	1
4	6	17
5	4	14
6	2	0

Table 5. Pyocin typing which revealed the epidemiology of a nursery outbreak of *P. aeruginosa*

Source	Pyocin production pattern
Seven sick infants	141 111 544
Ten healthy infants	141 111 544
Three sick infants	111 211 231
One healthy infant	111 211 231
One nurse	111 211 231
One oxygen bubbler	111 211 231
Five healthy infants	414 161 211
One nurse	414 161 211

pattern 141 111 544 was responsible for most of the problem; however, it was not detected in the environment or in nursery personnel. The conclusion was made that this is a virulent strain which was introduced into one of the infants (perhaps from a mother) and spread through the nursery by cross-infection. A second strain (bacteriocin production pattern 111 211 231) caused infections in three children and fecal carriage in another. This strain was traced to an oxygen bubbler used by the infants and to a nurse, who perhaps accidentally inoculated it into the bubbler, where it multiplied in the distilled water (13). A third strain (bacteriocin production pattern 414 161 211) caused fecal carriage in five infants, and the source was a nurse who also carried this strain in her gut. Thus, bacteriocin typing revealed the complete epidemiology of the outbreak (14).

VIII. Application of Bacteriocin Typing—Determining Cause of Cross-Infection

Table 4 shows the number of isolates of *P. aeruginosa* in an intensive care unit. From data such as these, it is usually difficult to distinguish trouble, such as cross-infections or a small outbreak, from normal variations in the numbers of isolates. To determine the amount of cross-infection attributable to *S. marcescens*, we asked several hospitals to send us all their *S. marcescens* isolates from patients for several months. We then compared all of the strains by determining their bacteriocin production patterns [these strains were also tested against nine additional *S. marcescens* indicator strains (8)]. Whenever a strain from one patient was found in another, it was designated as "cross-infection," and the "*S. marcescens* cross-infection rate" was defined as the number of cases in which cross-infections were involved, divided by the total number of cases, with all multiplied by 100.

Table 6 shows that the cross-infection rate varied greatly among different hospitals, all of which had over 300 beds. Hospital B was having a serious problem, while not a single case of cross-infection was evident in hospital C (however, only infections which were actually cultured could be compared). Hospital A also was having a serious problem, but knew it at the time. Hospital D had only two cases of cross-infection out of 42. Table 7 shows that a single strain was causing most of the problems in Hospital B, which almost could be considered as having a serious outbreak of urinary tract infections caused by the strain with bacteriocin production pattern 131 211. The other instance of cross-infection was due to a different strain (111 211). In this particular hospital, there was

Table 6. *Serratia marcescens* cross-infections in four large hospitals, as revealed by bacteriocin typing

Hospital	Per cent of *S. marcescens* infections which were due to cross-infection or a single source outbreak
A	61
B	93
C	0
D	5

Table 7. Epidemiology of *S. marcescens* infections in hospital B during a two-month period

Number of patients	Source	Bacteriocin production pattern	Streptomycin susceptibility
12	Urine	131 211	R[a]
2	Wound		
1	Urine[b]	111 211	S
1	Sputum		
1	Membrane	753 184	S
1	Urine	133 221	S

[a] Symbols: *R*, resistant; *S*, sensitive (Kirby-Bauer) method.

[b] This patient later became infected with resistant strains 131 and 211.

concern over the frequency of *S. marcescens* infections, but the hospital personnel were unaware of the problem. Bacteriocin typing could have answered their epidemiological questions. Unfortunately, this was a retrospective study, so the source(s) could not be determined.

IX. Bacteriocin Typing of *P. aeruginosa*

The possibility of differentiating *P. aeruginosa* by bacteriocins was first described by Holloway (15), and a number of different methods are in use today (7, 11, 16). The method perhaps in widest use is that of Gillies and Govan (7). This is a typical scrape and streak method, and its main advantage is its simplicity, which makes it applicable in any hospital. However, there are two disadvantages: it is hard to reproduce results, as with any scrape and streak method, and most patterns are so common that no epidemiological conclusions can be made unless the study is limited to a few isolates. The addition of five new indicator strains has improved the sensitivity; but, even with the added indicator strains, this method is not sensitive enough when large numbers of isolates are compared.

Farmer and Herman (11) described a method which was more sensitive in comparing large numbers of strains. They grew the strains in broth, induced bacteriocin-production with mitomycin C, and added the bacteriocins simultaneously to 27 indicator strains with a mechanical applicator. The epidemiological conclusions are usually definitive with this method, but more equipment and time are required. A number of improvements and shortcuts have been made, but it would not be wise to publish these until a standardized method can be proposed. Bacteriocin typing of *P. aeruginosa* is sensitive enough to determine the epidemiology of most situations, but only if the necessary time and effort are expended. Currently, there is a group working toward standardization, and hopefully, within the next few years, a standard method(s) will be available. This probably will consist of 1) determining the somatic antigen with commercially available antisera and then 2) subdividing the strains within these O groups with bacteriocin production, bacteriocin sensitivity, or bacteriophage susceptibility.

X. Typing *Proteus* by Bacteriocin Production

There are a number of methods for the "epidemiological fingerprinting" of *Proteus*, such as bacteriophage susceptibility (17), the Dienes reaction (1), serological typing (1), and bacteriocin production (6). However, none of these methods has been used widely or has undergone critical testing in determining the epidemiology of *Proteus* infections.

We obtained bacteriocin indicators for typing *Proteus* by the schema of Cradock-Watson through the courtesy of Dr. A. G. Towers, Cross-Infection Laboratory, Central Public Health Laboratory, Colindale, England.

The Cradock-Watson method is a typical scrape and streak procedure; unfortunately, the results were disappointing. Of 100 consecutive strains of *Proteus mirabilis* from hospital patients, only 50% produced bacteriocin against the Cradock-Watson indicators, and most of these fell into several common patterns. The Cradock-Watson method would be sensitive enough only if a particular outbreak strain happened to have a rare bacteriocin-production pattern. Like other scrape and streak methods, it was difficult to perform, and the results were difficult to reproduce.

In order to increase the number of typable strains and simplify the method, we have grown *Proteus* strains in broth and induced them with mitomycin C. The results have been promising, and a usable method for typing *P. mirabilis* by bacteriocin production should be forthcoming.

XI. Typing *Klebsiella-Enterobacter-Serratia* by Bacteriocin Production or Sensitivity

I recently proposed a standardized method for typing *S. marcescens* by bacteriocin production against nine indicator strains (8). Since that time, nine additional indicator strains have been added, and this improved method was used to study the epidemiology of *S. marcescens* infections in four large hospitals (Table 6). This method has been very sensitive in comparing strains, and in each hospital the epidemiology of infection was clearly evident.

Traub et al. (10) and Farmer (9) independently proposed schemata for differentiating *S. marcescens* by bacteriocin sensitivity. Traub et al. have used their method to study infections in his hospital and have reported good results. My experience has been more limited, since I prefer bacteriocin production as a marker. It would be easy to determine the bacteriocin sensitivity of unknown isolates against both sets of bacteriocins. This would enhance the sensitivity of the procedure. Fifty-five per cent of the *Klebsiella* and *Enterobacter* strains tested were also sensitive to the bacteriocins produced from *S. marcescens*. This fact suggests that if additional bacteriocin producers are selected which inhibit *Klebsiella* and *Enterobacter*, then a single method can be used to type the whole *Klebsiella-Enterobacter-Serratia* group. At present, however, there is no standard bacteriocin typing schema for *Klebsiella* or *Enterobacter*.

Acknowledgments

I thank Linda Farmer, Frances Hickman, John M. Hutson, Lois Faye Jones, Diana Presley, and John Zakanycz for their excellent assistance in these studies.

Literature Cited

1. De Louvois, J. Serotyping and the Dienes reaction on *Proteus mirabilis* from hospital infections. J. Clin. Pathol. 22: 263, 1969.
2. Fredericq, P. Colicins. Annu. Rev. Microbiol. 11: 7, 1957.
3. Ivanovics, G. Bacteriocins and bacteriocin-like substances. Bacteriol. Rev. 26: 108, 1962.
4. Reeves, P. The bacteriocins. Bacteriol. Rev. 29: 24, 1965.
5. Abbott, J. D., and R. Shannon. A method for typing *Shigella sonnei* using colicine production as a marker. J. Clin. Pathol. 11: 71, 1958.
6. Cradock-Watson, J. E. The production of bacteriocines by *Proteus* species. Zentbl. Bakt. Orig. 196: 385, 1965.
7. Gillies, R. R., and J. R. W. Govan. Typing of *Pseudomonas pyocyanea* by pyocine production. J. Pathol. Bacteriol. 91: 339, 1966.
8. Farmer, J. J., III. Epidemiological differentiation of *Serratia marcescens*: Typing by bacteriocin production. Appl. Microbiol. 23: 218, 1972.

9. Farmer, J. J., III. Epidemiological differentiations of *Serratia marcescens:* Typing by bacteriocin sensitivity. Appl. Microbiol. 23: 226, 1972.
10. Traub, W. H., E. A. Raymond, and T. S. Startsman. Bacteriocin (marcescin) typing of clinical isolates of *Serratia marcescens.* Appl. Microbiol. 21: 837, 1971.
11. Farmer, J. J., III, and L. G. Herman. Epidemiological fingerprinting of *Pseudomonas aeruginosa* by the production of and sensitivity to pyocin and bacteriophage. Appl. Microbiol. 18: 760, 1969.
12. Farmer, J. J. Improved bacteriophage-bacteriocin applicator. Appl. Microbiol. 20: 517, 1970.
13. Favero, M. S., L. A. Carson, W. W. Bond, and N. J. Peterson. *Pseudomonas aeruginosa:* Growth in distilled water from hospitals. Science 173: 836, 1971.
14. Falcão, D. P., C. P. Mendonca, A. Scrassolo, B. B. de Almeida, L. Hart, L. H. Farmer, and J. J. Farmer, III. Nursery outbreak of severe diarrhea due to multiple strains of *Pseudomonas aeruginosa.* Lancet 2: 38, 1972.
15. Holloway, B. W. Grouping *P. aeruginosa* by lysogenicity and pyocinogenicity. J. Pathol. Bacteriol. 80: 448, 1960.
16. Zabransky, R. J., and F. E. Day. Pyocine typing of clinical strains of *P. aeruginosa.* Appl. Microbiol. 17: 293, 1969.
17. France, D. R., and N. P. Markham. Epidemiological aspects of *Proteus* infections with particular reference to phage typing. J. Clin. Pathol. 21: 97, 1968.

5

Miscellaneous Facultatively Anaerobic Bacilli in Opportunistic Infections

Alexander von Graevenitz

Opportunists are often defined as organisms that cause infectious disease predominantly in "compromised hosts," i.e., in hosts with impaired local or general defense mechanisms. In "normal hosts," they are said to elicit either no symptoms at all or only a brief and mild response.

In the light of recent knowledge, however, two caveats to this definition have to be added:

1. Gastrointestinal and posttraumatic wound infections with bacteria generally regarded as "opportunists" have been observed in apparently "normal" hosts [e.g., infections with *Aeromonas* spp. (1)];

2. Some bacterial species (e.g., *Haemophilus* and *Listeria monocytogenes*) cause disease in both types of hosts, but an association with compromised defense mechanisms is quite conspicuous and more frequent than in infections with such "nonopportunists" as group A streptococci or *Shigella*.

The facultatively anaerobic rods that have been observed as opportunists can be divided into two groups. The first is a group of nonfastidious Gram-negative rods which are able to grow on enteric differential media and are fairly regularly encountered as opportunists (certain Enterobacteriaceae not covered elsewhere in this symposium, *Yersinia enterocolitica*, and *Aeromonas* spp.). The second is a more fastidious group of bacilli which do not grow on enteric differential media and in which opportunism is not regularly observed (the Gram-negative *Haemophilus influenzae* and *Haemophilus parainfluenzae*, as well as *Pasteurella multocida*, and the Gram-positive *L. monocytogenes*).

I. Nonfastidious, Gram-negative Opportunists

A. *Isolation and Identification*

The habitat of these bacteria may be the human gastrointestinal tract, from which endogenous infections may originate, or soil, water sources, food, or hospital equipment, which may be the source of exogenous infections.

Isolation of the nonfastidious Gram-negatives is traditionally accomplished on enteric differential plates, such as MacConkey agar, eosin methylene blue (EMB) agar, or desoxycholate agar. Their inhibitory qualities differ only slightly from each other; enterococci and yeasts may not be suppressed. On these media, Gram-negative rod colonies can be characterized by their ability to ferment lactose (and/or sucrose on EMB agar), but only a substantial degree of fermentation will result in a visible indicator change. Certain species ferment lactose on enteric agars fairly regularly, others vary in this ability, and some are consistently negative (see Table 1).

For final identification, the hospital laboratory cannot afford to use a large number of tests. Suitable tests should be 1) rapid, i.e., yielding reliable results after 24 or, maximally, 48 hr of incubation; 2) fairly consistent in their outcome for each species; and 3) economical, i.e., inexpensive and easy to perform.

For reasons of disease etiology, therapy, and epidemiology, species diagnoses are desirable; but, in many instances, a genus diagnosis has to suffice in the interest of speedy reporting. It may be supplemented later by speciation.

Table 1. Differential reactions of miscellaneous nonfastidious Gram-negative rods

Test	E. tarda	A. hinshawii	Salmonella spp.	C. freundii	C. diversus	Herbicola-Lathyri	Y. enterocolitica	Aeromonas spp.
Lactose fermentation on enteric media	−[a]	+/−	−	+/−	+/−	+/−	−	+/−
TSI agar - slant	K	A or K	K	A or K	A or K	A or K	A	A (or K)
- butt	AG	AG	AG (or A)[b]	AG (or A)	AG	A or AG	A (or AG)	A or AG
- H$_2$S	+	+	+[c]	+/−	−	−	−	−
Indole	+	−	−	−/+	+	−/+	+/−	+
Ornithine decarboxylase	+	+	+[d]	−/+	+	−	+	−
Motility	+	+	+[e]	+/(−)	+/(−)	+/(−)	+ (22°C)	+
Lysine decarboxylase	+	+	+[f]	−	−	−	−	−

[a] −, negative; +, positive; /, or (reaction of majority of strains listed first); K, alkaline; A, acid; G, gas; ( ), occasional strain.
[b] Mainly S. typhi and S. enteritidis bioser. gallinarum.
[c] Except S. enteritidis bioser. Paratyphi A, strains of S. cholerae-suis, and rare strains of S. enteritidis serotypes.
[d] Except S. typhi and S. enteritidis bioser. gallinarum.
[e] Except S. enteritidis bioser. gallinarum.
[f] Except S. enteritidis bioser. Paratyphi A.

In the experience of this laboratory, the following media and tests have been found most useful for a *preliminary* (but, in many cases, also final) identification (see Table 1):

>Triple sugar iron agar (TSI)
>Indole
>Ornithine decarboxylase (Falkow method)
>Motility
>Lysine decarboxylase (Falkow method)

Decarboxylase media may be prepared with 0.3% agar to make them semisolid for a motility check. A negative motility in such a medium, however, may be due to too much acidity or alkalinity and should be rechecked with a traditional hanging drop method. Lysine decarboxylase and H_2S production can be tested in lysine iron agar (Difco Laboratories, Detroit, Mich.), which is also helpful in the diagnosis of *Proteus*. While *Proteus mirabilis* and *Proteus vulgaris* rarely form H_2S in this medium, these species and *Proteus rettgeri* cause a burgundy-colored surface because of lysine deamination (2). For indole production, we found the motility-indole-ornithine medium (Difco Laboratories) less satisfactory than Trypticase (BioQuest, Cockeysville, Md.), presumably because the presence of glucose inhibits indole production.

Additional tests used for *selected* bacteria that cannot be diagnosed with the above tests include:

>Urease (Christensen's medium) ⎱ both used in a combined
>Phenylalanine deaminase   ⎰ medium
>Citrate utilization (Simmons' medium)
>Oxidase (Kovacs' technique)
>Voges-Proskauer reaction [PathoTec strips (Warner-Chilcott Laboratories, Morris Plains, N. J.)]
>Gelatin [Key strips (Key Scientific Products Co., Los Angeles, Calif.)]
>Beta-galactosidase [ONPG test; Key tablets (Key Scientific Products Co.)]
>Adonitol fermentation
>Deoxyribonuclease (not listed in the tables)

All tests are incubated for 24 hr at 37°C except: 1) the Voges-Proskauer and ONPG tests, which can be read within 4 hr; 2) the citrate test, which should be kept for 48 hr if negative after 24 hr; 3) the gelatin strips, which must be observed for about 5 days; and 4) the motility test for *Y. enterocolitica*, to be checked at 22°C. This number of tests, to be sure, constitutes a diagnostic minimum.

Sensitivity testing should be done on every pathogenically significant isolate. Two factors make prediction of susceptibility in this group of bacteria particularly difficult. One is the frequent application of antimicrobial agents to patients prior to the appearance of opportunists, and the other is the spread of R factors, especially in the intestine.

Only "intrinsic resistance," i.e., resistance that has been observed consistently since drug testing was introduced, can be predicted safely [e.g., resistance of *Aeromonas hydrophila* to ampicillin (1)].

B. Discussion of Species

1. *Edwardsiella tarda (3, 4)*. *E. tarda* has been isolated most often from stool specimens taken in connection with gastrointestinal disorders; very few fecal isolates from asymptomatic individuals have been reported [*E. tarda* grows on *Salmonella-Shigella* (SS) agar]. Nonenteric infections either occurred posttraumatically in normal hosts or were found in compromised hosts with leukemia, pancytopenia, or lupus erythematosus. Most strains tested have been sensitive to ampicillin, cephalothin, chloramphenicol, gentamicin, kanamycin, neomycin, streptomycin, and tetracycline but have been resistant to the polymyxin drugs, as have been two recent stool isolates (5) from this laboratory. Resistance to the polymyxins may be helpful in the diagnosis of *E. tarda* if sensitivity to other drugs prevails; it generally occurs together with resistance to either ampicillin, cephalothin, nitrofurantoin, or tetracycline in the genera *Proteus, Providencia,* and *Serratia* (5). Still, identification of *E. tarda* is easy if the tests mentioned in Table 1 are used.

2. *Arizona hinshawii (6–8)*. *A. hinshawii* has been isolated from stools of patients with gastrointestinal disorders, but it has been isolated also from asymptomatic individuals. It grows on SS agar. Extraintestinal infections include septicemia, arthritis, and localized tissue infections, mostly in compromised hosts with diabetes mellitus, sickle cell anemia, lupus erythematosus, or Letterer-Siwe disease.

As outlined in Table 2, there are some cross-reactions between *A. hinshawii* and *Salmonella* O antigens; however, of the most common human *Salmonella* groups (A–E), only O1, O6, and O7 antigens are related to certain *A. hinshawii* antigens (8–11).

Strains of Guckian, Byers, and Perry (7) and from our laboratory have been sensitive to all antimicrobials used against Enterobacteriaceae, while Washington (12) observed two strains that were resistant to ampicillin and cephalothin.

3. *Salmonella* species. Opportunistic *Salmonella* infections are known to occur in patients with malaria, relapsing fever, sickle cell anemia, bartonellosis, malignancies, after surgical interventions, and in very young and very old patients (13). They may be septicemic and show a predilection for bones, hematomas, aneurysms, and the meninges.

For the diagnosis of *Salmonella*, it is important to keep in mind that biochemical tests have to be done on *several* suspicious colonies from selective enteric plates. For screening, triple sugar iron agar plus lysine iron agar proved, in our experience, to be a good combination. Lactose-positive *Salmonella* strains are extremely rare (11). *Salmonella enteritidis* bioser. Paratyphi A and strains of *Salmonella cholerae-suis* and of few *S. enteritidis* serotypes are H_2S-negative (11); furthermore, some *Salmonella* species give aberrant decarboxylase reactions (see Tables 2 and 3, which list differential diagnostic considerations). Biochemical tests should precede serotyping, and H typing should not be done from enteric plates but from Kligler's or triple sugar iron agar. Aside from the possibility of the presence of a Vi antigen in *Salmonella typhi* and *S. enteritidis* bioser. Paratyphi C, which would cause O inagglutinability, certain cross-reactions with *A. hinshawii* and with *Citrobacter freundii* may occur in *Salmonella* (11).

Antimicrobial sensitivities of *Salmonella* strains cannot be predicted. A report from 1969 on 292 strains (14) lists 21% as resistant to one or more of eight drugs commonly used against

Table 2. Differential diagnosis of H$_2$S-positive *Salmonella* species

Test	*Salmonella* spp.	*A. hinshawii*	*C. freundii*	*P. vulgaris*	*P. mirabilis*
Lysine decarboxylase	+	+	−	−	−
Ornithine decarboxylase	+	+	−/+	−	+
Phenylalanine deaminase	−	−	−	+	+
Urea	−	−	+/−	+	+/(−)
ONPG	−	+	+	−	−
TSI slant	K	A (or K)	A (or K)	A (or K)	K

Table 3. Differential diagnosis of H$_2$S-negative *Salmonella* species (rare ones excepted)

Test	*Salmonella enteritidis* bioser. Paratyphi A[a]	*C. freundii* (H$_2$S −)	*P. mirabilis*	*S. cholerae-suis* (H$_2$S −)[a]	*Enterobacter hafniae*
Lysine decarboxylase	−	−	−	+	+
Ornithine decarboxylase	+	−/+	+	+	+
Phenylalanine deaminase	−	−	+	−	−
Urea	−	+/−	+/(−)	−	−
ONPG	−	+	−	−	+

[a] Confirmation by serology.

Enterobacteriaceae; 15% were resistant to streptomycin, 13.5% to ampicillin and carbenicillin (linked resistance?), 8.2% to tetracycline, and 3.3% each to the cephalosporins and to kanamycin. Resistance of the most common species, *S. enteritidis* ser. typhimurium, against each antibiotic is five times more frequent than that of the other serotypes together. Resistance to chloramphenicol and to polymyxin B is not observed; the former type of resistance is still rare in the United States (15).

4. *Citrobacter freundii (8, 16).* C. *freundii* may be found in stool specimens of normal individuals (17); its role in the pathogenesis of diarrheal disease is not clear. Outside the intestinal tract, it is most often found in the urines of patients with underlying urological disorders and/or a history of previous instrumentation (8). Next in frequency are isolates from the respiratory tract, where *C. freundii* appears most often in mixed flora and as a secondary invader which rarely contributes to pneumonitis (8, 18, 19). Cases of septicemia, meningitis, osteomyelitis, and endocarditis have also been reported in compromised hosts (8).

For the identification of *C. freundii*, it is important to know that about 16% of the strains do not form H_2S in triple sugar iron agar and that one-third of the H_2S-negative strains—but very few of the H_2S-positive ones—also produce indole (16). The lysine decarboxylase reaction is always negative. Tables 4 and 5 list the differential-diagnostic considerations.

C. freundii strains are most often resistant to the cephalosporins and sensitive to carbenicillin, colistin, gentamicin, and nitrofurantoin, while susceptibility to ampicillin as well as to other broad-spectrum drugs may vary widely (8, 12, 20–22).

5. *Citrobacter diversus (Levinea malonatica,* atypical *Enterobacter cloacae, Padlewskia).* The taxonomy of this species [genus? (23)] has been the subject of a recent review by Ewing and Davis (24), who proposed the name *Citrobacter diversus.* The characteristic biochemical reactions are listed in Tables 1 and 4. Important are positive indole, ornithine, and citrate reactions and negative H_2S and lysine tests. Adonitol fermentation and (not listed) KCN inhibition differentiate this species from *C. freundii.*

In our experience, the organism is at least as frequent as *C. freundii* in human specimens, particularly from the urinary and respiratory tracts, where it may assume primary or secondary

Table 4. Differential diagnosis of H_2S- and lysine-negative, indole-positive, nonfastidious Gram-negative rods

Test	C. freundii	C. diversus	Herbi-cola-Lathyri	Aero-monas spp.	E. coli	Y. entero-colitica	Proteus morganii	P. rettgeri	Provi-dencia spp.	Shigella A–C
TSI - slant	A or K	A or K	A or K	A (or K)	A (or K)	A	K	K	K	K
Motility	+/(−)	+/(−)	+/(−)	+	+/−	+ (22°C)	+/(−)	+/(−)	+	−
Ornithine decarboxylase	+	+	−	−	+/−	+	+	−	−	−[a]
Urea	+/−	+/−	+/−	−	−	+	+	+	−	−
Phenylalanine deaminase	−	−	−/+	−/+w[b]	−	−	+	+	+	−
Voges-Proskauer reaction, 37°C	−	−	+/−	+/−[c]	−	−	−	−	−	−
Gelatin	−	−	+D/(−)	+	−	−	−	−	−	−
Citrate	+	+	−/+	+/−	−	−	−	+	+	−
Oxidase	−	−	−	+	−	−	−	−	−/+w	−
Adonitol (A)	−	+	−	−	−	−	−	+	+[d]	−
Yellow pigment	−	−	+/−	−	−	−	−	−	−	−

[a] Exception: group C, type 13.
[b] W, weak; D, delayed.
[c] A. punctata does not form acetoin from glucose.
[d] Providencia alcalifaciens +; Providencia stuartii −.

importance. The data of Washington, Yu, and Martin (25) are in agreement with this observation. Furthermore, in contrast to *C. freundii* and *Enterobacter* spp., *C. diversus* is sensitive to the cephalosporins but resistant to ampicillin and carbenicillin (25, 26).

6. The *Herbicola-Lathyri* bacteria (various *Erwinia* spp. (27), *Enterobacter agglomerans*). These bacteria have only lately been recognized as potential human pathogens. Their taxonomy is still under discussion, along with the question of whether the genus *Erwinia* should be maintained as defined 55 years ago and whether part or all of its ill-defined "species" belong to the family Enterobacteriaceae. The *Herbicola-Lathyri* bacteria comprise many of the *Erwinia* species listed in the seventh edition of *Bergey's Manual* (27), as well as some former *Xanthomonas* and *Pseudomonas* species which have been recognized as fermenters (28). Ewing and Fife (29) have proposed the species name "*Enterobacter agglomerans*;" the term "*Herbicola-Lathyri* bacteria" will be used here without prejudice.

Key characteristics of the *Herbicola-Lathyri* bacteria are negative reactions for H_2S, decarboxylases, and adonitol fermentation, and, in 80% of the strains (29), a delayed gelatin liquefaction. Formation of yellow pigment, symplasmata, biconvex bodies, and fermentative gas occurs only in part of the strains. Motility is due to peritrichal flagella. Further reactions and differential-diagnostic considerations are listed in Tables 1, 4, and 5.

Herbicola-Lathyri bacteria are ubiquitous in nature and were isolated from human sources as early as the 1930's ("*Bacterium typhi flavum*"; see Ref. 28). Growth on SS agar is variable. Many human isolates seem to have no pathogenic significance. Notable exceptions are blood isolates and pure isolates from the urinary tract or from pus observed in compromised hosts (30). Many cases of septicemia were recorded in the United States between 1970 and 1971 as a result of contamination in the closure area of intravenous infusion bottles; young patients without predisposing factors, as well as old, debilitated patients, were affected (31).

Herbicola-Lathyri bacteria show variable susceptibility to ampicillin, carbenicillin, cephalothin, and nitrofurantoin but have generally been sensitive to chloramphenicol, colistin, nalidixic acid,

Table 5. Differential diagnosis of H_2S- and lysine-negative, indole-negative, nonfastidious Gram-negative rods

Test	C. freundii	Herbicola-Lathyri	Klebsiella ozaenae (lysine −)	Klebsiella rhino-scleromatis	Shigella spp.[a]	Y. enterocolitica
TSI - slant	A or K	A or K	A or K	A or K	K	A
Motility	+/(−)	+/(−)	−	−	−	+ (22°C)
Ornithine decarboxylase	−	−	−	−	−[b]	+
Urea	+/−	+/−	−/(+)	−	−	+
Voges-Proskauer reaction, 37°C	−	+/−	−	−	−	−
Gelatin	−	+D/(−)	−	−	−	−
Citrate	+	−/+	+/−	−	−	−
Adonitol (A)	−	−	+	−	−	−

[a] Confirmation by serology.
[b] Exceptions: group C, type 13, and group D.

gentamicin, kanamycin, and tetracycline (28, 32; unpublished observations).

7. *Y. enterocolitica (4, 10).* The taxonomic position of *Y. enterocolitica* is not clear as of this writing (family Brucellaceae or Enterobacteriaceae). The bacterium is well characterized; its portal of entry seems to be the gastrointestinal tract, with the main transmitting agent apparently being pork. In one series, it was cultured from nearly 1% of all routine stool specimens by means of an enrichment in selenite cystine broth with 40 µg of novobiocin per ml (33). Growth occurs on enteric differential and selective media (SS agar); colonies are smaller than those of Enterobacteriaceae and often are visible only after 48 hr of incubation. Diagnostically important are motility by peritrichal flagella—present at 22°C, lost at 37°C—and a positive urease reaction. Most North American isolates have been indole positive (34). The differential diagnosis is listed in Tables 1, 4, and 5. From *Yersinia pseudotuberculosis*, *Y. enterocolitica* can be differentiated by its positive ornithine test and the acid slant on triple sugar iron agar (*Y. pseudotuberculosis* does not ferment sucrose). *Yersinia pestis* is nonmotile and biochemically inert.

Most diseases caused by *Y. enterocolitica* present as enterocolitis, mesenteric lymphadenitis, or erythema nodosum in normal hosts. In compromised hosts (suffering from diabetes, chronic alcoholism, or leukemia) or in old-age patients, septicemia and, rarely, meningitis and arthritis have been observed.

Y. enterocolitica is sensitive to most antimicrobials used against Enterobacteriaceae; ampicillin and cephalothin, however, are often ineffective.

8. *Aeromonas species (1, 35).* Aeromonads belong to the family Pseudomonadaceae. They show polar monotrichous flagellation, are fermentative, and give positive oxidase and DNase tests. The latter reactions serve to differentiate them from *Escherichia coli* (see Table 4). Most strains show beta-hemolysis, which differs from *E. coli* hemolysis in the ratio of zone diameter to colony diameter (3:1 or higher in *Aeromonas*, 2:1 or lower in *E. coli*). Oxidase-positive *Vibrio* species (*Vibrio cholerae*, *Vibrio alginolyticus*, and *Vibrio parahaemolyticus*) may also show beta-hemolysis and DNase activity but are lysine- and ornithine-positive.

The species *A. hydrophila* and, rarely, *Aeromonas punctata* (which does not produce acetoin from glucose) have been found in human infections (1, 36). They may be found in stools of normal individuals as well as in stools of patients with gastrointestinal symptoms, especially during the summer months. In our experience, small numbers of colonies on enteric plates (including SS agar) are not associated with diarrheic disease. Localized infections may be water-borne, similar to gastrointestinal ones.

The finding of aeromonads in blood and in respiratory and urinary tracts has been confined mostly to compromised hosts, with septicemia occurring in leukemics as well as in patients with Laënnec's cirrhosis (1, 35–37).

Aeromonads are resistant to ampicillin, vary in their susceptibility to cephalothin, and occasionally are resistant to colistin (1, 37). They are sensitive mostly to chloramphenicol, gentamicin, kanamycin, nalidixic acid, nitrofurantoin, and tetracycline (1, 35).

II. Fastidious Opportunists

A. *Haemophilus influenzae* and *Haemophilus parainfluenzae*

Isolation of hemophili has to take into consideration 1) their growth requirements (see Table 6), and 2) possible overgrowth by resident flora in cultures taken from their normal habitat, i.e., the oropharynx.

Although red blood cells are a good source of V and X factors, hemophili grow poorly or not at all on common blood agars, partly because of the anti-V activity of sheep and human blood. Such activity is minimal in 5% horse or rabbit blood, which can be used in isolation media without further addition of V factor and which offer the only means of differentiating hemolytic from nonhemolytic hemophili. To differentiate the non-X-requiring species from the others, a satellite plate on tryptic [Trypticase (BioQuest)] soy agar (Difco Laboratories) is necessary.

V and X factors may also be supplied by Fildes Enrichment (Difco Laboratories) (a peptic-acid digest of sheep blood); by Supplement B or C (both made by Difco Laboratories); or by

Table 6. Differential diagnosis of *Haemophilus* species

Requirement for	*H. influenzae*	*H. para-influenzae*	*Haemophilus haemo-lyticus*	*H. parahae-molyticus*	*Haemophilus aphro-philus*[a]	*Haemophilus paraphro-philus*	*Actinobacillus actinomycetem comitans*[b]
X factor	+	−	+	−	−/(+)	−	−
V factor	+	+	+	+	−	+	−
Beta hemolysis (rabbit or horse blood agar)	−	−	+	+	−	−	−

[a] Does not grow in dry air; requires moist air or 10% CO_2 for growth.
[b] Requires 10% CO_2 for growth. Differs from *H. aphrophilus* in lactose and sucrose fermentation (negative in *A. actinomycetem comitans*).

heated blood with added yeast extract or IsoVitaleX (BioQuest) (chocolate agar). For selection of hemophili from the oropharynx, five units of bacitracin per ml should be added to the plates (38). For enrichment from body fluids, addition of rabbit blood to tryptic digest broths is recommended. Blood cultures are to be subcultured to chocolate agar.

The differential diagnosis of the hemophili is outlined in Table 6 (39). Part of *H. influenzae* and *H. parainfluenzae* infections have been found to be associated with impaired host defenses, such as in children with meningitis (40) and in adults (41) with diabetes mellitus, alcoholism, head trauma, spinal anesthesia, or inadequate drainage of sinusitis or otitis, as well as with bronchopneumonia in adults with chronic lung disease (42). The role of defense factors has received more attention lately because correlation of *Haemophilus* infections with low bactericidal serum titers has not stood up to close scrutiny (43). However, the bulk of respiratory infections with *Haemophilus* spp. in children still is nonopportunistic; and the frequency of these infections, as well as of nonopportunistic respiratory infections in adults, has increased recently (44).

In vitro, most strains of *H. influenzae* and *H. parainfluenzae* are sensitive to commonly used antimicrobial agents, including penicillin (which is not recommended for treatment). Methicillin, oxacillin, lincomycin, vancomycin, bacitracin, and, sometimes, the cephalosporins are ineffective (45).

B. *P. multocida*

This bacterium is carried in the oropharynx of a wide variety of animals. The usual human infection occurs through a dog or cat bite. *P. multocida* has also been isolated from the respiratory tract of individuals in whom it led to complications of preexisting chronic disease (chronic bronchitis, bronchiectasis), resulting in exacerbation of bronchitis, pneumonitis, or even empyema (46).

The diagnosis is easy: oxidase and indole reactions are positive, the urease reaction is negative [*Pasteurella pneumotropica* is urease positive; *Pasteurella haemolytica* and *Pasteurella ureae* are urease positive and indole negative (39)]. Of 465 strains examined by the

Table 7. Differential diagnosis of *L. monocytogenes*

Test	*L. monocytogenes*	*Erysipelothrix insidiosa*	aerobic *Corynebacterium* spp.	*Kurthia* spp.
Catalase	+	−	+	+
Motility 22°C	+	−	−	+
Glucose (A)	+	+	+	−
Nitrate reduction	−	−	+/−	−

Center for Disease Control in Atlanta, Ga., only 269 gave typical fermentation patterns [i.e., fermentation of glucose, xylose, mannitol, and sucrose; no fermentation of lactose and maltose (34)].

P. multocida is sensitive to penicillin, erythromycin, chloramphenicol, tetracycline, the polymyxins, kanamycin, nitrofurantoin, ampicillin, and cephalothin. Sensitivity to streptomycin and to the sulfonamides varies (46).

C. L. monocytogenes (See Ref. 47)

Only a few features of *Listeria* deserve mention here.

L. monocytogenes is probably ubiquitous. It has been isolated from animals, vegetation, and soil (48), as well as from human feces [between 10 and 30% were found to be carriers in several series taken from individuals working in egg product factories and slaughterhouses (49)].

In order to isolate the organism from heavily contaminated specimens, selection and enrichment methods must be used: nalidixic acid-blood agar for selection (49) and/or Gray's refrigeration and holding procedure (50) are preferred at present. The typical beta-hemolysis may be absent, particularly in strains that are not pathogenic for mice (48). Most important diagnostically are "tumbling" motility at 22°C, anaerogenic fermentation of glucose, catalase activity, and nitrate reduction (see Table 7). In addition, urea is not hydrolyzed and salicin is not fermented.

Most *Listeria* strains are sensitive to penicillin, ampicillin, erythromycin, chloramphenicol, tetracycline, streptomycin, and kanamycin but may be resistant to lincomycin (unpublished observation) or cephalothin; the polymyxins are ineffective (47, 51).

The long-held belief that listeriosis is a typical opportunistic infection occurring mainly in newborns and in older compromised hosts with lymphoproliferative disorders, leukemia, or a history of steroid or X-ray treatment or transplantation (9, 51) needs revision. In a recently published series of 11 cases, only 5 showed *Listeria* as an opportunist (52). The subject obviously calls for further immunological studies.

Literature Cited

1. von Graevenitz, A., and A. H. Mensch. The genus *Aeromonas* in human bacteriology. Report of 30 cases and review of the literature. New Engl. J. Med. 278: 245, 1968.
2. Johnson, J. K., L. J. Kunz, W. Barron, and W. H. Ewing. Biochemical differentiation of the Enterobacteriaceae with the aid of lysine-iron agar. Appl. Microbiol. 14: 212, 1966.
3. Bockemuehl, J., R. Pan-Urai, and F. Burkhardt. *Edwardsiella tarda* associated with human disease. Pathol. Microbiol. 37: 393, 1971.
4. Sonnenwirth, A. C. Bacteremia with and without meningitis due to *Yersinia enterocolitica*, *Edwardsiella tarda*, *Comamonas terrigena*, and *Pseudomonas maltophilia*. Ann. N. Y. Acad. Sci. 174: 488, 1970.
5. von Graevenitz, A., and M. Nourbakhsh. Antimicrobial resistance of the genera *Proteus*, *Providencia*, and *Serratia* with special reference to multiple resistance patterns. Med. Microbiol. Immunol. 157: 142, 1972.
6. Edwards, P. R., M. A. Fife, and C. H. Ramsey. Studies on the *Arizona* group of Enterobacteriaceae. Bacteriol. Rev. 23: 155, 1959.
7. Guckian, J. C., E. H. Byers, and J. E. Perry. *Arizona* infection of man. Report of a case and review of the literature. Arch. Intern. Med. 119: 170, 1967.
8. Fields, B. N., M. M. Uwaydah, L. J. Kunz, and M. N. Swartz. The so-called *"Paracolon"* bacteria. A bacteriologic and clinical reappraisal. Amer. J. Med. 42: 89, 1967.
9. Louria, D. B., A. Blevins, and D. Armstrong. Listeria infections. Ann. N. Y. Acad. Sci. 174: 545, 1970.
10. Mollaret, H. H.: (a) L'infection humaine à *"Yersinia enterocolitica."* Pathol. Biol. 14: 981, 1966. (b) L'infection humaine à *"Yersinia enterocolitica"* en 1970, à la lumière de 642 cas récents. Aspects cliniques et perspectives épidémiologiques. Pathol. Biol. 19: 189, 1971.
11. Edwards, P. R., and W. H. Ewing. Identification of Enterobacteriaceae. 3rd Ed. Burgess Publishing Co., Minneapolis, 1972.
12. Washington, J. A. Antimicrobial susceptibility of Enterobacteriaceae and nonfermenting Gram-negative bacilli. Proc. Staff Meet. Mayo Clin. 44: 811, 1969.
13. Black, B. H., L. J. Kunz, and M. N. Swartz. Salmonellosis—a review of some unusual aspects. New Engl. J. Med. 262: 811, 864, 921, 1960.
14. Winshell, E. B., C. Cherubin, J. Winter, and H. C. Neu. Antibiotic resistance of *Salmonella* in the Eastern United States. Antimicrob. Ag. Chemother. 86, 1969.
15. Gill, F. A., and E. W. Hook. *Salmonella* strains with transferable antimicrobial resistance. JAMA 198: 1267, 1966.

16. Davis, B. R., and W. H. Ewing. "The Biochemical Reactions of *Citrobacter freundii.*" Center for Disease Control, Atlanta, 1966.
17. Popovici, M., L. Szégli, C. Racovitză, E. Bădulescu, D. Florescu, M. Negut, E. Thomas, and S. Marek. Ueber die aetiologische Bedeutung und Haeufigkeit der Keime der Citrobactergruppe bei Enteritiden. Zentbl. Bakt. Abt. I Orig. 204: 112, 1967.
18. Slifkin, M., and C. Engwall. The clinical significance of *Citrobacter intermedius.* Amer. J. Clin. Pathol. 52: 351, 1969.
19. Washington, J. A., P. Yu, and W. J. Martin. Hydrogen sulfide-negative variant of *Citrobacter.* Appl. Microbiol. 20: 587, 1970.
20. Duval, J., G. Atlan, H. Gaudin, A. Kerzoncuf, P. Mathieu-Saint-Laurent, and M. Mora. Niveau et évolution de la résistance des bacilles à Gram négatif. Pathol. Biol. 17: 825, 1969.
21. Slocombe, B., and R. Sutherland. Beta-lactamase activity and resistance to ampicillin, carbenicillin, and cephaloridine of *Klebsiella, Enterobacter,* and *Citrobacter.* Antimicrob. Ag. Chemother. 78, 1969.
22. Washington, J. A. In vitro susceptibility of Gram-negative bacilli to carbenicillin. Proc. Staff Meet. Mayo Clin. 47: 332, 1972.
23. Young, V. M., D. M. Kenton, B. J. Hobbs, and M. R. Moody. *Levinea,* a new genus of the family Enterobacteriaceae. Internatl. J. Syst. Bacteriol. 21: 58, 1971.
24. Ewing, W. H., and B. R. Davis. Biochemical characterization of *Citrobacter diversus* (Burkey) Werkman and Gillen and designation of the neotype strain. Internatl. J. Syst. Bacteriol. 22: 12, 1972.
25. Washington, J. A., P. Yu, and W. J. Martin. Biochemical and clinical characteristics and antibiotic susceptibility of atypical *Enterobacter cloacae.* Appl. Microbiol. 17: 843, 1969.
26. Lund, M. E., J. M. Matsen, and D. J. Blazevic. Characterization and antibiotic susceptibility of H_2S-negative *Citrobacter* and atypical *Klebsiella-Enterobacter.* Bacteriol. Proc. 123, 1972.
27. Breed, R. S., E. G. D. Murray, and R. N. Smith. Bergey's Manual of Determinative Bacteriology. 7th Ed. Williams & Wilkins, Baltimore, 1957.
28. von Graevenitz, A. *Erwinia* species isolates. Ann. N. Y. Acad. Sci. 174: 436, 1970.
29. Ewing, W. H., and M. A. Fife. *Enterobacter agglomerans* (Beijerinck) comb. nov. (the *Herbicola-Lathyri* bacteria). Internatl. J. Syst. Bacteriol. 22: 4, 1972.
30. Meyers, B. R., E. Bottone, S. Z. Hirschman, and S. S. Schneierson. Infections caused by microorganisms of the genus *Erwinia.* Ann. Intern. Med. 76: 9, 1972.
31. "Nosocomial bacteremias associated with intravenous fluid therapy—

USA." In Morbidity and Mortality Weekly Report, Center for Disease Control, Atlanta, 20 (Suppl.): 9, 1971.
32. Thornsberry, C., C. N. Baker, and A. Balows. In vitro susceptibility of the *Herbicola-Lathyri* bacteria to antimicrobials. Proc. Intersci. Conf. Antimicrob. Ag. Chemother. 109, 1971.
33. van Noyen, R., and J. Vandepitte. L'isolement de *Yersinia enterocolitica* par une technique usuelle de coproculture. Ann. Inst. Pasteur 114: 463, 1968.
34. Weaver, R. E. "Gram-negative Organisms: An Approach to Identification." Center for Disease Control, Atlanta, 1971.
35. Slotnick, I. J. *Aeromonas* species isolates. Ann. N. Y. Acad. Sci. 174: 503, 1970.
36. Zajc-Satler, J. Morphological and biochemical studies of 27 strains belonging to the genus *Aeromonas* isolated from clinical sources. J. Med. Microbiol. 5: 263, 1972.
37. Abrams, E., C. H. Zierdt, and J. A. Brown. Observations on *Aeromonas hydrophila* septicaemia in a patient with leukemia. J. Clin. Pathol. 24: 491, 1971.
38. Ederer, G. M., and M. L. Schurr. Optimal bacitracin concentration for selective isolation medium for *Haemophilus*. Amer. J. Med. Tech. 37: 304, 1971.
39. King. E. O. "The Identification of Unusual Pathogenic Gram-negative Bacteria." Center for Disease Control, Atlanta, 1964 (revised 1967).
40. Hable, K. A., G. B. Logan, and J. A. Washington. Three *Haemophilus* species. Pathogenic activity. Amer. J. Dis. Child. 121: 35, 1971.
41. Snyder, S. N., and S. Brunjes. *Hemophilus influenzae* meningitis in adults: Review of the literature and report of 18 cases. Amer. J. Med. Sci. 250: 658, 1965.
42. Tillotson, J. R., and A. M. Lerner. *Hemophilus influenzae* bronchopneumonia in adults. Arch. Intern. Med. 121: 428, 1968.
43. Feigin, R. D., D. Richmond, M. W. Hosler, and P. G. Shackelford. Reassessment of the role of bactericidal antibody in *Hemophilus influenzae* infection. Amer. J. Med. Sci. 262: 338, 1971.
44. Quintiliani, R., and P. J. Hymans. The association of bacteremic *Haemophilus influenzae* pneumonia in adults with typable strains. Amer. J. Med. 50: 781, 1971.
45. Sabath, L., L. L. Stumpf, S. J. Wallace, and M. Finland. Susceptibility of *Diplococcus pneumoniae, Haemophilus influenzae,* and *Neisseria meningitidis* to 23 antibiotics. Antimicrob. Ag. Chemother. 53, 1970.
46. Maneche, H. G., and H. W. Toll. Pulmonary cavitation and massive hemorrhage caused by *Pasteurella multocida*. Report of a case. New Engl. J. Med. 271: 491, 1964.

47. Bojsen-Møller, J. Human listeriosis. Epidemiological and clinical studies Acta Pathol. Microbiol. Scand. B. 229 (Suppl.): 1, 1972.
48. Welshimer, H. J., and J. Donker-Voet. *Listeria monocytogenes* in nature. Appl. Microbiol. 21: 516, 1971.
49. Kampelmacher, E. H., and L. M. van Noorle Jansen. Isolation of *Listeria monocytogenes* from faeces of clinically healthy humans and animals. Zentbl. Bakt. Abt. I Orig. 211: 353, 1969.
50. Gray, M. L. *Listeria monocytogenes* and listeric infection in the diagnostic laboratory. Ann. N. Y. Acad. Sci. 98: 686, 1962.
51. Buchner, L. H., and S. S. Schneierson. Clinical and laboratory aspects of *Listeria monocytogenes* infection, with a report of ten cases. Amer. J. Med. 45: 904, 1968.
52. Medoff, G., L. J. Kunz, and A. N. Weinberg. Listeriosis in humans: An evaluation. J. Infect. Dis. 123: 247, 1971.

6

Anaerobic Bacteria:
Culture and Identification

*Earle H. Spaulding, Valerie Vargo,
Thomas C. Michaelson,
Myroslawa Korzeniowski,
and Robert M. Swenson*

Interest in the role of anaerobic bacteria and the human host has increased sharply during the last few years. Two technological developments were responsible for this new interest. First, with the introduction of the commercial GasPak apparatus in 1966 (1), anaerobic incubation became a practical routine procedure for the first time in hospital clinical microbiology laboratories.

The second development actually began in 1950, when Hungate (2) described a method with which for the first time he was able to isolate fastidious and highly oxygen-sensitive microorganisms from gastric contents of ruminant animals. A sine qua non of his method was the complete exclusion of air, not only during collection and transport of the specimen, but also during all the laboratory manipulations. This exclusion was accomplished by means of roll tubes (stoppered test tubes with a thin inner coating of agar).

This research was supported by a grant from the Upjohn Company, Kalamazoo, Michigan, and by funds from the Temple University Health Sciences Center, Philadelphia, Pennsylvania.

Contact with oxygen even for a minute or two rendered some strains nonviable. Loesche (3) recently (1969) provided some perspective for viewing oxygen sensitivity when he suggested that anaerobes exhibit two patterns, namely, *strict* anaerobes, which do not grow at O_2 tensions greater than 0.5%, and *moderate* anaerobes, which show good growth at tensions up to 3%. It is worth noting at this point that most strains which have been recovered from human infections to date belong to the latter category. Furthermore, Hungate (4) discovered that some strains could not grow unless the culture media were prepared entirely under anaerobic conditions. He called such media "*pre*reduced, *a*naerobically *s*terilized (PRAS)." This observation by Hungate can be explained by the concept of "organic peroxides," which may form in certain types of media upon oxidation (5).

The impact of the Hungate methodology upon medical microbiology was markedly delayed and came about largely through the work of W. E. C. Moore, who had established an anaerobe laboratory at the Virginia Polytechnic Institute and State University (VPI). It was his paper in 1969 (6) which brought wide-scale attention of the infectious disease community to the need for adapting the new roll tube methodology (7) to the study of anaerobic bacteria, both as part of the normal microbial flora and as participants in the pathogenesis of human infections. However, it should be pointed out that for several years before this time, Finegold (8) had been publishing a series of reports upon the frequent presence of anaerobes in human infection and describing various laboratory methods for their isolation and identification (9).

In 1970, McMinn and Crawford (10) reported that they had isolated twice as many anaerobes from a series of clinical specimens by the Hungate roll tube method as by conventional methods. And, in 1971, Gordon, Stutman, and Loesche (11) demonstrated the superiority of roll tubes over anaerobic jars for isolating anaerobes from gingival crevices of man.

In the meantime, Freter and associates (12) had described a glove box (anaerobic chamber) procedure that used anaerobically prestored, but not PRAS, media which produced very high normal flora counts from the human gingiva and mouse cecum, both of which contain fastidious, highly O_2-sensitive anaerobes.

Anaerobic Bacteria

We started a special Anaerobe Laboratory at Temple University in 1969, with two initial objectives in mind: 1) to determine whether the Hungate type of anaerobic methodology would produce from clinical specimens many more anaerobes than the routine method that our Diagnostic Laboratory was using at the time, and 2) to provide a basis for deciding whether our clinical microbiology laboratory should adopt the Hungate roll tube methodology. We set up an informal anaerobe group, composed of two infectious-disease clinicians, two infection-control nurses, and laboratory personnel. It was decided to collect test specimens from patients identified as appropriate by one of the four clinical people, the collection being personally supervised by one of them. Two specimens were collected at the same time, one destined for the Anaerobe Laboratory and the other for the Diagnostic Laboratory (Clinical Microbiology Laboratories of the Temple University Hospital). Thus, a comparative study of the procedures used in these two laboratories was started in June, 1970, and the major steps are contrasted in Table 1.

Table 1. Comparison of primary culture methods, 1970–1972 study

	AC-PS-AC (Anaerobe Laboratory)	versus	GasPak (Diagnostic Laboratory)
Collection	Gassed-out stoppered tube		Aerobic tube
Transport	Pickup by laboratory		Routine
Medium	BHI-S + blood agar (prestored anaerobic)[a]		Trypticase soy 5% sheep blood agar
Incubation	Anaerobic chamber, 48 or 72 hr		GasPak 24 + 24 hr
Identification	Speciation (VPI)[b]		Gram stain and subculture

[a] Brain heart infusion agar, supplemented (VPI Manual, 1972), plus 5% sheep blood.
[b] VPI Manual, 1972 (15).

I. Methods Used by the Anaerobe Laboratory

During its first 8 months of operation, the Anaerobe Laboratory experimented with a variety of collection, isolation, and identification methods, but the Anaerobe Laboratory procedure described below has been used since June, 1970, except as indicated otherwise.

A. Collection of Specimens

We adopted the recommendation of Dr. Finegold that all specimens, except solid tissues, be collected by aspiration with needle and syringe (13). This can be done without exposing the specimen to air. With very few exceptions, the specimens were collected in such a manner as to avoid as much as possible any contamination with normal microbial flora, including use of such procedures as transtracheal aspiration, culdocentesis, etc.

B. Transport

Anaerobic transport is accomplished by use of an empty, gassed-out, O_2-free tube (14). Anaerobic collection tubes and bottles are now available commercially (Hyland Division of Travenol Laboratories, Inc., Costa Mesa, Calif.; Robbins Laboratories Division, Scott Laboratories, Inc., Fiskeville, R. I.).

We also use a broth collection tube which is the same type of tube as the anaerobic collection tube and which contains one ml of PRAS-Brain Heart Infusion Supplemented Broth (Difco Laboratories, Detroit, Mich.) (15). This is the basal medium used in our laboratory and is abbreviated as "PRAS-BHI-S" broth. PRAS-BHI-S agar, however, is made with Brain Heart Infusion from the BBL Division of BioQuest (Cockeysville, Md.). Either commercial product is satisfactory for both broth and agar. The broth collection tube is needed when the area to be sampled is too dry to be aspirated or the specimen is very scanty. When used properly, broth can be withdrawn, used to flush the area, and returned to the tube without oxidizing the resazurin oxidation-reduction indicator in the medium.

A messenger from the Anaerobe Laboratory, usually present when the specimen was collected, delivered the collection tube specimen (but not the swab specimen) promptly to that laboratory.

C. Culture

We decided that roll tubes were not convenient for our applications and constructed a rigid glove-box anaerobic chamber, which allowed us to use agar plates. Primary culture is carried out on BHI-S agar, to which is added 5% sheep blood. At first, we prepared this as a PRAS medium, which meant that plates had to be poured inside the anaerobic chamber (AC), but we soon abandoned this practice as impractical. Instead, the basal agar medium is prepared aerobically, with the addition of cysteine and blood after autoclaving. As soon as they have solidified, the freshly poured agar plates are passed into the AC, where they are stored until the control plate of medium (resazurin but no blood) becomes colorless (at least −40 mv). This takes 24–48 hr in the atmosphere of our chamber. The procedure and equipment just described are essentially those used by Aranki et al. (12). We designate media prepared this way as PS (prestored). They are not anaerobically sterilized.

We prepare all of our PRAS media according to the VPI Manual (15); however, this is a time-consuming, laborious, and expensive process. Unless a laboratory has an extensive facility for media preparation, we recommend that PRAS media be purchased. Many types of commercially prepared PRAS media are now available (Hyland; Robbins; McGaw Laboratories, Glendale, Calif.).

Upon receipt in the Anaerobe Laboratory, the specimen tube is passed into the AC, an aliquot aspirated with needle and syringe, and inoculated to the surface of one PS-BHI-S blood agar plate. The specimen is then passed out of the AC and inoculated to one aerobic Trypticase soy blood plate and one tube of PRAS-BHI-S broth as a backup. The latter is rarely needed (an example is growth in this broth tube but none on either the primary aerobic or anaerobic plates), but we continue the practice as worthwhile.

D. Incubation

We now have two glove-box anaerobic chambers, the newer one being the larger, a four-port, collapsible model described by Aranki et al. (12) and available commercially (Coy Manufacturing Co., Ann Arbor, Mich.). It has been eminently satisfactory. We fill it with a gas mixture of 85% N_2, 10% H_2, and 5% CO_2. Whereas our first AC was maintained at 37°C, the large one is kept at ambient temperature, and cultures are placed in an incubator situated within the chamber. This is a more satisfactory arrangement.

E. Identification

Culture plates can be examined at any time without interfering with anaerobiosis. Although incubation usually continues for 7–10 days, examination for growth begins at 24 hr and continues daily. Colony types are compared with those on the comparable aerobic plate, and appropriate subcultures are made to another plate of the same medium for purity. If the subculture growth appears to be only one colony type, a single colony is picked from a tube of PRAS-BHI-S (1972 VPI Manual), which is brought out of the AC and incubated. When growth develops, this is subcultured to two Trypticase soy agar plates for incubation aerobically and in a candle jar. Strains which grow in both plates are not anaerobes. Those growing in the candle jar are considered to be microaerophilic (for the accurate use of this term, see Ref. 3) and are identified. Most isolates, however, are obligate anaerobes. These are speciated by the morphological and cultural criteria, biochemical tests, and gas-liquid chromatographic methods described in the VPI Manual.

II. Methods Used by the Diagnostic Laboratory

The methods which were being used at our institution for the collection and culturing of clinical specimens in June, 1970, are described below, and these were continued without change until May, 1972, when the comparative study was stopped. We believe that they are representative of the methods that were in general use in June, 1972, and probably are still in use in many laboratories. The routine methods currently used at Temple University are discussed later in this chapter.

A. Collection and Transport of Specimens

Most of the specimens destined for the Diagnostic Laboratory were obtained with a swab or were fluids or exudates. The collection tubes were aerobic.

Transport to the Diagnostic Laboratory was via the regular delivery system; the average transit time is estimated as having been 1–2 hr.

B. Diagnostic Laboratory Culture Procedure

Upon receipt in the laboratory, specimens were inoculated promptly to a tube of thioglycolate medium and in duplicate to commercially prepared Trypticase soy 5% sheep blood agar plates, which were used three to seven days after delivery by the manufacturer. The freshly inoculated aerobic plates were placed in the incubator without delay; the others (anaerobic) were placed in jars but sometimes remained exposed to air for as long as 2 hr before the jars were prepared for anaerobic incubation.

The GasPak system was used, but the packets of palladium GasPak catalyst were not always reactivated by heat before reuse. After 24 hr of incubation, all jars were opened and the culture plates were examined for growth. A minority of anaerobic cultures were discarded at this time; the others remained in contact with air for an estimated average of 1–2 hr before being placed in the GasPak for a second incubation of 24–48 hr.

C. Identification

Colonies on anaerobic plates which differed in appearance from any colony type on the comparable aerobic plate were subcultured to agar for aerobic incubation and smeared to a slide for Gram staining. If there was no growth aerobically, the microscopic examination served as the basis for reporting the isolate as an anaerobic coccus or a *Bacteroides* (any Gram-negative bacillus was so labelled) or an anaerobic Gram-positive bacillus. *Actinomyces israeli* was identified by traditional methods. Clostridia were not designated by species, except for *Clostridium perfringens*, which was identified by microscopic examination of a large colony surrounded by double-zone hemolysis.

III. Results of Comparative Study

A total of 700 paired specimens were considered comparable. When the Diagnostic Laboratory specimens were lost or otherwise unsatisfactory, both specimens were excluded from this study.

Many paired blood cultures were collected in the beginning of the study. The Anaerobe Laboratory prepared its own metal-capped, perforable-stoppered bottles containing 50 ml of PRAS-BHI-S broth which received a 5-ml sample of blood. At that time, the Diagnostic Laboratory employed aerobic and anaerobic, Vacutainer-tubed Trypticase soy broth (BioQuest, Cockeysville, Md.). Before long, however, the Diagnostic Laboratory adopted routinely the use of supplemented peptone broth blood culture medium in Vacutainer tubes (Becton-Dickonson Co., Rutherford, N. J.), at which time comparison of blood cultures was discontinued.

This study extended from June, 1970, to May, 1972. Most of the specimens were from wounds or abscesses or consisted of body fluids. A summary of the results appears in Table 2. The AC-PS-AC method produced 268 specimens (38%) positive for anaerobes and a total of 584 anaerobe isolates, whereas the corresponding figures for the Diagnostic Laboratory's GasPak procedure were 95 (14%) and 103, respectively. Thus, the Anaerobe Laboratory obtained almost three times as many positive specimens and nearly six times as many isolates than did the Diagnostic Laboratory.

It appears, therefore, that diagnostic laboratories which employ similar aerobic collection-GasPak procedures will fail to detect the presence of anaerobic bacteria nearly two-thirds of the time, and

Table 2. Anaerobic bacteria from clinical specimens, June, 1970, to May, 1972

Total 700	AC-PS-AC (Anaerobe Laboratory)	versus	GasPak (Diagnostic Laboratory)
No of specimens			
No growth	200		
Negative for anaerobes	232		
Positive for anaerobes	268[a]		95[b]
% positive	38	2.8 times	14
No. of anaerobe isolates	584		103
Ratio		5.7 times	

[a] Includes 18 reported as "no growth" by Diagnostic Laboratory.
[b] Includes five positive only in Diagnostic Laboratory.

only one time in five or six will they detect a mixture of anaerobes when it is present.

These results fulfilled the first objective of this study, for the AC-PS-AC procedure had, indeed, grown many more anaerobes from clinical specimens than the Diagnostic Laboratory's GasPak. But they, in turn, raised another question, i.e., "Were these differences largely due to the better collection method, the richer culture medium, the anaerobic chamber-versus-GasPak incubation, or some other factor?"

We assumed that each of the steps in the AC-PS-AC method was superior to its GasPak counterpart, and so we undertook studies to evaluate each of them. The collection and transport of specimens for anaerobic culture, as commonly practiced today, is not conducive to the survival of highly O_2-sensitive bacteria. Indeed, some workers think that this step may be the most important factor in increasing the number of anaerobic isolates (16). We have results from 11 anaerobe-positive pairs of swab and collection-tube specimens obtained simultaneously and brought immediately to the Anaerobe Laboratory, where they were processed together by the AC-PS-AC procedure. Both the swab and collection-tube specimens were positive in all instances, but the swabs produced only 19 anaerobic isolates, whereas the collection tubes produced 26. If this small sample is a correct indication, one can expect at least one-third more isolates from collection-tube specimens than from swabs, even though they are cultured within 15 min after collection.

Other aspects in the Diagnostic Laboratory's routine anaerobe procedure which have been examined in a preliminary way are the nature of the primary culture medium and the manner in which culture plates are handled after inoculation, including the GasPak procedure itself. A few specimens, some as swabs and others in collection tubes, have been used to compare two different, commercially prepared agar bases. These were the Trypticase soy blood agar plates in routine use in the Diagnostic Laboratory and the BHI-S agar base (VPI formulation), containing 5% sheep blood, that was delivered at the same time. To date, only five positive specimens have been so compared, but we obtained 12 anaerobe isolates from Trypticase soy blood agar, as opposed to 17 from BHI-S blood agar.

GasPak, flush jar, and anaerobic chamber incubations were also compared in yet another small series; there was no clear superiority of one method over the others. Our results agree, therefore, with those recently reported by Rosenblatt et al. (16) and by Killgore et al. (17), both of which indicate that GasPak incubation may be as effective as an anaerobic chamber for the isolation of anaerobes from clinical specimens not contaminated with normal flora.

There are three additional steps which can be taken to increase the number of anaerobes isolated in by GasPak. All are readily applicable to any laboratory using this procedure. The first step is to protect inoculated plates from unnecessary exposure to air. In the 1970–1972 study, freshly inoculated plates were placed in a lidded jar until it was ready for GasPak. This variable exposure to air, averaging 1–2 hr in that study, can be almost eliminated by placing a double-vented lid (BioQuest) on this jar and flushing it with O_2-free gas each time a plate is added.

The second improvement is always to use freshly reactivated (heated) catalyst; the third is to maintain continuous 48- to 72-hr incubation, as opposed to opening jars after 24 hr. Because clinicians need culture reports in 24 hr, clinical laboratories often examine and report on anaerobic cultures after only 24 hr of incubation. Therefore, we decided to compare the effect of 24- versus 48-hr primary GasPak incubations upon the number of anaerobes which could be isolated. The results pointed clearly to a third improvement which would yield increased numbers of anaerobic isolates. Some specimens were swabs, whereas others were contained in anaerobic collection tubes. They were streaked to duplicate plates of commercially prepared BHI-S sheep blood agar

Table 3. GasPak: Length of incubation versus no. of anaerobe isolates

	Jar A		Jar B	
No. of days	1	2	3	5–7
No. of positive specimens	15	24	26	26
No. of anaerobic isolates	25	71	78	88[a]

[a] Includes nine B. melaninogenicus isolates not detected at three days.

plates and were placed promptly in separate GasPak jars containing freshly reactivated catalyst. One jar (A) was opened at 24 hr; the colonies then were examined and subcultured for aerobic growth and were speciated by VPI methods. The other jar (B) was not opened for 48 hr; after examination and subculture, these plate cultures were reincubated for a total of five to seven days. The results are contained in Table 3. Jar A produced only 15 anaerobe-positive cultures and 25 different isolates, whereas 71 anaerobes (2.8 times as many) were recovered from 25 specimens after 48 hr of incubation in jar B. The total number of isolates in jar B increased to 78 after three days of incubation and to 88 (mostly *Bacteroides melaninogenicus*) after five to seven days of incubation.

Thus, no single one of the differences between the GasPak (Diagnostic Laboratory) and the AC-PS-AC (Anaerobe Laboratory) procedures (Table 1) accounts for the greatly increased number of anaerobes which were isolated by the latter procedure in the 1970–1972 comparative study. Rather, it appears that each step in the latter procedure may be an improvement over its counterpart, i.e., anaerobe collection tube versus aerobic swabs, use of a richer medium for primary isolation, careful avoidance of exposure to air of fresly inoculated plates, etc. Our studies indicate, however, that the most important single factor is the way in which the GasPak procedure is carried out. The simple step of continuing primary GasPak incubation for 48 instead of 24 hr increased the number of anaerobe-positive specimens by two-thirds and increased the number of isolates 2.5- to 3-fold.

The results presented in this paper clearly suggest five practicable steps which clinical laboratories using GasPak incubation can take to increase the number of anaerobic isolates from clinical specimens. These five steps are listed together in Table 4. Since May, 1972, when the 1970–1972 comparative study was stopped, the procedure shown in Table 4 has been used routinely in our Diagnostic Bacteriology Laboratory. The enriched medium is commercially prepared BHI-S blood agar. In the third step of the procedure, the freshly inoculated plates are placed at once in a jar fitted with a double-vented lid which can be connected to a tank of O_2-free gas (in our case, 85% N_2, 10% H_2, 5% CO_2), which is run slowly through the jar for 5–10 min. The purpose of storage in

Table 4. Routine procedure for primary isolation of anaerobes from clinical specimens

1. Collect specimens anaerobically (gassed-out tubes)

2. Use enriched medium for primary culture

3. Store freshly inoculated plates in flush jar to protect them from exposure to air until ready for GasPak

4. Use freshly reactivated catalyst in GasPak procedure

5. Incubate GasPak jars two or three days without opening

a flushed-out jar is the same as that of the method described by Martin (18), who employs a continuous stream of CO_2. This step avoids killing the more O_2-sensitive anaerobes from prolonged exposure to air. When the jar is ready for GasPak, the vented lid is replaced by the usual type.

The importance of heat reactivation of catalyst *each time* it is used does not seem to be generally recognized. Retained moisture, and especially absorption of H_2S on the surfaces of the palladium-coated pellets, can reduce considerably the catalytic activity, which, however, can be restored with dry heat at 160°C for 1.5 hr, as recently emphasized by Sutter et al. (13). The importance of the fifth step of the procedure has already been discussed.

We are asking ourselves the obvious question, "How does the recommended procedure compare with AC-PS-AC procedure?" Although we do not have good comparative data, we expect the difference between them to be much smaller than in the 1970–1972 series. Additional reason to expect this is found in recent reports (16, 17), which agree in that the GasPak method produced results equivalent to those with more complex systems. Our current view, therefore, is that an anaerobic chamber is a valuable tool for research in anaerobic bacteriology, especially for the study of the normal flora, but that it is not needed in the clinical laboratory.

There is another important question, i.e., "How important is it to isolate all the anaerobic species which can be recovered by the AC-PS-AC procedure?" We doubt that anyone is willing to answer this question at the present time. It may be helpful, however, to look at the species distribution of 639 isolates obtained in the Anaerobe Laboratory from infected sites (Table 5).

As expected, *Bacteroides* predominated, with *Bacteroides fragilis* and *B. melaninogenicus* accounting for two-thirds of the isolates. Nearly half of all isolates were Gram-negative, nonsporulating bacilli (*Bacteroides* and *Fusobacterium*). However, it should also be noted that the cocci accounted for more than 30%. Thus, all the types appearing in the column on the right in Table 5 account for only 20%.

Some anaerobic species are known to occur often under circumstances which incriminate them strongly as etiological agents of infection. It follows, therefore, that a satisfactory, routine, anaerobic culture method must be able consistently to recover these species. In this category are *B. fragilis*, *B. melaninogenicus*, and certainly *C. perfringens*. Examination of our 1970–1972 data suggests that *B. fragilis* will be isolated most of the time and that *C. perfringens* will be isolated practically every time. However, the results of the improved GasPak study indicated that *B. melaninogenicus* will be missed more than one-half the time unless the total incubation time is at least three and preferably five days (Table 3).

The speciation of anaerobic bacteria is still in a state of flux. In general, the VPI procedures are followed in laboratories competent to work with prereduced media and to carry out gas-liquid chromatography. However, the 1972 edition of the VPI Anaerobe Laboratory Manual (15) contains many changes in species and even in generic designations, in comparison to the 1970 edition. Although both satisfactory PRAS media and relatively inexpensive but adequate gas-liquid chromatography equipment are available commercially, they cannot be added to the operation of the average clinical microbiology laboratory without considerable commitment of time. Laboratories that are not prepared to adopt at least one of these procedures may use the simple classification followed by our Diagnostic Laboratory in its routine laboratory reports.

1. Subculture each type of colony to three blood agar plates, one for anaerobic incubation, one for aerobic, and one for a candle jar (CO_2). A Gram-stained smear, Kopeloff modification, (VPI Manual, 1972) is also examined.

Table 5. Anaerobe isolates from clinical specimens, June, 1970, to May, 1972

Bacteroides spp.			*Eubacterium* spp.	
fragilis	29		*lentum*	10
melaninogenicus	82		Other	26
Other (11)	62			19
	50	223		55
Fusobacterium spp.			*Propionibacterium* spp.	
fusiforme	4		*acnes*	2
Other (9)	15		Other (4)	5
	42	61		5
				12
Gram-negative bacteria (not identified)		6	*Lactobacillus* spp.	
			catenaforme	7
Peptococcus spp.			Other (2)	8
asaccharolyticus	3			4
magnus	23			19
prevotii	21		*Bifidobacterium*	7
	46	93	*Actinomyces*	5
			Gram-positive nonsporulating bacillus	12
Peptostreptococcus spp.				24
anaerobius	9		*Clostridium* spp.	
intermedius	34		*perfringens*	3
	30	73	Other (10)	9
				13
Anaerobic coccus	10			25
Microaerophilic streptococcus	20	30	Total	639
Veillonella		18		

2. If growth occurs only on the anaerobic plate, it is an obligate anaerobe. Growth on both the anaerobic and CO_2 plates, but no growth aerobically, means it can be reported as microaerophilic.
3. Obligately anaerobic Gram-negative bacilli are probably *Bacteroides*. Reincubation for two to three days may reveal the black colonies of *B. melaninogenicus*.
4. Gram-positive bacilli must be examined closely for spore production by microscopic examination, preferably of a three- to seven-day subculture on a PRAS chopped meat slant. Nonsporulating bacilli are not easily identified; report simply as "a Gram-positive, nonsporulating anaerobic bacillus."
5. Anaerobic, Gram-negative cocci can be called "*Veillonella* species."
6. Gram-positive cocci can be reported as "anaerobic streptococcus" if there is growth on the anerobic subculture plate but not on the CO_2 plate, and as "microaerophilic streptococcus" if there is growth in CO_2.

IV. Summary of Results

The apparent superiority of the AC-PS-AC procedure is not due solely to technological advances but also—and probably much more so—to the human factor. Persistent efforts must be made to persuade clinicians to use properly one of several types of anerobe collection tubes or bottles which are commercially available. Also, the need for careful performance of anaerobic culture techniques must be recognized by microbiologists.

It is particularly important that bench-level personnel realize why full exploitation of these techniques requires the painstaking and time-consuming task of examining primary cultures thoroughly but quickly for different colony types, preparing and examining many stained smears, and making both aerobic and CO_2 subcultures to determine if, in fact, the organism is an obligate anaerobe, a microaerophile, or a facultative species. Unless the comparable aerobic culture is negative, colonies suspected of containing anaerobes should not be reported as such until these subcultures have been incubated.

Readers will find the recently published manual by Sutter et al. (13) very useful as a guide for good anaerobic culture methods in the clinical laboratory.

Acknowledgments

We acknowledge with gratitude the invaluable participation in this study by Rose Vitagliano, R. N., and Delores Dolan, R. N.; also the interest and cooperation of Dr. Kenneth R. Cundy and Evalyn Bernhardt; and especially the technical assistance of Elaine Forsch and Maria Carolina Martinez.

Literature Cited

1. Brewer, J. H., and D. L. Allgeier. Safe self-contained carbon dioxide-hydrogen anaerobic system. Appl. Microbiol. 14: 985, 1966.
2. Hungate, R. E. The anaerobic mesophilic cellulolytic bacteria. Bacteriol. Rev. 14: 1, 1950.
3. Loesche, W. J. Oxygen sensitivity of various anaerobic bacteria. Appl. Microbiol. 18: 723, 1969.
4. Hungate, R. E. A roll tube method for cultivation of strict anaerobes. In J. R. Norris and D. W. Ribbons (eds.), Methods in Microbiology. Vol. 3B, p. 117. Academic Press, New York, 1969.
5. Smith, L. D., and L. V. Holdeman. The Pathogenic Anaerobic Bacteria. Charles C Thomas, Springfield, Ill., 1968, p. 13.
6. Moore, W. E. C., E. P. Cato, and L. V. Holdeman. Anaerobic bacteria of the gastrointestinal flora and their occurrence in clinical infections. J. Infect. Dis. 119: 641, 1969.
7. Moore, W. E. C. Techniques for routine culture of fastidious anaerobes. Internatl. J. Syst. Bacteriol. 16: 173, 1966.
8. Finegold, S. M. Infections due to anaerobes. Med. Times 96: 174, 1968.
9. Finegold, S. M. Isolation of anaerobic bacteria. In Manual of Clinical Microbiology. American Society for Microbiology, Bethesda, 1970, p. 265.
10. McMinn, M. T., and J. J. Crawford. Recovery of anaerobic microorganisms from clinical specimens in prereduced media versus recovery by routine clinical laboratory methods. Appl. Microbiol. 19: 207, 1970.

11. Gordon, D. F., F. Stutman, and W. J. Loesche. Improved isolation of anaerobic bacteria from the gingival crevice area of man. Appl. Microbiol. 21: 1046, 1971.
12. Aranki, A., S. A. Syed, E. B. Kenney, and R. Freter. Isolation of anaerobic bacteria from human gingiva and mouse cecum by means of a simplified glove box procedure. Appl. Microbiol. 17: 568, 1969.
13. Sutter, V. L., H. R. Attebery, J. E. Rosenblatt, K. S. Bricknell, and S. M. Finegold. Anaerobic Bacteriology Manual. U.C.L.A. Extension Division, Los Angeles, 1972. 89 p.
14. Attebery, H. R., and S. M. Finegold. Combined screw-cap and rubber-stopper closure for Hungate tubes (pre-reduced, anaerobically-sterilized roll tubes and liquid media). Appl. Microbiol. 18: 558, 1969.
15. Holdeman, L. V., and W. E. C. Moore, Anaerobe Laboratory Manual. V.P.I. Anaerobe Laboratory. Virginia Polytechnic Institute and State University, Blacksburg, Va., 1972. 130 p.
16. Rosenblatt, J. E., A. M. Fallon, and S. M. Finegold. Recovery of anaerobes from clinical specimens. Abstr. Annu. Meet. Amer. Soc. Microbiol., 1972, p. 94.
17. Killgore, G. E., S. E. Starr, V. E. Del Bene, D. N. Whaley, and V. R. Dowell, Jr. Comparison of three anaerobic systems for isolation of anaerobic bacteria from clinical specimens. Abstr. Annu. Meet. Amer. Soc. Microbiol., 1972, p. 94.
18. Martin, W. J. Practical method for isolation of anaerobic bacteria in the clinical laboratory. Appl. Microbiol. 22: 1168, 1971.

7

Antibiotic Susceptibility Testing of Anaerobic Bacteria

Tracy D. Wilkins

Improvements in the anaerobic methods used in clinical laboratories have resulted in the isolation of many more anaerobes from infections than were isolated by previous methods. As a result, clinical laboratories are asked for antibiotic susceptibility data on many more anaerobic bacteria than in the past. The purpose of this chapter is to assess the current status of the methodology used for susceptibility testing of anaerobes, perhaps with more emphasis on the deficiencies of the techniques than on the good points.

I. Antibiotics Used

In any antibiotic susceptibility testing procedure, all of the available antibiotics cannot be tested on every organism; therefore, decisions must be made as to which antibiotics should be tested with anaerobic isolates. Unfortunately, many antibiotics which are very effective against facultative and aerobic pathogens are not

---

The research on antibiotic susceptibility testing, performed at the V.P.I. Anaerobe Laboratory, was supported by U. S. Public Health Service Grant No. 14604 from the National Institute of General Medical Sciences.

effective, at least in vitro, against anaerobic bacteria. These ineffective antibiotics include the aminoglycosides (streptomycin, kanamycin, neomycin, and gentamycin), the polymyxins, and the sulfonamides. Among the more effective antibiotics for anaerobes are chloramphenicol, clindamycin (7 chloro-lincomycin), the penicillin group, the cephalosporins, erythromycin, and tetracycline. The results of susceptibility tests performed at the Virginia Polytechnic Institute (V.P.I.) Anaerobe Laboratory with these more effective antibiotics on random clinical isolates from our local hospital are shown in Table 1. The patterns of resistance among the different species were approximately the same as those reported recently in a much more extensive study by Martin, Gardner, and Washington (1) at the Mayo Clinic.

The broadest spectrum antibiotic that we have tested with anaerobes is chloramphenicol. None of the 113 clinical isolates was resistant to the attainable blood level of this drug (12 µg per ml), and Martin et al. (1) reported that only three strains of 601 clinical isolates were resistant to chloramphenicol. Chloramphenicol does have side-effects which may restrict its use; however, with controlled dosage in hospitals, this antibiotic should be very effective for treatment of severe anaerobic infections.

Erythromycin also has a broad spectrum of activity against anaerobes, but different laboratories have reported widely differing degrees of activity. This antibiotic is much less active at pH values of less than 7.0. Since the majority of anaerobes require some CO_2 for growth, most in vitro tests are performed in an atmosphere of 10% CO_2, which lowers the pH of the media. However, the activity of this antibiotic does not decrease equally for different species as the pH is lowered. The exact cause of this phenomenon has not been found, but, where possible, erythromycin should be tested at pH ranges near neutrality.

Clindamycin has recently gained prominence for its broad spectrum of activity against anaerobic bacteria, and our tests confirm this activity. However, resistant organisms are routinely encountered, especially in the genus *Clostridium* (2). Resistant organisms do occur among other anaerobic genera, but at lower frequency. I hope that clindamycin will not be misused for "shotgun"-type therapy of all types of anaerobic infections, since the number of

Table 1. Resistance of 113 anaerobic clinical isolates

Species	No. of isolates	Chloramphenicol	Clindamycin	Erythromycin	Penicillin	Tetracycline
Bacteroides fragilis	23	0	0	1	23	14
Bacteroides species[b]	17	0	1	0	3	2
Peptostreptococcus intermedius	18	0	0	0	2	2
Peptostreptococcus anaerobius	5	0	0	0	0	1
Peptococcus magnus and *Peptostreptococcus micros*	8	0	0	0	0	1
Other anaerobic cocci[b]	8	0	0	1	1	2
Fusobacterium species[b]	8	0	0	3	0	0
Clostridium perfringens	6	0	3	0	0	1
Clostridium ramosum	4	0	0	0	1	2
Clostridium species[b]	3	0	2	0	0	0
Fusobacterium species[b]	0	0	0	0	0	0
Lactobacillus species[b]	7	0	0	0	0	0
Propionibacterium acnes	2	0	0	0	0	0
Total	113	0	6	5	28	25

[a] Resistant to following concentrations per ml: chloramphenicol = 12.5 µg; clindamycin = 1.6 µg; erythromycin = 3.1 µg; penicillin = 2 U; and tetracycline = 6.2 µg.
[b] Represent identified species, of which there were fewer than three isolates of each species.

resistant strains undoubtedly would then increase and reduce the efficacy of the antibiotic.

Penicillin resistance is restricted primarily to strains of *Bacteroides fragilis* at the present time. At least 95% of the strains of this species are resistant to clinically useful levels of penicillin, ampicillin, cephalosporins, and the penicillinase-resistant penicillins. For the other anaerobic bacteria, penicillin is a very effective antibiotic. Since ampicillin and cephalothin do not have a spectrum of activity demonstrably different from that of penicillin, routine susceptibility testing of ampicillin and cephalothin does not seem to be necessary for anaerobic organisms.

Tetracycline has an intriguing history that suggests the possible presence of a transferable resistance factor in anaerobes. Tetracycline used to be an excellent broad spectrum antibiotic for almost all types of anaerobic infections. *B. fragilis* strains were uniformly susceptible to this antibiotic, and since *B. fragilis* is penicillin resistant, tetracycline was the drug of choice for treatment. Now, the majority of the *B. fragilis* isolates in the United States are resistant to useful levels of tetracycline, and resistance appears to be increasing among the other species of anaerobes. Fortunately, resistance to tetracycline is easy to detect by antibiotic susceptibility tests, since the organisms are either very resistant or very susceptible; very few anaerobes have been isolated that have intermediate susceptibilities. Thus, almost any susceptibility test designed for use with anaerobes accurately will predict tetracycline resistance, even though the same test may be highly inaccurate with other antibiotics.

Since there are always exceptions to any general rules, treating patients with antibiotics on the basis of species identification without confirmatory susceptibility tests can lead to problems in response. The tests need to be rapid so that they may be completed before a positive identification can be made, thus resulting in better treatment of patients. Unfortunately, standard methods used for testing the antibiotic susceptibility of aerobic and facultative organisms cannot be used for anaerobes without modifications. Much of the theory of antibiotic susceptibility testing of anaerobic bacteria is the same as for aerobes, but there are several additional factors that must be considered.

It is obvious that the tests must be conducted in an anaerobic environment, but since anaerobes vary greatly in oxygen tolerance, many can be tested by methods in which not all of the manipulations are anaerobic. The growth rates of anaerobes also vary greatly between different species, so it is difficult to design a single test that will give valid results for most anaerobic bacteria. Growth rates are influenced not only by the nature of each distinct species, but also by the degree of anaerobiosis of the medium and its nutrient value. In general, anaerobes are nutritionally more fastidious than most facultative pathogens and thus require more complex media for good growth.

II. Methods for Antibiotic Susceptibility Testing

Because most anaerobic bacteria require complex nutrients in the growth media, the standardized Bauer-Kirby disc diffusion test with Mueller-Hinton agar medium does not give adequate growth of many anaerobes. Simple modification of this method by addition of blood to the medium also gives poor results with anaerobes (3, 4). Recently, Zabransky, Johnston, and Hauser (5) reported that more extensive modification of the Bauer-Kirby method by using "nutritionally fortified" Mueller-Hinton medium and seeding the inoculum as a thin agar layer mixed with blood gave more accurate results, but further details of the method have not been published yet.

Mueller-Hinton agar medium was originally selected for susceptibility testing of facultative bacteria because of its relatively defined composition in addition to its lack of sulfonamide antagonists. However, extensive modification of this medium by the addition of complex substances eliminates all of the original reasons for choosing this medium. A more logical approach would seem to be to find a complex medium which supports good growth of anaerobic bacteria and then to develop a disc diffusion test using this medium. Unfortunately, complex media differ somewhat in composition from batch to batch, but at the present time, in the absence of a usable, defined medium, this variation must be accepted.

Dr. Vera Sutter and her colleagues (6) tested several media for the ability to support good growth of anaerobes and found that

Brucella agar medium (Pfizer Inc., New York, N. Y.) with 5% sheep blood and 0.5 µg of menadione per ml was much superior to Mueller-Hinton medium with blood. Using this medium, these workers have developed a method which is very similar to the Bauer-Kirby procedure. In this procedure, three to four colonies are picked into thioglycolate broth (BBL-135C; BBL Division of BioQuest, Cockeysville, Md.) supplemented with hemin, $NaHCO_3$, and menadione. After growth has occurred, the culture is diluted aerobically in *Brucella* broth to the turbidity standard used in the Bauer-Kirby test. The inoculum is then swabbed onto the surface of freshly made plates of supplemented *Brucella*-blood agar medium. After the antibiotic discs are applied, the agar plates are incubated in a GasPak anaerobic jar overnight. The zones of inhibition are measured as seen by using reflected light from the top surface of the plate.

With all disc diffusion methods that use a single concentration disc for each antibiotic, the degree of susceptibility is related to the diameter of the zone of inhibition. The mere presence or absence of an inhibition zone cannot be used as a criterion of susceptibility. Research laboratories must determine which zone diameters correspond to the categories of susceptible and resistant. This is done by determining minimal inhibitory concentrations (MIC's) of each antibiotic for a large number and variety of organisms and then plotting these values against the zone diameters obtained with the test method. The interpretative zone diameter "breakpoints" are assigned for each antibiotic on the basis of the concentration of antibiotic that can be attained safely in the patient's body fluids. Such determinations have been initiated by Dr. Sutter and co-workers, but, so far, only a few species have been tested in detail. In their first publication (6), these data were presented for *B. fragilis* and tetracycline. In more recent work, *Clostridium perfringens* (7) and some fusobacteria (8) have been tested against a number of antibiotics. As more species are tested, the interpretative zone diameters undoubtedly will change to some degree, but approximate interpretative values have been determined and are shown in Table 2. *C. perfringens* strains have uniformly smaller zones of inhibition around the antibiotic discs than the Gram-negative anaerobes tested, presumably because of the very rapid growth rate of this organism. Other species may

Table 2. Interpretative zone diameters currently suggested for use with the method of Sutter et al. (6, 8)

Antibiotic	Disc potency	Resistant	Equivocal	Susceptible
Chloramphenicol	30μg			>20
Clindamycin	2μg	<9	9-14	>14
	10μg	<15	15-25	>25
Erythromycin	15μg	<17	17-26	>26
Lincomycin	2μg		6-15	>15
	10μg	<10	10-24	>24
Penicillin[a]	2 U		6-22	>22
	10 U	<13	13-27	>27
Tetracycline	30μg	<16	16-28	>28
Vancomycin	30μg	<15	15-21	>21

[a] 80% inhibition used as end point for *Fusobacterium varium* and *Fusobacterium mortiferum*.

routinely produce either smaller or larger zones and may require different interpretative values. So far, the method has been tested only for use with the fastest growing and most oxygen-tolerant anaerobes. Further research will indicate what percentage of clinical isolates can be accurately tested with this method. Oxygen-sensitive species will be killed to varying degrees during the aerobic dilution and during swabbing of the plates; the extent to which this will interfere with the accuracy of the test is not known.

A disc diffusion method for testing the more aerotolerant anaerobic bacteria has been developed (9). Anaerobes grow better in pour plates than they do on the surface of agar media, probably because of some degree of protection from atmospheric oxygen. The use of pour plates had been suggested earlier for antibiotic susceptibility tests on anaerobes (10). We standardized the procedure and determined interpretative zone diameters. In this method, a single colony is picked into prereduced chopped meat carbohydrate broth, and the organism is allowed to grow to maximal turbidity overnight at 37°C. Freshly made or prereduced brain heart infusion medium (BBL) supplemented with 0.5% yeast extract, hematin, menadione, and 2.5% agar (Difco Laboratories, Detroit, Mich.) is then melted and cooled to 50°C before addition of 1.5 ml of the overnight culture to 10 ml of the agar medium in a stoppered tube. The inoculum then is rapidly mixed with the agar medium by two inversions and poured into 90-mm Petri dishes. As soon as the agar hardens (2–3 min), antibiotic discs are added from a commercial dispenser, and the plates are placed immediately into a GasPak anaerobic jar. In emergencies, two sets of agar plates can be incubated, and one set can be opened after only 6–8 hr. Such results are always confirmed, however, by another set of plates examined after overnight incubation (37°C).

Standardization of the inocula to a set turbidity did not yield equal numbers of cells of each anaerobic species because of large size differences between species. Dilution of the inoculum in aerobic dilution fluid may result in the killing of many cells, and this effect can nullify any benefits of standardization. A very large inoculum should be used so that the cells can reduce the agar medium rapidly and start growing quickly with very little lag phase.

In tests on the common anaerobic species isolated in clinical laboratories, this method can be used effectively for approximately 75% of common clinical isolates. It should not be used for extremely slow-growing anaerobes or organisms that grow only to a very low turbidity. Also, approximately 30% of the *C. perfringens* isolates produce zones that are uniformly smaller than those of other anaerobes, so, currently, this method is not recommended for use with *C. perfringens*. With these restrictions, the interpretative zone diameters given in Table 3 are used in our laboratory for susceptibility testing of clinical isolates. As more data become available, these interpretative values may be modified to increase the accuracy of the method.

The large inoculum incorporated in a pour plate allows growth of some organisms that do not grow well on the surface of agar plates in anaerobe jars. However, the large inoculum used in the pour plates does cause some problems. The zones of inhibition obtained with this method are sometimes cloudy, and it is difficult for technicians trained to record only zones of complete inhibition in the Bauer-Kirby test to disregard this background growth. We

Table 3. Interpretive zone diameter breakpoints currently used in the V.P.I. Anaerobe Laboratory[a]

Antibiotic	Resistant	Intermediate	Sensitive
Penicillin-G	<15[a]	15-17	>17
Ampicillin	<15	15-17	>17
Cephalothin	<15	15-18	>18
Carbenicillin	<15	15-18	>18
Tetracycline	<15	15-16	>16
Clindamycin	<15	15-17	>17
Erythromycin	<12	12-15	>15

[a] Zone diameter in mm.

recommend using a high-intensity lamp for transmitted light and a black background in order to see the zones well. The largest and most obvious zone of inhibition is measured, even though this may not be a zone of complete inhibition of growth. In case of doubt, the result should not be reported.

Each of the disc diffusion methods described for use with anaerobes has one major deficiency; during some portion of the test, the organisms are exposed to oxygen. An obvious way to alleviate this problem is to perform all manipulations inside an anaerobic glove box. However, the zones obtained may be smaller when the test is performed in this manner, since the organisms can initiate growth immediately. Until comparative tests are performed, interpretation of zone diameters obtained by use of a glove box should not be based on the zone diameter breakpoints described for use on the bench top.

Determinations of MIC's are the standard to which other methods are compared. For most clinical laboratories, performance of MIC tests is not practical, since these tests require considerable time and materials. However, if large numbers of anaerobes are processed each day, MIC determinations could be made. The most rapid procedure is the agar dilution method, as described by

Finegold, Harada, and Miller (11) and used on a large scale by Martin et al. (1) at the Mayo Clinic. In general, at least 20 organisms have to be available for testing each day in order to make this test practical.

Some laboratories are performing partial MIC determinations in which only one, two, or three concentrations of each antibiotic are tested. These concentrations are chosen to approximate clinically useful levels of each antibiotic, and the organism is reported as susceptible or resistant to these concentrations. Such tests do not provide as much information as a complete MIC, but the reduced amount of time and labor involved in this modification could make it a clinically useful test.

Complete or partial MIC's also can be performed inside an anaerobic glove box either by the plate technique or by either macro- or micro-tube-dilution procedures. Such procedures could be clinically useful only in rather large clinical laboratories or research laboratories in which large numbers of anaerobes are tested each day.

A simple method for estimating the antibiotic susceptibility of anaerobes in a completely anaerobic atmosphere has been examined by this author. Basically, the method consists of using antibiotic discs as carriers of antibiotics into tubes of prereduced brain heart infusion broth media opened under O_2-free CO_2. The antibiotic rapidly diffuses from the discs, and the medium then contains the approximate clinically useful level of that antibiotic. Resistance or susceptibility to each antibiotic is determined by the amount of growth in each tube, as compared with a control culture without antibiotic. A similar procedure was originally proposed by Schneierson (12) for testing facultative bacteria and was modified by Abramson and Smibert (13) for testing spirochetes. Recently, this idea also has been adapted for use in the automated antibiotic susceptibility testing device published by Isenberg, Reichler, and Wiseman (14) and scheduled for marketing by Technicon Instruments, Tarrytown, N.Y. Commercial production of this machine will require production of antibiotic discs with very closely controlled contents, which would further improve the anaerobic broth-disc method that I have been testing. The automated machine also could be modified for testing anaerobic bacteria, but the cost of such modifications seems prohibitive at the present time. In the future, when automation becomes more prevalent in susceptibility testing, it may be feasible to test both anaerobes and aerobes on the same equipment. If possible, this type of equipment should be produced with the possibility in mind of adding accessories that would permit testing of anaerobes in the future.

III. Summary of Current Status

Methodology for antibiotic susceptibility testing of anaerobic clinical isolates has progressed considerably in the last year, but difficulties still exist. At the present time, the methods described in this chapter allow separation of the definitely resistant organisms from the definitely susceptible organisms, but organisms with intermediate susceptibility presently could be judged either resistant or susceptible. In the hands of experienced technicians, these methods are considerably more accurate than judgments based only on the normal susceptibility of each species, but, if improperly performed, the results can be misleading. The most common error is the use of either different media or different procedures from those used to develop the standard zone diameter breakpoints. Clinical laboratories must refrain from altering any detail of methods or from combining parts of several methods unless they are willing and able to do the research necessary to prove that such modifications do not adversely affect the results.

In the next few years, many different methods will be published for testing the antibiotic susceptibility of anaerobic bacteria. Some of these methods will undoubtedly work, and others will give inaccurate results; some methods will be practical for use in clinical laboratories, and others will be impractical. Eventually, an amalgam of the best approaches obtained from several methods will probably evolve as the "standard method," and perhaps at that time, involvement by governmental agencies in the standardization process will be practical. At the present time, involvement of the Food and Drug Administration would tend only to stifle experimentation in a new field of research.

The final criterion of any method of antibiotic susceptibility testing must come from tests in clinical laboratories and from the correlation of these results with clinical response of patients. Although laboratories are hesitant to try any techniques which have not been extensively tested, someone must test these methods at the clinical level. Methods that might be very useful for large clinical laboratories may be completely impractical for small laboratories, and vice-versa. I am optimistic that we can use wisely the experience gained from susceptibility testing of facultative pathogens to shorten the years of development and testing normally required for new clinical tecnniques.

Acknowledgments

I am grateful to Dr. Vera Sutter for permission to reproduce the zone diameter breakpoints given in the *Anaerobic Bacteriology Manual* prepared for the Clinical Microbiology Technique Workshop, September 16–17, 1972, at U.C.L.A. (Sutter, V. L., H. R. Atteberry, J. E. Rosenblatt, K. S. Bricknell, and S. M. Finegold, authors).

The excellent technical assistance of Teresa Thiel during this work is appreciated.

Literature Cited

1. Martin, W. J., M. Gardner, and J. A. Washington, II. In vitro antimicrobial susceptibility of anaerobic bacteria isolated from clinical specimens. Antimicrob. Ag. Chemother. 1: 148, 1972.
2. Williams, K. J., M. Brandish, and A. T. Willis. Some observations on clindamycin. Med. Labr. Technol. 29: 233, 1972.
3. Thornton, G. F., and J. A. Cramer. Antibiotic susceptibility of *Bacteroides* species. Antimicrob. Ag. Chemother. 1970: 509, 1971.
4. Bodner, S. J., M. G. Koenig, L. L. Treanor, and J. S. Goodman. Antibiotic susceptibility testing of *Bacteroides*. Antimicrob. Ag. Chemother. 2: 57, 1972.
5. Zabransky, R. J., J. Johnston, and K. Hauser. A diffusion test for antibiotic susceptibility testing of anaerobic bacteria. Proceedings of the 12th Interscience Conference on Antimicrobial Agents and Chemotherapy (Abstr.), September 26–29, Atlantic City, 1972. p. 68.
6. Sutter, V. L., Y.-Y. Kwok, and S. M. Finegold. Standardized antimicrobial disc susceptibility testing of anaerobic bacteria. I. Susceptibility of *Bacteroides fragilis* to tetracycline. Appl. Microbiol. 23: 268, 1972.

7. Sapico, F. L., Y.-Y. Kwok, V. L. Sutter, and S. M. Finegold. Standardized antimicrobial disc susceptibility testing of anaerobic bacteria. II. In vitro susceptibility of *Clostridium perfringens* to nine antibiotics. Antimicrob. Ag. Chemother. 2: 320, 1972.
8. Sutter, V. L., and S. M. Finegold. Antibiotic susceptibility testing of anaerobes. *In* A. Ballows (ed.), Current Techniques for Antibiotic Susceptibility Testing. Charles C Thomas, Springfield, Ill. (In press)
9. Wilkins, T. D., L. V. Holdeman, I. J. Abramson, and W. E. C. Moore. Standardized single-disc method for antibiotic susceptibility testing of anaerobic bacteria. Antimicrob. Ag. Chemother. 1: 451, 1972.
10. Merritt, E. S. A simple method for determination of the antibiotic-sensitivity of anaerobic organisms. Amer. J. Clin. Pathol. 38: 203, 1962.
11. Finegold, S. M., N. E. Harada, and L. G. Miller. Lincomycin: Activity against anaerobes and effect on normal human fecal flora. Antimicrob. Ag. Chemother. 1965: 639, 1966.
12. Schneierson, S. S. A simple rapid disc-tube method for determination of bacterial sensitivity to antibiotics. Antibiotics Chemother. 4: 125, 1954.
13. Abramson, I. J., and R. M. Smibert. A method of testing antibiotic sensitivity of spirochaetes, using antibiotic discs. Brit. J. Vener. Dis. 48: 269, 1972.
14. Isenberg, H. D., A. Reichler, and D. Wiseman. Prototype of a fully automated device for determination of bacterial antibiotic susceptibility in the clinical laboratory. Appl. Microbiol. 22: 980, 1971.

8

In Vitro Susceptibility Tests of Opportunistic Pathogens: A Clinical Appraisal

Robert M. Swenson

Effective chemotherapy of infections is dependent on many variables. Among these are the site of infection, nature of the causative organism, antimicrobial agent employed, and a variety of factors involved in the host's response to the infection. Of all these, the inherent susceptibility of the infecting microorganism to antimicrobial agents is subject to direct in vitro measurement and provides a reference point for selecting an appropriate antibiotic.

Since the introduction of antibiotics over 25 years ago, the susceptibilities of many organisms have been tested. Many species have remained remarkably homogeneous in their sensitivity to antibiotics. Examples of such organisms are *Streptococcus pyogenes* and *Treponema pallidum*, which remain exquisitely susceptible to penicillin. Indeed, this finding is so uniform that, although there are simple procedures available, many laboratories do not even test the former organism for susceptibility to penicillin. However, the susceptibilities of other organisms have changed with time and have varied from hospital to hospital. Notable examples of this are the *Staphylococcus aureus* and many of the Gram-negative bacilli now commonly encountered as nosocomial pathogens. Thus, antibiotic susceptibility testing has become an increasingly major part of the work of the clinical microbiology laboratory.

Robert M. Swenson

I. Methods of Susceptibility Testing

A. Broth Dilution Technique

This is a simple titration of the minimal concentration of the drug required to inhibit or kill the microorganism. The reproducibility and accuracy of the procedure depend on the degree of standardization of the test and the size of the dilution steps employed.

The most commonly employed method is based on that described soon after the advent of penicillin (1). In this procedure, a standardized inoculum is seeded into tubes of broth containing decreasing concentrations of antibiotic. After 18–24 hr, the tubes are examined, and the lowest concentration of antibiotic which inhibits visible growth of bacteria is designated as the minimal inhibitory concentration (MIC). The minimal bactericidal concentration (MBC) can be determined in a similar way by subculturing known volumes from each tube to media free of antibiotic, so that the chemotherapeutic will diffuse away from any remaining viable organisms.

This method can provide a precise MIC and MBC, but it is expensive in terms of both materials and personnel time required. For these reasons, it is not routinely employed in the laboratory. However, this method remains important today for two reasons. First, in severe infections with nosocomial pathogens, it is frequently quite helpful to have a precise MIC or MBC of the infecting bacteria. Second, many nosocomial pathogens (e.g., fungi) can be tested only by modifications of this method.

B. Agar Dilution Technique

These techniques correlate well with broth dilution techniques (2, 3). Varying concentrations of antibiotic are incorporated into solid media. Standardized inocula are seeded onto the surface of the media, and the minimal inhibitory concentrations are read after an appropriate incubation period.

However, these techniques suffer from many of the problems of broth techniques, and, in order to be made economically feasible, a large number of tests must be carried out daily.

These techniques are necessary, however, for testing slower-growing organisms, such as *Nocardia* and *Actinomyces*, for which diffusion tests are inadequately standardized (4). They are also important in obtaining quantitative data on the susceptibilities of organisms to new chemotherapeutics and in determining interpretive standards for diffusion tests.

C. Disc Diffusion Technique

In this procedure, the organism to be tested is exposed on an agar medium to a diffusion gradient of the antibiotic arising from a filter paper disc. Susceptibility is then determined by measuring the size of the zone of inhibition around the disc and relating this to the minimal inhibitory concentration. Although many modifications of this procedure have been employed, there are presently only two acceptable standardized diffusion techniques. The first was developed by Ericsson and colleagues in Sweden (5), and the other was developed by Kirby et al. (6) at the University of Washington. The details of these procedures are beyond the scope of this monograph and may be found in the references noted above.

II. Technical Considerations of Disc Diffusion Tests

Since the disc diffusion technique is the most commonly employed procedure for susceptibility testing of bacteria, the remainder of the discussion is confined to this procedure.

A great many factors influence the size of the zone of inhibition around an antibiotic disc. These factors *must* be held constant or variation in test conditions will affect the results markedly. Some of these important factors are listed below.

A. Medium

Variations in peptones, pH, dextrose content, and concentrations of cations may cause considerable variability in the zone sizes. A notable example of this is the presence of sulfonamide antagonists in many media.

Occasionally, these effects may be extremely subtle. For example, Gilbert and co-workers (7) have recently described the effects of variations in magnesium and calcium ion content on zone sizes obtained with strains of *Pseudomonas aeruginosa* tested against gentamicin. As the concentration of Mg^{++} in the medium was increased, zone sizes decreased, and the MIC, as determined in dilution tests, was increased. Similar but less striking results were seen when the Ca^{++} content of the agar was examined. When commercial lots of Mueller-Hinton agar were assayed, the Mg^{++} content varied from 2.6–4.3 mg per 100 ml. Twenty strains of *P. aeruginosa* were tested on plates prepared from the low-Mg^{++} agar. All had zone diameters in the sensitive range. However, when the high-Mg^{++} agar was used, 80% of strains appeared resistant. When other Gram-negative bacilli were tested against gentamicin, this effect was not nearly as marked. Similarly, when kanamycin, a closely related antibiotic, was tested against susceptible Gram-negative bacilli, little effect was noted.

B. Inoculum

Variations in inoculum size considerably affect the results of tests. Heavier inocula give higher MIC's and smaller zone sizes.

C. Instability of Antibiotics

Incubation of some labile antibiotics may increase the apparent resistance of an organism. Notable examples of this are the aminoglycoside antibiotics, when they are incubated anaerobically.

D. Variations in Medium Depth and Agar Content

Thinner plates and lower agar content tend to produce larger zone sizes.

In Vitro Susceptibility Tests

E. Nature of the Organism Tested

In general, standardized disc diffusion procedures are available only for the rapidly growing aerobic and facultative bacteria.

Recently, a diffusion technique was developed for anaerobic bacteria (8), but this procedure is not yet generally accepted. Finally, there are no standardized susceptibility tests for the fungi.

Despite these problems, a standardized disc diffusion procedure *can* provide reliable, reproducible results. For example, in the recently published World Health Organization collaborative study on antibiotic sensitivity testing (9), three different laboratories tested organisms isolated from patients in their own hospital by using standardized agar dilution and disc diffusion techniques. For all antibiotics tested, the slope and position of the calculated regression line relating MIC and zone size were remarkably similar. Thus, it was demonstrated that different laboratories could achieve similar results, provided that a standardized procedure was carefully followed.

However, it is exceedingly important that the laboratory perform these procedures as carefully as possible. If this is not done, there will be significant variability in results from day to day. Some idea of the magnitude of this problem is provided by the study of Petralli and co-workers (10) on the method of quality control of antibiotic susceptibility testing at their hospital. This particular study involves the use of a computer for continuous evaluation. To form a basis for this evaluation, Petralli et al. compiled a frequency distribution of zone sizes for each organism and antibiotic tested for the previous six months. The resulting histogram then was divided into those zones which occurred frequently and those which occurred infrequently. With these data, whenever a zone for a disc susceptibility test was found to fall into one of the infrequently occurring zones, it was submitted for restudy, inasmuch as this occurrence was so statistically unlikely as to most likely represent an error. Restudy consisted of three phases: first, confirmation of the fact that the secretary had transcribed the report correctly; second, examination of the plate to verify the original reading; and finally, repetition of the test.

During the 10-month period of the study, the susceptibility results of 7590 isolates were examined. A total of 1498 zones from 1125 isolates were rejected. In 594 instances, correction of the error resulted in a significant change in the report (e.g., change in identification of the organism or its antibiotic susceptibility pattern). This represents one important error for every 13 reports issued. The mistakes occurred at many points in the procedure and included such things as secretarial error, technician plating and reading errors, use of impure inoculum, and identification error. Thus, without an adequate quality control program, a given laboratory cannot provide reproducible results on a day-to-day basis.

III. Interpretation of Zone Size–MIC Values

Once a zone size or MIC has been obtained, this must be interpreted in terms of whether the organism should be considered susceptible or resistant to the antimicrobial agent in question. Such determinations have been made in several ways, such as those listed below.

A. By Relating the Susceptibility of the Tested Strain to Other Members of the Species

A good example of this is the sensitivity of *S. aureus* to penicillin. The MIC's and zone sizes form a bimodal distribution in which one group has low MIC's and large zones, while the other group has high MIC's and small zones. The former is considered susceptible and the latter is considered resistant. However, this method is less applicable to the Gram-negative bacilli, since they usually do not give this bimodal distribution (11).

B. By Evaluating Clinical Effectiveness on the Basis of the Experience with the Antibiotic in Question

Again, this method is not particularly applicable to the Gram-negative nosocomial pathogens, since the morbidity and mortality from infections with these organisms are so high even when an "appropriate" antimicrobial agent is employed.

C. By Relating the MIC of the Organism to Blood Levels Attainable with Usual Dosage Schedules of the Antibiotic to be Employed

This is the most commonly used method today. It is very important to realize that most of these determinations are made on the basis of blood levels and that the antibiotic level in other body fluids may be quite different. For example, urine levels of ampicillin and cephalosporins greatly exceed blood levels. It has been well documented (12) that because of this phenomenom, the organisms often can be eradicated from the urinary tract even though they would be considered resistant on the basis of antibiotic levels in the blood. Because of this circumstance, Stamey et al. have suggested that different criteria of susceptibility be set up for treatment of urinary tract infections.

The converse of this is also true. Virtually all antibiotics penetrate poorly into the cerebrospinal fluid. For this reason, bacteria may be considered susceptible, but the clinical response may be exceedingly poor because of the low levels of antibiotic attainable in the cerebrospinal fluid. These are just two occurrences that necessitate the physician's being able to interpret the results of susceptibility in light of the clinical findings in the case under consideration.

IV. Correlation of Microbial Susceptibility and Clinical Response

As noted above, the outcome of a given infection is dependent on many variables. Thus, it is not surprising that there is marked variability in the correlation of in vitro susceptibility with clinical response. In some circumstances, it is quite good. For example, in primary and secondary syphilis, the organism (*T. pallidum*) remains exquisitely sensitive to penicillin, and the clinical response is excellent. However, in most instances, the correlation is not nearly so good. In one study (13), there was a 40%

mortality with staphylococcal bacteremia, even though the organisms were susceptible to penicillin, the antibiotic with which the patients were treated. Similar observations have been made in studies of bacteremia with Gram-negative bacilli (14, 15). The correlation is even worse with some other opportunistic pathogens. In our own observations of patients with *Candida* endocarditis, the mortality is 90%, even though the infecting organisms all have been susceptible in vitro to both amphotericin B and 5-fluorocytosine.

This lack of correlation in the case of the opportunistic pathogens is explainable by the fact that, in the case of infections with these organisms, the normal host response mechanisms are significantly impaired. Thus, the efficacy of the antimicrobial agent is markedly reduced, since an effective therapeutic response is dependent on both the action of the antimicrobial agent and the host's own response to the infection.

This is not meant to imply that susceptibility testing is not important in this situation. Indeed, it is probably more important than with infections in the uncompromised host, since, in this situation, the chemotherapeutic agent is unaided by the usual host defense mechanisms. Thus, choosing what will be the most potent antimicrobial agent is extremely important.

Literature Cited

1. Rammelkamp, C. H., and T. Maxon. Resistance of *Staphylococcus aureus* to the action of penicillin. Proc. Soc. Exp. Biol. Med. 51: 386, 1942.
2. Jackson, G. G., and M. Finland. Comparison of methods for determining sensitivity of bacteria to antibiotics in vitro. Arch. Intern. Med. 88: 446, 1951.
3. Bauer, A. W., C. E. Roberts, and W. M. M. Kirby. Single disc versus multiple disc and plate dilution techniques for antibiotic sensitivity testing. Antibiotics Annu. 574, 1960.
4. Orfanakis, M. G., H. G. Wilcox, and C. B. Smith. In vitro studies of the combined effect of ampicillin and sulfonamides on *Nocardia asteroides* and results of therapy in four patients. Antimicrob. Ag. Chemother. 1: 215, 1972.
5. Ericsson, H., G. Tunevall, and K. Wickman. The paper disc method for

determination of bacterial sensitivity to antibiotics. Scand. J. Clin. Lab. Invest. 12: 414, 1960.
6. Bauer, A. W., W. M. M. Kirby, J. C. Sherris, and M. Turck. Antibiotic susceptibility testing by a standardized single disc method. Amer. J. Clin. Pathol. 45: 493, 1966.
7. Gilbert, D. N., E. Kutscher, P. Ireland, J. A. Barnett, and J. P. Sanfrod. Effect of concentrations of magnesium and calcium on the in vitro susceptibility of *Pseudomonas aeruginosa* to gentamicin. J. Infec. Dis. 124 (Suppl.): 537, 1971.
8. Wilkins, T. D., L. V. Holdeman, I. J. Abramson, and W. E. C. Moore. Standardized single-disc method for antibiotic susceptibility testing of anaerobic bacteria. Antimicrob. Ag. Chemother. 1:451, 1972.
9. Ericsson, H. M., and J. C. Sherris. Antibiotic sensitivity testing: Report of an international collaborative study. Acta. Pathol. Microbiol. Scand. B (Suppl.): 217, 1971.
10. Petralli, J., E. Russell, A. Kataoka, and T. C. Merigan. On-line computer control of antibiotic sensitivity testing. New Engl. J. Med. 283: 735, 1970.
11. Petersdorf, R. G., and J. C. Sherris. Methods and significance of in vitro testing of bacterial sensitivity to drugs. Amer. J. Med. 39: 766, 1965.
12. Stamey, T. A., D. A. Govan, and J. M. Palmer. The localization and treatment of urinary tract infections. The role of bactericidal levels as opposed to serum levels. Medicine 44: 1, 1965.
13. Abboud, F. M., and B. A. Waisbren. Correlation between in vitro studies and response to antibiotic therapy in staphylococcic bacteremia. Arch. Intern. Med. 104: 226, 1959.
14. Bryant, R. E., A. H. Hood, C. E. Hood, and M. G. Koenig. Factors affecting mortality of Gram-negative bacteremia. Arch. Intern. Med. 127: 120, 1971.
15. Myerowitz, R. L., A. A. Medeiros, and T. F. O'Brien. Recent experience with bacillemia due to Gram-negative organisms. J. Infect. Dis. 124: 239, 1971.

9

Identification and Ecology of Yeasts of Medical Importance

Donald G. Ahearn

I. Introduction

Yeasts are fungi that typically exist as microscopic, single cells which reproduce by budding. Dependent upon cultural conditions, many yeasts may form extensive true- or pseudomycelium. Yeasts with this capacity frequently are referred to as "yeast-like." Thus, the general categorization of a fungus with the yeasts is arbitrary. The yeasts comprise a heterogeneous, taxonomic group which includes over 400 recognized species, representing the Hemiascomycetes, the Heterobasidiomycetes, and the Deuteromycetes. They are ubiquitous in nature, occurring from the polar to the tropic regions and from terrestrial to oceanic environments. Their metabolism may be oxidative and fermentative or strictly oxidative. Although they are noted for their activity against diverse carbohydrates, various yeasts readily may metabolize such compounds as hydrocarbons, proteins, lipids, and nucleic acids.

A few yeasts, such as *Candida albicans* and *Torulopsis glabrata*, are associated closely with man and other warm-blooded animals. If the host is physiologically stressed, e.g., with diabetes, cancer, or immunological defects, the yeasts may become adventitious pathogens. Recent advances in surgical and chemotherapeutic procedures, such as developments permitting organ transplant and heart surgery and the increased use of immunosuppressants, broad spectrum antibiotics, and oral progestational agents have been accompanied by an increased incidence of yeast infections. Moreover, there has been increased involvement with species other than the most commonly reported pathogens, *C. albicans* and *Cryptococcus neoformans*.

II. Methods

A variety of procedures and classification schemes have been advocated for the identification of yeasts. Most of these will give satisfactory results with adequately trained personnel and proper laboratory facilities. Unfortunately, these conditions generally do not exist within the mycological area of most clinical laboratories. The following represents a selection and modification of methods which should suffice in the medical laboratory for the definitive species determination of the clinically important yeasts. A variety of excellent and valid procedures for yeast identification are available in greater detail in Lodder (1) and Wickerham (2).

A. Isolation

A modified Sabouraud's agar, containing 20 g of dextrose, 10 g of neopeptone, and 20 g of agar per liter, or Wickerham's yeast extract-malt extract agar, containing 3 g of malt extract, 3 g of yeast extract, 5 g of peptone, 10 g of dextrose, and 20 g of agar per liter, is adequate for the isolation of most yeasts. In general, a medium containing dextrose, trace elements, vitamins, and ammonium sulfate or peptone readily will allow most yeasts to grow, other than certain *Pityrosporum* sp. For these latter yeasts, fatty acids (e.g., myristic acid) must be supplied. The addition of 10 ml of Tween 80 or olive oil per liter of isolation medium and an incubation temperature of 32°C generally will permit the growth of *Pityrosporum* sp. To inhibit bacterial contaminants, one may employ heat-stable antibiotics; chloramphenicol, 0.05–0.5 g per liter; or gentamicin, 0.02–0.4 g per liter. I add gelatin capsules of antibiotic to the isolation medium prior to autoclaving and, frequently, used paired media with and without antibiotics. The ease in handling the capsules more than offsets their higher cost. Using capsules and the above media, the higher concentrations of antibiotics have not proven unduly inhibitory for common, animal-associated yeasts. The main advantage of the higher concentrations is the ready recovery of yeasts from bacteria-laden urine and stool specimens. Mycosel agar (BBL Division of BioQuest, Cockeysville, Md.) and Mycobiotic agar (Difco Laboratories, Detroit, Mich.) are used frequently to isolate fungi from clinical specimens, but these media are inappropriate for the isolation of many yeasts. *C. albicans* typically is resistant to over 0.5 g per liter of cycloheximide, but only occasional strains of the other common, animal-associated species (e.g., *Candida tropicalis, Candida parapsilosis, Cryptococcus albidus*) will grow at this concentration. Most strains of *C. neoformans* are particularly sensitive to cycloheximide.

The pH of the isolation medium may be lowered to between 4.5 and 5.5 with the addition of 10 ml of a 10% solution of lactic acid (85% strength) per liter, as an alternative to the use of antibiotics. The lactic acid is sterilized by filtration and added to the autoclaved medium when it has cooled to about 50°C. If a pH near 4.5 is employed, it may be necessary to increase the agar concentration to 23–25 g per liter to ensure adequate solidification.

Isolation media may be incubated at temperatures of between 20 and 35°C. Most pathogenic yeasts grow well at 37°C, although a few strains of *C. neoformans* of proven pathogenicity give only negligible growth at 37°C on dextrose-peptone or blood agars. All primary isolates should be streaked on isolation agar to ensure culture purity prior to studying all diagnostic characteristics other than germ tubes. Infection by multiple species is possible; therefore, all discrete colonies, as distinguished by gross colony and microscopic morphology, should be isolated for study. For microscopic examination of cell morphology, suspend the yeast cells in a drop of water. If the culture is from cerebral spinal fluid or if *C. neoformans* is suspected, examine the cells in a nigrosine or India ink suspension prepared in a 10% formalin solution.

B. Germ Tubes

The formation of germ tubes provides a rapid, reliable procedure for the identification of *C. albicans* and its variant, *Candida stellatoidea* (3–6). Bovine or pooled human serum, plasma or tissue culture Medium 199 (7), or egg albumin (8) are suitable for the formation of germ tubes. Germ tubes may be produced by certain strains of *C. albicans* at different temperatures (28–38°C) and in a variety of media ranging in complexity from 1.0% water agar (found with rare rough colony types) to combinations of amino acids in phosphate buffer or defined tissue culture medium. The latter and various sera, including bovine, horse, swine, chicken, sheep, and human, have proved to be 100% effective in inducing germ tubes. This accuracy, however, may not be achieved in initial screening procedures with cells of varying growth states. Cells older than 96 hr or those exposed to antibiotics may not produce germ tubes readily.

Preliminary screening for germ tubes may be accomplished by transferring cells directly from isolation medium to serum. For best results, yeasts should not be permitted to grow more than 96 hr on the isolation agar prior to the germ tube test. The serum and cells are incubated at 37°C for 2–3 hr, and the cell sediment is examined microscopically.

A simple, economical screening test for *C. albicans* is as follows. Cells from representative yeast colonies on the isolation agar are transferred into about 0.3 ml of pooled human serum contained in clean, nonsterile, 12- × 75-mm test tubes via the tip of a clean plastic tube. The serum may be predispensed into the test tubes and kept frozen until used. The plastic tubes, prepared by dividing commercial cocktail straws (3- to 4-mm bore diameter) into about 100-mm lengths, are left immersed in the sera during a 2- to 3-hr incubation at 37°C. The straws are then employed to transfer a drop of the serum-cell suspension to slides for unstained, wet-mount, microscopic examination. The yeast cells of *C. albicans* produce thin germ tubes 3–4 μ in diameter and up to 20 μ in length. The germ tubes, unlike pseudohyphal cells, are not constricted at their point of origin (4, 5). *C. albicans* produces both germ tubes and pseudohyphal elements (marked constriction at their point of origin), but only the germ tubes are diagnostic.

Identification and Ecology of Yeasts

Inexperienced personnel may mistake germinating arthrospores of *Geotrichum candidum* or *Trichosporon* sp. for germ tubes of *C. albicans*. In some instances, colonies may have formed hyphal elements on the isolation agar. These may be mistaken for germ tubes when observed in serum. For this reason, if obvious germ tubes are not evident, the germ tube test should be repeated with young budding cells from a broth culture at a concentration to give 10^5-10^7 cells per ml of serum. A known isolate of *C. albicans* and an isolate of *C. tropicalis* should be included in each germ tube test as controls.

C. Pseudomycelium and Chlamydospore Production

Corn meal agar or yeast morphology agar (Difco) are adequate for the induction of hyphae. Tween 80 (15 ml in 85 ml of distilled water, filter sterilized, and added to the above media prepared with 900 ml of distilled water) may be used to stimulate chlamydospore formation. Four to eight yeasts may be cut into the agar medium in a Petri dish. The cuts are made several millimeters longer than a sterile coverslip, which is placed over the cut. After two to four days of incubation at 22–26°C, the yeasts may be examined either with low magnification through the back of the unopened plate or with higher magnification through the coverslip. Most of the common candidas readily produce pseudohyphae, but, with slower-growing forms, the plates should be examined over a period of at least 10 days.

Bile agar (Difco), containing 10 g of oxgall and 20 g of agar per liter, gives a rapid and profuse production of chlamydospores that generally are positive with *C. albicans* in 24–48 hr at 22–26°C (9). Inoculate the oxgall medium with a thin surface streak slightly longer than a cover glass; cover the streak with a sterile cover glass. This medium is not appropriate for the formation of hyphae. Occasional strains of *C. tropicalis* produce profuse numbers of chlamydospores on oxgall agar.

D. Induction of Perfect Stages

The yeast extract-malt extract isolation agar will induce certain strains to produce ascospores; however, no single medium or incubation temperature is appropriate for inducing the perfect stage of all yeasts. The common species of *Saccharomyces*, *S. cerevisiae*, the bread and wine yeast, and *Saccharomyces uvarum* (syn. *Saccharomyces carlbergensis*), the beer yeast, are among the more common perfect yeasts found in clinical specimens. These species and *Kluyveromyces fragilis*, the perfect stage of *Candida pseudotropicalis*, generally will form ascospores on malt agar (malt extract, 50 g; agar, 30 g per liter) at 20–30°C. Diamalt (Standard Brands, New York, N.Y.) may be used as the malt extract. Ascospores may be observed best by microscopic examination of the cells in water. Heterobasidiomycetous yeasts (10) may produce teliospores and true hyphae subsurface in the malt agar. More detailed information on the sexual stages of yeasts may be found in Lodder (1).

E. Assimilation Tests

Yeast nitrogen base and yeast carbon base (Difco), prepared according to the defined formulas of Wickerham (2), are most suitable for the assimilation tests. The yeast nitrogen base (6.7 g) and 5 g of the appropriate carbohydrate (glucose, galactose, sucrose, lactose, maltose, raffinose, trehalose, melibiose, inositol, and cellobiose) are dissolved in 100 ml of distilled water. The yeast carbon base (11.2 g) is supplemented with 0.8 g of KNO_3. These concentrated bases are sterilized by filtration. The bases may be solidified with 20 g of agar in 900 ml of distilled water. The agar solution is sterilized separately by autoclaving. Cotton-stoppered test tubes or steel- or plastic-capped tubes are used for the agar slants. Screw-capped tubes should not be used for the assimilation tests. Slants containing the basal medium without the carbon or nitrogen should be employed as controls for each yeast tested. The use of agar slants facilitates handling and storage in the clinical laboratory. Moreover, the positive slants may be examined visually for possible contaminants, which could give erroneous determinations.

Broth assimilation tests may be employed (add 0.5 ml of base to 4.5 ml of sterile water in a capped test tube). Ideally, the broth tests are incubated with agitation. A roller drum (TC5; New Brunswick Scientific Company, New Brunswick, N. J.) gives good agitation with the tubes incubating on a 10- to 20-degree angle. Inocula for broth tests should be checked for purity after inoculation of the assimilation tests by spot inoculation of an isolation agar plate. Broth medium generally gives more distinct and rapid results. False positive results, attributable to impurities present in the agar, are avoided.

Inocula for the carbohydrate assimilation tests are prepared by transferring a few cells to 5 ml of the yeast nitrogen broth containing 1.0 mg of glucose per liter. Cells are starved in yeast carbon base for the nitrogen assimilation test. After 24–36 hr of incubation at 22–26°C, about 0.01 ml of cell suspension (one drop) is used for inoculating the assimilation tests. If liquid assimilation tests are employed, the inoculum for the carbohydrate test may be introduced into the yeast carbon base medium with KNO_3. After 24 hr of growth, a loopful of cells is transferred to a second tube of yeast carbon base with KNO_3. The nitrate assimilation results are read from this second tube in 48 hr. The carbon assimilation tests for each yeast are read after at least 96 hr of incubation by comparison of growth on the various carbohydrates with growth of the same yeast on glucose. The nitrate assimilation medium contains 1.0% glucose; therefore, if the yeast utilized KNO_3, growth will be heavy. Frequently, weakly positive growth on KNO_3 is obtained because endogenous nitrogen has not been sufficiently reduced.

F. Fermentation Tests

The basal fermentation broth contains 5.5 g of yeast extract, 7.5 g of peptone, and sufficient bromcresol purple (about 0.4 g per liter) to give a purple color. The fermentation base is dispensed, 4 ml per tube, into 16- × 125-mm, screw-capped test tubes containing gas inserts; the medium is sterilized by autoclaving. The carbohydrates, in 6% solutions (except for raffinose at 12%), are sterilized separately by filtration, and 2.0 ml are aseptically added to each tube. Sugars routinely tested for fermentation are glucose, galactose, sucrose, maltose, and raffinose. The fermentation tubes may be inoculated with a cell suspension prepared directly from the stock slant. If the same cell preparation used for inoculating the assimilation tests is employed, the inoculum should be 0.1–0.2 ml. The caps should be securely tightened during the 10-day incubation period, with incubation in static culture at 22–26°C. Positive fermentation is recorded for the production of gas only. To detect false negatives attributable to supersaturation of the broth, all tubes giving an acid reaction should be shaken lightly and the cap vented. This procedure frequently is followed by bubbling of the broth, denoting fermentation. All positive fermentations of a carbohydrate are accompanied by a positive assimilation of the carbohydrate; however, sugars may be assimilated without being fermented.

G. Urease Test

Christensen's urea agar (Difco; Ref. 11) or Littman's urea agar (12) are suitable for determining the presence of the classical "urease" enzyme. This enzyme liberates ammonia from urea, resulting in a rise of the pH of the medium and a change of the phenol red indicator from yellow to red. Christensen's urea agar contains 1 g of peptone, 1 g of dextrose, 5 g of NaCl, 2 g of KH_2PO_4, 20 g of urea, 0.012 g of phenol red, and 15 g of agar per liter. The agar slants should have a pH of about 6.8 and show no orange or red coloration. Littman's medium contains 1 g of thiotone, 5 g of dextrose, 5 g of NaCl, 3 g of KH_2PO_4, 3 g of NA_2HPO_4, 10 g of urea, 0.01 g of phenol red, and 12 g of agar per liter; the pH is about 6.0. For both media, the urea is filter sterilized in a separate solution and added to the autoclaved base when it has cooled to about 50°C. Urea agar slants are inoculated with a 0.1-ml cell suspension and incubated for at least five days at 22–26°C. Littman's urea agar supports a more luxuriant yeast growth and often gives the most intense urease reaction, whereas Christensen's agar is commercially available and typically gives a rapid urease reaction with *C. neoformans*. All species of *Cryptococcus* and *Rhodotorula* and strains of *Candida*, *Trichosporon*, and other genera are urease positive.

The production of urease, the ability to grow at 37°C, and the production of a brown pigment on bird seed (*Guizotia abyssinica*) agar (13) are characteristic of typical strains of *C. neoformans*. However, a few strains give negative or negligible reactions for these tests, whereas occasional strains of *Cryptococcus laurentii* and *C. albidus* are positive for all three tests.

H. Animal Inoculation

Pathogenicity for mice may be employed as an adjunct test for the identification of *C. neoformans*. If the clinical situation demands, white mice (we use four test animals) are inoculated intracerebrally with a 0.05- to 0.1-ml saline suspension of cells from the youngest available culture. The cell suspension should contain approximately 10^8 cells per ml. The cerebral hemispheres of those animals that die are exposed and then are scraped lightly with an inoculating needle, and the adhering tissue is mixed on a slide with the formalin-nigrosine solution for miscrosopic examination. Strains of *C. neoformans* vary in their pathogenicity for mice; mice may die within two days or they may survive many weeks. Therefore, this test is performed in conjunction with the assimilation tests, and the most rapidly available results are employed.

I. Serological Techniques

The slide-agglutination procedure of Sweet and Kaufman (14) for *Candida* sp. and the fluorescent-antibody reagent of Pidcoe and Kaufman (15) for *C. neoformans* are particularly valuable for the rapid presumptive identification of the medically important yeasts. The slide-agglutination procedure does not permit the identification of rough strains and does not distinguish directly *C. albicans* type A from *C. tropicalis*. The fluorescent-antibody reagent provides the most accurate rapid identification of *C. neoformans*. Unfortunately, these serological reagents are rarely available in clinical laboratories.

III. Ecology of Principal Pathogens

A. C. albicans

This yeast, which normally occurs as an obligate commensal of the gastrointestinal and urinary-genital tracts of man, is the most common etiological agent of yeast infections. The species is associated more frequently with females than with males. In my studies of apparently normal cases, considering varied types of samples given, I have found a 26% incidence with females (308 samples) and a 12% incidence with males (92 samples). The association with females is higher during pregnancy and with the use of birth control pills than at other times. Infections range in severity from superficial skin diseases to systemic mycoses. The pathology of candidiasis and factors predisposing to infection have been described in detail by Winner and Hurley (16). Probably the most common type of infection by *C. albicans* is vaginitis. *C. albicans* occurs infrequently on healthy human skin; however, skin lesions associated with the yeast may be slight enough to go unnoticed. In this regard, certain cases of supposedly chronic vaginitis may be reinfections by the sexual partner. *C. albicans* is rarely isolated from other than warm-blooded animals. Its relatively rare occurrence in water and soil generally has been linked to recent contamination by human or animal excrement.

B. C. tropicalis and C. parapsilosis

These yeasts occur within the mouth, intestinal tract, and vagina and on the skin, but they are not obligate commensals, nor do they cause infections often. In association with man, *C. tropicalis* frequently occurs in the mouth and intestinal tract and on the more sheltered areas of human skin. *C. parapsilosis* is associated less frequently with these areas, but is more often isolated from the skin of the hand, arms, and face. Both of these yeasts are widespread in nature. *C. tropicalis* occurs particularly in regions of high organic content, whereas *C. parapsilosis* may be found more frequently in low-nutrient waters and soils. *C. tropicalis* appears to be somewhat more virulent than *C. parapsilosis*. Moreover, *C.*

tropicalis has been implicated in vaginitis, and both species have been proven to cause endocarditis and fungemia. During the past five years, I have identified 90 yeast isolates from the blood of patients residing in various geographical areas of the United States. These included: *C. parapsilosis*, 28 isolates; *T. glabrata*, 24 isolates; *C. tropicalis*, 13 isolates; *C. neoformans*, five isolates; and *C. albicans*, four isolates. Sixteen of the individuals whose blood yielded *C. parapsilosis* were either drug addicts or patients who had histories of intravenous injections. It is important to determine the species of yeast involved in fungemia, inasmuch as this disease, caused by the less invasive species (*C. parapsilosis*, *Rhodotorula rubra*), may respond to treatment for the generalized symptoms without the use of the potentially dangerous polyene antibiotics.

C. T. glabrata

This yeast also may be categorized as an obligate commensal of warm-blooded animals, but it has a host-free survival index greater than that of *C. albicans*. *T. glabrata* is most commonly associated with the vagina and urinary tract and may be infective in both instances. It is frequently a pathogen when diabetes mellitus is a predisposing factor. *T. glabrata* is associated most frequently with females; its presence in male urine in high numbers suggests a serious, underlying debilitation (5).

D. C. neoformans

This yeast is a neurotropic pathogen of man and other animals. During recent years in the United States, it has been diagnosed as one of the major lethal fungi. Meningitis is the most commonly diagnosed mycosis caused by *C. neoformans*, but the primary infection is probably pulmonary. Systemic dissemination with fungemia and, rarely, the development of skin lesions may occur. In most instances, cryptococcosis is associated with impaired hosts, yet underlying debilitations are not always evident. In nature, *C. neoformans* occurs in high densities in pigeon droppings and occasionally in soil (17). Staib (18) has demonstrated

Table 1. Characteristics of yeast isolates

	Dextrose	Galactose	Lactose	Maltose	Sucrose	Melibiose	Cellobiose	Trehalose	Raffinose	Melezitose	Inositol[a]	Rhamnose[a]	Erythritol[a]	Xylose[a]	Urease	Hyphae	Germ tubes	KNO$_3$
C. albicans	F	VF	–	F	+[b]	–	–	VF	–	V	–	–	–	+[c]	–	+	+	–
C. stellatoidea	F	VF	–	F	–	–	–	V	–	–	–	–	–	+	–	+	+	–
C. tropicalis	F	F	–	F	F	–	V	F	–	+	–	–	–	+	–	+	–	–
Candida krusei	F	–	–	–	–	–	–	–	–	–	–	–	–	–	V	+	–	–
C. pseudotropicalis	F	F	F	–	F	–	+	–	F	–	–	–	–	V	–	+	–	–
Candida guilliermondii	F	VF	–	+	F	VF	+	F	F	+	–	V	–	+	–	–	–	–
R. rubra	+	+	+	+	+	–	V	+	+	+	–	–	–	+	+	+	–	–
Trichosporon cutaneum	+	V	+	V	V	V	V	V	V	V	V	V	V	V	+	+	–	–
Trichosporon pullulans	+	+	+	+	+	V	+	+	V	+	V	+	+	+	+	+	–	+
C. laurentii	+	+	+	+	+	V	+	+	V	V	+	+	V	+	+	R	–	–
C. neoformans	+	+	–	+	+	–	+	+	V	+	+[c]	+	V	+	+	R	–	–

Cryptococcus terreus	+	V	–	V	–	–	+	+	–	V	–	+	+	R	–	+
C. albidus	+	V	V	+	+	V	+	+	+	V	V	+	+	R	–	+
S. cerevisiae	F	F	–	F	F	–	–	V	VF	–	–	–	–	RA	–	–
T. glabrata	F	–	–	–	–	–	–	F	–	–	–	–	–	–	–	–

[a] Tested for assimilation only; F, fermentation and assimilation positive; VF, positive assimilation with variable fermentation; +, positive assimilation; V, strain variation in assimilation; R, occasional to rare hyphal elements; A, ascospores.
[b] Rarely fermented.
[c] Rarely negative.

that *C. neoformans* can survive for prolonged periods and that it utilizes dandelions and hay as growth substrates. The guanine-plus-cytosine content of the deoxyribonucleic acid, i.e., about 50% (19), the production of extracellular deoxyribonuclease (20), and the production of hyphal stages similar to those of *Leucosporidium* (21) all indicate a basidiomycetous nature for *C. neoformans*. In contrast, *C. albicans* has a guanine-plus-cytosine content of about 35%, lacks an extracellular deoxyribonuclease, and is not known to produce a stage with clamp connections. These characteristics suggest that *C. albicans* is ascomycetous.

IV. Classification

Tests with yeasts in most clinical laboratories are limited to those for the induction of mycelium and chlamydospores and the urease reaction. At a minimum, the rapid and economical germ tube test should be added to this regimen. Germ tubes are produced only by *C. albicans* and *C. stellatoidea*. This latter yeast, also a potential pathogen, is of relatively rare occurrence, generally being isolated from the vagina. *C. stellatoidea* may be considered an alphaglucosidase-negative variant of *C. albicans* (6). The sucrose assimilation test or the rapid procedure of Kamaya (22) may be

Table 2. Key to asporogenous clinical yeast isolates

1. Germ tubes positive	2
Germ tubes negative	3
2. Sucrose positive	*C. albicans*
Sucrose negative	*C. stellatoidea*
3. Pseudohyphae absent or sparse	4
Pseudohyphae well developed	8
4. Inositol positive (*Cryptococcus*)	5
Inositol negative (*Torulopsis*)	17
5. Potassium nitrate positive	6
Potassium nitrate negative	7

Table 2, continued

6. Maltose and sucrose positive	*C. albidus*
Maltose variable, sucrose negative	*C. terreus*
7. Maltose, sucrose, and dulcitol positive; lactose and melibiose negative	*C. neoformans*
Maltose, sucrose, and lactose positive; melibiose and dulcitol variable	*C. laurentii*
Maltose and sucrose positive; lactose, melibiose, and dulcitol negative	*Cryptococcus uniguttalatus*
8. Arthrospores produced (*Trichosporon*)	9
Arthrospores not produced (*Candida*)	10
9. Potassium nitrate negative; lactose and melibiose positive	*T. cutaneum*
Potassium nitrate positive; lactose positive; melibiose variable	*T. pullulans*
10. Potassium nitrate positive	*Candida* sp.
Potassium nitrate negative	11
11. Lactose positive and fermented	*C. pseudotropicalis*
Lactose negative	12
12. Raffinose positive and melibiose positive	*C. guilliermondii*
Raffinose negative	13
13. Trehalose positive	14
Trehalose negative	15
14. Cellobiose positive; maltose fermented	*C. tropicalis*
Cellobiose negative	16
15. Glucose positive; galactose, sucrose, and maltose negative	*C. krusei* complex
16. Maltose and sucrose fermented	*C. tropicalis*
Maltose fermentation negative; sucrose fermentation variable (generally negative)	*C. parapsilosis*
Maltose fermented; sucrose negative (repeat germ tube test)	*C. albicans*
17. Only glucose and trehalose fermented	*T. glabrata*

used to distinguish the variety. The use of oxgall agar gives the best and most rapid production of chlamydospores. It should be noted that some isolates of *C. albicans* give negligible production of chlamydospores and, in rare instances, even of hyphae. Only a few strains of *C. tropicalis* will produce chlamydospores on oxgall agar, and these chlamydospores are smaller and atypical of those observed in *C. albicans*. Clinical isolates of *C. tropicalis* typically assimilate cellobiose, whereas *C. albicans* and *C. parapsilosis* do not assimilate this sugar.

Germ-tube-negative yeasts should be inoculated onto urea slants, which normally are read over a five-day period. Cryptococci frequently give a positive reaction in 24 hr. The urease test is not specific, but a positive reaction, in conjunction with cell morphology and the clinical syndrome, may justify a presumptive identification. Definitive identification of the clinical yeasts usually is dependent upon the results of the assimilation and fermentation tests and morphological studies (Table 1).

The presence or absence of pseudomycelium or hyphae on corn meal agar is a major classification characteristic. Species of *Cryptococcus*, *Torulopsis*, and many sexual yeasts rarely produce pseudohyphae, whereas *Candida*, *Trichosporon*, and many *Pichia* and *Hansenula* sp. produce profuse pseudohyphae. *C. tropicalis* and *Trichosporon* sp. (arthrospore producers) typically produce heavy mycelium within 24–36 hr. The experienced technician may utilize the distinctive morphology of the common medical yeasts for presumptive identifications (for detailed species descriptions, see Ref. 1). A key to the common medical yeasts is presented in Table 2. Unless fermentation is specified within the key, the physiological reactions refer to assimilation tests.

Literature Cited

1. Lodder, J. (ed.). The Yeasts. North Holland Publishing Co., Amsterdam, 1970.
2. Wickerham, L. J. Taxonomy of yeasts. U. S. Dept. Agric. Tech. Bull. 1029: 1, 1951.
3. Taschdjian, C. L., J. J. Burchall, and P. J. Kozinn. Rapid identification of

Candida albicans by filamentation in serum and serum substitutes. Amer. J. Dis. Child. 99: 212, 1960.
4. Mackenzie, D. W. R. Morphogenesis of *Candida albicans* in vivo. Sabouraudia 3: 225, 1964.
5. Ahearn, D. G., J. R. Jannach, and F. J. Roth. Speciation and densities of yeasts in human urine specimens. Sabouraudia 5: 110, 1966.
6. Fell, J. W., and S. A. Meyer. Systematics of yeast species in the *Candida parapsilosis* group. Mycopathol. Mycol. Appl. 32: 176, 1967.
7. Morgan, J. F., H. J. Morton, G. M. Healy, and R. C. Parker. Nutrition of animal cells in tissue culture. VI. Low toxicity of barium. Proc. Soc. Exp. Biol. Med. 78: 880, 1951.
8. Buckley, H. R., and N. van Uden. The identification of *Candida albicans* within two hours by the use of an egg white slide preparation. Sabouraudia 4: 205, 1963.
9. Marcano, C., and M. Feo. Investigacion de levaduras en vulva y vagina. Mycopathol. Mycol. Appl. 47: 275, 1972.
10. Fell, J. W: Yeasts with heterobasidiomycetous life cycles. *In* D. G. Ahearn (ed.), Recent Trends in Yeast Research, p. 67. Georgia State University, Atlanta, 1970.
11. Christensen, W. B. Urea decomposition as a means of differentiating *Proteus* and *Paracolon* cultures from each other and from *Salmonella* and *Shigella* types. J. Bacteriol. 52: 461, 1946.
12. Littman, M. An improved method for detection of urea hydrolysis by fungi. J. Infect. Dis. 101: 51, 1957.
13. Shields, A. B., and L. Ajello. Medium for selective isolation of *Cryptococcus neoformans*. Science 151: 208, 1966.
14. Sweet, C. E., and L. Kaufman. Application of agglutinins for the rapid and accurate identification of medically important *Candida* species. Appl. Microbiol. 19: 830, 1970.
15. Pidcoe, V., and L. Kaufman. Fluorescent-antibody reagent for the identification of *Cryptococcus neoformans*. Appl. Microbiol. 16: 271, 1968.
16. Winner, H. I., and R. Hurley. *Candida albicans*. Little, Brown and Co., Boston, 1964.
17. Emmons, C. W. Pathogenic yeasts. Antonie van Leeuwenhoek 35 (Suppl. Yeast Symposium): 113, 1969.
18. Staib, F. Plants as a substratum for growth of *Cryptococcus neoformans*. Zentbl. Bakt. Hyg., Abt. I. Orig. A218: 486, 1971.
19. Meyer, S. A., and H. J. Phaff. Taxonomic significance of the DNA base composition in yeasts. *In* D. G. Ahearn (ed.), Recent Trends in Yeast Research, p. 1. Georgia State University, Atlanta, 1970.
20. Cazin, J., T. R. Kozel, D. M. Lupan, and W. R. Burt. Extracellular deoxyribonuclease production by yeasts. J. Bacteriol. 100: 760, 1969.

21. Shadomy, H. J. Clamp connections in two strains of *Cryptococcus neoformans*. *In* D. G. Ahearn (ed.), Recent Trends in Yeast Research, p. 67. Georgia State University, Atlanta, 1970.
22. Kamaya, T. Simple rapid identification of *Candida albicans* with emphasis on the differentiation between *Candida albicans* and *Candida stellatoidea*. Mycopathol. Mycol. Appl. 32: 105, 1968.

10

Serodiagnosis of Opportunistic Mycoses

Morris A. Gordon

I. Introduction

Diagnostic serology of cryptococcosis, established and reliable, is based upon testing for capsular polysaccharide antigen as well as for antibody. The rapid slide latex agglutination test for detection of antigen in disseminated cryptococcosis is highly sensitive and specific. Results of both the charcoal-particle card agglutination test and the tube agglutination test for cryptococcal antibody correlate well with the presence of localized active cryptococcosis or less acute central nervous system disease.

Serology of candidiasis is very useful, but not yet fully standardized. Candidiasis is difficult to diagnose by conventional nonserological methods, but indications of active infection can be obtained by measurement of specific antibody either by immunodiffusion in agar gel or by a significant change in agglutinin titer. Some promising new techniques include determination of indirect fluorescent-antibody titer; immunoelectroosmophoresis, which is more sensitive than immunodiffusion (ID), as well as very rapid; slide latex agglutination, more sensitive than ID, but with more cross-reactions; and a proposed assay for "interfering factor." Serum antibody levels do not seem to provide an index of host resistance to invasion by either *Candida* or *Cryptococcus*, since resistance is based very largely upon cellular immunity.

Immunodiffusion is specific and provides a high degree of sensitivity for the diagnosis of aspergillosis. An index of the severity of the *Aspergillus* invasion is given by the number and intensity of precipitin lines formed.

Precipitins detectable by immunodiffusion appear in cases of rhinocerebral mucormycosis. Both agglutinins and precipitins have been detected in human torulopsosis.

II. Cryptococcosis

Of all the opportunistic mycoses, cryptococcosis is associated with the best-defined immunoserology, including excellent diagnostic and prognostic tests for active infection. The peculiar attribute of cryptococcal serology is that it depends largely upon detection of *antigen*, rather than antibody, in host fluids. As the population of encapsulated *Cryptococcus neoformans* cells in the body increases, capsular polysaccharaide neutralizes and exceeds specific antibody. The latter can be demonstrated early in the evolution of a case of cryptococcal meningitis, cerebral abscess, or disseminated disease, as well as throughout the course of an infection that remains localized in the skin or lungs. However, as the disease progresses, cryptococcal cells multiply rapidly, thus flooding the body with the highly antigenic capsular material. Although the production of host antibody may continue, it is soon neutralized by the abundant antigen, the excess of which is then detectable in such body fluids as blood serum, cerebrospinal fluid, and urine. Antigen titers continue to increase in the absence of specific chemotherapy. However, with adequate treatment (amphotericin B or 5-fluorocytosine), they generally drop two-fold in about two weeks and four-fold in a month; they often become undetectable after six weeks. At that point, antibody may become demonstrable again.

A. Antigen Detection

In practice, most cases of cryptococcosis that come to medical attention are in a relatively advanced stage, so that antigen, rather than antibody, is in excess. For this reason, and because the test for antigen is simpler and more rapid than that for antibody, tests for antigen are done first, and only if it is not detected are tests performed for antibody. Very seldom are both found in the same specimen, and then usually in very low titers.

The standard method for detection and measurement of cryptococcal antigen in body fluids is the slide latex agglutination (SLA) procedure, in which test specimens are mixed with a stable reagent consisting of uniform latex particles coated with rabbit anticryptococcal globulin. After 3 min of agitation, the slide is read for clumping. This test is highly sensitive and highly specific for cryptococcal infection; the only significant source of nonspecific reactions is serum containing high-titered rheumatoid factor (1). This difficulty may be overcome by pretreatment of serum with a disulfide-reducing agent, which splits the IgM antibody and thus keeps it from reacting with the globulin-coated latex. This is the only cryptococcosis test for which reagents are commercially available (Industrial Biological Laboratories, Rockville, Md.). Cryptococcal antigen may also be detected and titrated by a quantitative complement-fixation procedure (2).

B. Antibody Detection

Of the several methods for determination of cryptococcal antibody, the tube agglutination procedure (3) appears to be most specific for active infection. The charcoal-particle card agglutination technique (4) is rapid and somewhat more sensitive, but it may result in nonspecific reactions in the lowest dilutions of serum. The indirect fluorescent-antibody technique (5) appears to be still more sensitive, in that it yields a higher number of positive sera; however, many of these reactions are achieved at the expense of specificity, since, in a relatively large number of cases, there is no other evidence of cryptococcal infection.

Skin test materials for delayed hypersensitivity to *C. neoformans* have been tried experimentally (6, 7), but they are not yet developed to a state at which they might be of diagnostic value.

C. Immunoserology

While circulating antibodies are detectable in a minority of cases, they appear to play an inconsequential role in protecting the host or resolving an infection, despite the fact that the capsular polysaccharide antigen against which they are directed apparently acts as a virulence factor, in various ways, in cryptococcosis of experimental animals (8–15). Rabbit anticryptococcal gammaglobulin enhances the protection provided by amphotericin B against experimental cryptococcosis of mice (16), but a number of studies indicate that the defense is predominantly a matter of cellular immunity (17–19).

III. Candidiasis

Candidiasis is the opportunistic mycosis most in need of definitive serology, since it is so difficult to diagnose clinically with conventional cultural methods. The fact that *Candida albicans* is a constituent of the normal human flora renders its routine cultural isolation a matter of questionable significance; at the same time, it sets up a screen of "normal" *Candida* antibodies in a large part of the population. *Candida* serology is employed widely, however, as an aid in diagnosis, with the most common and useful techniques being immunodiffusion and yeast-cell agglutination.

A. Immunodiffusion Techniques

Immunodiffusion, or double-diffusion in agar gel, is a sensitive technique which, when it employs "somatic" antigen, provides a high degree of specificity for deep-seated candidiasis. Taschdjian and colleagues (20, 21) demonstrated antibody to "somatic" antigen (saline extract of disrupted *C. albicans* cells) in 85–90% of patients with systemic candidiasis. They concluded that precipitins are highly specific for systemic candidiasis and that false positives are found only in cases of candidal granuloma and in autoimmune endocrinopathies associated with cutaneous and mucocutaneous candidiasis (22). False negatives were found in some leukemic patients (see Ref. 23), in those in terminal stages of disease, and in those who were totally anergic. Pepys et al. (24), however, found precipitins to protein antigens of *C. albicans* type A in some cases of asthma. They detected a strong correlation between such precipitin reactions and the production of type III skin and inhalation test reactions to *Candida* antigens.

Stickle et al. (25) agreed with Taschdjian in finding ID to be 95% sensitive for detection of systemic candidiasis. They also noted an extremely high specificity, with the only noncandidal reaction being elicited in a case of torulopsemia. However, results of *Candida* ID tests must be accepted with caution, in view of additional reports which indicate a lack of absolute specificity (26, 27) and insufficient sensitivity (27). In our own laboratories, in a limited series of cases, we have found no apparent false positives with the ID test, but we are not certain that we have not missed some cases.

Studies by Taschdjian et al. (21) have indicated that prolonged storage of sera may result in a loss of 75–100% of precipitating antibody, so that older sera might yield a deceptively high proportion of false negative reactions. It has also been reported (20, 27) that *Candida* antibody titers tend to decrease with remission of disease as serum proteins (i.e., elevated gamma-globulin) return to normal.

A refinement of gel double-diffusion, "immunoelectroosmophoresis" (IEOP), is more sensitive than ID as well as more economical, in terms of time and reagents (28). In a rather extensive series of candidiasis cases, Remington, Gaines, and Gilmer (29), using a form of IEOP which they called "counterimmunoelectrophoresis," obtained neither false positive nor false negative reactions. Hellwege, Fischer, and Bläker (30), however, concluded that demonstration of precipitating antibodies by IEOP is not absolute proof of *Candida* infection. They pointed out that false negative results might also be expected in anergic patients with severe candidiasis and in patients with other antibody deficiencies.

B. Yeast-cell Agglutination

Candida agglutinins are so common in the general population (31) that their absence in anyone over 10 years of age is considered to support a diagnosis of immunological deficiency (H. Meuwissen, personal communication, 1972). However, titers above an established level, depending upon the test system, or those showing a four-fold or more increase in a given case generally are accepted as indicative of systemic candidiasis. Although Taschdjian and her colleagues (32) found a rise in agglutinin titers as sensitive as a positive precipitin test in detection of systemic candidiasis in six of their eight patients with acute leukemia, their experience with other patients (21, 33) led them to conclude that, in general, this is not so. Preisler et al. (27) also found the agglutination test of particular value in acute leukemia and recommended serial determinations of agglutinating antibody titers as the most reliable means for diagnosing visceral candidiasis in patients known to have increased susceptibility to fungal infections. However, their results indicate not only a lack of sensitivity, but a number of apparently false positive reactions, chiefly in patients suffering from other systemic mycoses. In another series (23), these investigators determined that a four-fold rise in agglutinin titer was specific for visceral candidiasis (diagnosed postmortem), but that there were many false negative results. The endocarditis study of Murray, Buckley, and Turner (26) suggested that agglutination of *Candida* species, in addition to *C. albicans*, particularly *Candida parapsilosis*, afforded more positive evidence of endocarditis than did agglutination of *C. albicans* alone.

C. Miscellaneous Methods

Other promising serological techniques for aid in diagnosis of candidiasis include the indirect fluorescent-antibody (IFA) and SLA tests. Antibodies reactive in the IFA test were found to be common, up to certain serum levels, in the normal population and in *Candida* carriers; higher titers were considered good indicators of candidiasis (21, 34—36). The SLA test had both diagnostic and prognostic value, but was less specific than ID in a comparative study (25). In one series of investigations (37) interfering factor appeared to be a better indicator of the presence of infection caused by *Candida* than either agglutinins or precipitins.

Lehner, Buckley, and Murray (38), in comparing fluorescent, agglutinating, and precipitating antibodies to *C. albicans* in a limited number of cases, concluded that they could not make a differential diagnosis between endocarditis (i.e., systemic candidiasis) and mucocutaneous candidiasis by any of the three tests. In fact, they found that, contradictory to some of their reports and those of others (39, 40), precipitins were formed in 6 of 10 patients with chronic mucocutaneous candidiasis. Their immunoabsorption studies suggested that all three serological tests estimate antibodies to mannans rather than to proteins, and they felt that the specificity ascribed to precipitins probably is due to their belonging to the IgG class of immunoglobulins, unlike the agglutinins, which are found in IgG, IgM, and IgA. They suggested that IFA is a more reliable test than either precipitation or agglutination and that a rise in IFA anti-IgG titer to a level of 1:64 or greater should be indicative of systemic candidiasis. The studies of Hellwege et al. (30) support this argument: they found that agglutinating antibodies resulting from simple *Candida* colonization belonged mainly to IgM, whereas infections causing a rise in agglutinin titers induced predominantly the synthesis of IgG antibodies.

D. Immune Defenses

Although immunological deficiencies may inhibit production of *Candida* agglutinins, the opportunism of *C. albicans* rests primarily upon a deficiency in or suppression of cellular immune defenses (41–43). Investigations of chronic mucocutaneous candidiasis have revealed a spectrum of such immunodeficiencies (38). Lehrer and Cline (17) found that, although serum factors are necessary for optimal phagocytosis of *C. albicans*, they are not directly candidacidal. Neutrophils were found to play an important part in resistance to candidiasis; myeloperoxidase is an important participant. Thymus-dependent cellular immunity may be stimulated by infusion of competent viable lymphocytes, but since there may be danger to the recipient in case of histoincompatibility, it has been recommended that massive transfer-factor therapy be employed (44). The roles of clumping factor and interfering factor in defense against candidiasis (45) have yet to be defined clearly.

IV. Torulopsosis

Little is known about the diagnostic serology of torulopsosis, a rather uncommon disease (46). Since *Torulopsis glabrata* is part of the normal human flora (47), it may be predicted safely that anti-*Torulopsis* agglutinins will be found in a large proportion of the normal population. It is a simple matter to produce high-titered antiserum (agglutinins) to this species in rabbits in response to injection of killed cells (48). Recently, in a case of apparent *Torulopsis* meningitis in which budding, yeast-like organisms resembling *T. glabrata* were found in cerebrospinal fluid, an agglutinin titer of 1:640 and precipitin titers as high as 1:16 were obtained with the patient's serum (P. J. Kozinn, personal communication, 1971).

Benham (49) reported that *T. glabrata* possesses antigens in common with *C. albicans*. This fact has since been confirmed by several groups of workers (48, 50, 51), and, as noted above (25), in a case of torulopsemia, the patient's serum reacted with antigen of *C. albicans*.

V. Aspergillosis

Although other methods have been proposed, the most widely used and generally accepted serological technique for diagnosis of aspergillosis is immunodiffusion. One of the earliest studies of aspergillosis utilizing the gel double-diffusion procedure was that of Pepys et al. (52), in which the antigen employed was a cell-sap preparation of *Aspergillus fumigatus*. Filtrate antigens are now most commonly used, although we have found that cell-sap preparations give comparable results. A suitable antigen is available commercially from Bencard, Brentford, England, but most workers use a nonstandardized, homemade product, such as our partially purified, acetone-precipitated aspergillin. Others (53, 54) have quantitated their product by carbohydrate content. We favor the ID pattern recommended by Proctor (55), in which the patient's serum is placed in a well opposing two antigen wells, one being approximately one-tenth of the volume of the other; both wells contain undiluted serum, but, in effect, they provide a 10-fold dilution. Proctor's rationale for this procedure is that better resolution is given by a relatively strong antigen in a small well than by a weaker one in a large well.

Both the number and the intensity of precipitin bands are significant for interpretation of the degree or severity of involvement with *A. fumigatus* in a given case (36, 54, 56). Elicitation of three or four bands is practically diagnostic for either invasive aspergillosis or aspergilloma, although some aspergillomas may produce fewer than three bands. Few reactions occur with asthmatic sera; those from patients with allergic bronchial aspergillosis generally produce one or two distinct bands.

There are distinctive combinations of skin-test response and precipitin activity corresponding to the various types of aspergillus involvement (36, 54, 57–59). Very few sera from asthmatics without pulmonary eosinophilia yield precipitin bands, but these patients commonly produce reaginic antibody, resulting in immediate skin-test reactivity. The essential features of allergic bronchial aspergillosis are asthma, expectoration of brown plugs, eosinophilia of peripheral blood and sputum with characteristic lung infiltration, and occurrence of aspergillus mycelium in sputum and bronchial aspirate. Typically, these patients show type I (reaginic) skin activity and, in some cases, type III (Arthus); the sera of 50–60% of such cases evoke strong precipitin bands. Of sera from patients with aspergilloma or invasive aspergillosis, 90% or more give multiple strong precipitin bands, and most display intense, delayed skin reactions, although few have reaginic antibody. Very few, if any, false positive precipitin results have been found in these studies. A recent report (60) cites lack of detectable antibody response to *A. fumigatus* in 15 leukemic patients with "widespread invasive aspergillosis." However, in all of these patients, the serum was obtained within the last three weeks of life; one patient had leukopenia and aplastic anemia, while the rest had malignant disease and were immunosuppressed.

Species other than *A. fumigatus* (primarily *Aspergillus flavus*, *Aspergillus niger*, *Aspergillus terreus*, and *Aspergillus nidulans*) occasionally cause disease, and there is some degree of species specificity. Thus, antigens of *A. fumigatus* frequently will react with sera of patients infected with a heterologous species, but they have been found to miss some of these cases (54, 57, 58). A battery consisting of antigens of *A. fumigatus*, *A. flavus*, and *A. niger* probably would detect all significant *Aspergillus* infections.

Patients' response to chemotherapy is reflected in a reduction and, often, a disappearance of serological reactivity (53, 54). The same reduction follows surgical removal of aspergillomas (36, 57).

There are few reports of the use of techniques other than ID for serological diagnosis of aspergillosis. Walter and Jones (61) compared immunoelectrophoresis with the complement-fixation procedure and advocated use of the latter. Drouhet (36) also employed immunoelectrophoresis and remarked upon its species specificity, but Longbottom and Pepys (57) found it less sensitive than ID. In the same publication, Drouhet recommended a "gradient" method for ID, in which serum is placed in a central trough and antigen is placed in lateral wells at graded distances from the trough. In general, he found the indirect fluorescent-antibody technique useful and more sensitive than immunoelectrophoresis.

VI. Mucormycosis

There is not much information available concerning diagnostic serology of mucormycosis. Utilizing cellular antigens of *Rhizopus*, *Mucor*, and *Absidia*, we have detected antibody, by means of immunodiffusion, in some cases of rhinocerebral mucormycosis but not in others. In this limited series of cases, however, the appearance of precipitins appeared to correlate with the severity of the disease. In one case in which *Rhizopus oryzae* was cultured, the appearance of precipitins to *Mucor* sp. preceded that of antibody to the homologous species.

VII. Immunoelectroosmophoresis

Bussard (62) introduced the technique of "electrosyneresis" by combining electrophoresis with immune precipitation in agar gel. The method depends upon the fact that while most antigens, as well as serum proteins other than gamma-globulin, migrate toward the anode in an electric field, antibodies in general are displaced toward the cathode by the resulting electroosmotic flow. Therefore, if serum specimens to be tested for antibody are placed in anodic wells and test antigens are placed in opposing cathodic wells, their convergent migration results in an immune precipitate. Gocke and Howe (63) termed their analogous technique "counterimmunoelectrophoresis," while we employ the modification called "immunoelectroosmophoresis," developed by Prince and Burke (64) for detection of Australia antigen. The test is very rapid, i.e., final results are readable in 1–4 hr, depending upon the test system, and it appears in general to be significantly more sensitive than immunodiffusion. Gocke and Howe (63) found it to be 10 times more sensitive than ID for detection of Australia antigen in serum. This increased sensitivity has been confirmed by use of several fungal antigen-antibody systems, including histoplasmosis, candidiasis, and aspergillosis (28). In our experience, IEOP is also more sensitive in detecting farmer's lung antibody, thus confirming the findings of Jameson (65).

Optimal results with IEOP depend upon several factors in the test procedure. Any of several types of electrophoresis equipment may be employed. We have abandoned the Beckman Durrum cell (Beckman Instruments, Inc., Fullerton, Calif.), which we formerly used, in favor of a Gelman electrophoresis chamber (Gelman Instrument Co., Ann Arbor, Mich.). With the former apparatus, the slides tended to heat up during the flow of current and therefore required an ice bath; the agar tended to pile up at one end of the slide unless extreme care was taken to level the apparatus; and the buffer precipitated at the anode. We use a discontinuous barbital buffer system, pH 8.6, ionic strength 0.05, applying 1 mA per cm (or 2.5 mA per 1- × 3-inch slide) at about 40 v for 4 hr. Agarose appears to be the better substrate for histoplasma antigen-antibody reactions, while ion agar gives more clear-cut results with cryptococcal materials. However, the method is considerably less sensitive than slide latex agglutination for detection of cryptococcal antigen.

As noted above, others also have employed IEOP successfully for serology of candidiasis. However, additional experience is needed with this and other mycotic systems before the technique can be accepted as a routine diagnostic procedure.

Literature Cited

1. Bennett, J. E., and J. W. Bailey. Control for rheumatoid factor in the latex test for cryptococcosis. Amer. J. Clin. Pathol. 56: 360, 1971.
2. Bennett, J. E., H. F. Hasenclever, and B. S. Tynes. Detection of cryptococcal polysaccharide in serum and spinal fluid: Value in diagnosis and prognosis. Trans. Assoc. Amer. Physicians 77: 145, 1964.
3. Gordon, M. A., and D. K. Vedder. Serologic tests in diagnosis and prognosis of cryptococcosis. JAMA 197: 961, 1966.
4. Gordon, M. A., and E. Lapa. Charcoal particle agglutination test for detection of antibody to *Cryptococcus neoformans:* A preliminary report. Amer. J. Clin. Pathol. 56: 354, 1971.
5. Vogel, R. A. The indirect fluorescent antibody test for the detection of antibody in human cryptococcal disease. J. Infect. Dis. 116: 573, 1966.
6. Salvin, S. B., and R. F. Smith. An antigen for detection of hypersensitivity to *Cryptococcus neoformans.* Proc. Soc. Exp. Biol. Med. 108: 498, 1961.
7. Muchmore, H. G., F. G. Felton, S. B. Salvin, and E. R. Rhoades, Delayed hypersensitivity to cryptococcin in man. Sabouraudia 6: 285, 1968.
8. Drouhet, E., G. Segretain, and J.-P. Aubert. Polyoside capsulaire d'un champignon pathogène *Torulopsis neoformans.* Relation avec la virulence. Ann. Inst. Pasteur 79: 891, 1950.
9. Drouhet, E., and G. Segretain. Inhibition de la migration leucocytaire in vitro par un polyoside capsulaire de *Torulopsis (Cryptococcus) neoformans.* Ann. Inst. Pasteur 81: 674, 1951.
10. Gadebusch, H. H. Active immunization against *Cryptococcus neoformans.* J. Infect. Dis. 102: 219, 1958.
11. Gadebusch, H. H., P. A. Ward, and E. P. Frenkel. Natural host resistance to infection with *Cryptococcus neoformans.* III. The effect of cryptococcal polysaccharide upon the physiology of the reticuloendothelial system of laboratory animals. J. Infect. Dis. 114: 95, 1964.

12. Abrahams, I., and T. G. Gilleran. Studies on actively acquired resistance to experimental cryptococcosis in mice. J. Immunol. 85: 629, 1960.
13. Bulmer, G. S., and M. D. Sans. *Cryptococcus neoformans*. III. Inhibition of phagocytosis. J. Bacteriol. 95: 5, 1968.
14. Bennett, J. E., and H. F. Hasenclever. *Cryptococcus neoformans* polysaccharide: Studies of serologic properties and role in infection. J. Immunol. 94: 916, 1965.
15. Murphy, J. W., and G. C. Cozad. Immunological unresponsiveness induced by cryptococcal capsular polysaccharide assayed by the hemolytic plaque technique. Infect. Immun. 5: 896, 1972.
16. Gordon, M. A., and E. Lapa. Serum protein enhancement of antibiotic therapy in cryptococcosis. J. Infect. Dis. 114: 373, 1964.
17. Lehrer, R. I., and M. J. Cline. Interaction of *Candida albicans* with human leukocytes and serum. J. Bacteriol. 98: 996, 1969.
18. Louria, D. B., T. Kaminski, and G. Finkel. Further studies on immunity in experimental cryptococcosis. J. Exp. Med. 117: 509, 1963.
19. Goren, M. B. Experimental murine cryptococcosis: Effect of hyperimmunization to capsular polysaccharide. J. Immunol. 98: 914, 1967.
20. Taschdjian, C. L., P. J. Kozinn, A. Okas, L. Caroline, and M. A. Halle. Serodiagnosis of systemic candidiasis. J. Infect. Dis. 117: 180, 1967.
21. Taschdjian, C. L., P. J. Kozinn, M. B. Cuesta, and E. F. Toni. Serodiagnosis of candidal infection. Amer. J. Clin. Pathol. 57: 195, 1972.
22. Taschdjian, C. L., P. J. Kozinn, and E. F. Toni. Opportunistic yeast infections, with special reference to candidiasis. Ann. N. Y. Acad. Sci. 174: 606, 1970.
23. Preisler, H. D., H. F. Hasenclever, A. A. Levitan, and E. S. Henderson. Serologic diagnosis of disseminated candidiasis in patients with acute leukemia. Ann. Intern. Med. 70: 19, 1969.
24. Pepys, J., J. A. Faux, J. L. Longbottom, D. S. McCarthy, and F. E. Hargreave. *Candida albicans* precipitins in respiratory disease in man. J. Allergy 41: 305, 1968.
25. Stickle, D., L. Kaufman, S. O. Blumer, and D. W. McLaughlin. Comparison of a newly developed latex agglutination test and an immunodiffusion test in the diagnosis of systemic candidiasis. Appl. Microbiol. 23: 490, 1972.
26. Murray, I. G., H. R. Buckley, and G. C. Turner. Serological evidence of *Candida* infection after open-heart surgery. J. Med. Microbiol. 2: 463, 1969.
27. Preisler, H. D., H. F. Hasenclever, and E. S. Henderson. Anti-*Candida* antibodies in patients with acute leukemia. Amer. J. Med. 51: 352, 1971.
28. Gordon, M. A., R. E. Almy, C. H. Greene, and J. W. Fenton, II. Diagnostic mycoserology by immunoelectroosmophoresis: A general, rapid, and sensitive microtechnic. Amer. J. Clin. Pathol. 56: 471, 1971.

29. Remington, J. S., J. D. Gaines, and M. A. Gilmer. Demonstration of *Candida* precipitins in human sera by counterimmunoelectrophoresis. Lancet i: 413, 1972.
30. Hellwege, H. H., K. Fischer, and F. Bläker. Diagnostic value of *Candida* precipitins. Lancet ii: 386, 1972.
31. Winner, H. J. A study of *Candida albicans* agglutinins in human sera. J. Hyg. 53: 509, 1955.
32. Rosner, F., F. D. Gabriel, C. L. Taschdjian, M. B. Cuesta, and P. J. Kozinn. Serologic diagnosis of systemic candidiasis in patients with acute leukemia. Amer. J. Med. 51: 54, 1971.
33. Kozinn, P. J., C. L. Taschdjian, M. S. Seelig, L. Caroline, and A. Teitler. Diagnosis and therapy of systemic candidiasis. Sabouraudia 7: 98, 1969.
34. Lehner, T. Immunofluorescence study of *Candida albicans* in candidiasis carriers and controls. J. Pathol. Bacteriol. 91: 97, 1966.
35. Esterly, N. B. Serum antibody titers to *Candida albicans* utilizing an immunofluorescent technic. Amer. J. Clin. Pathol. 50: 291, 1968.
36. Drouhet, E. Aspects actuels des mycoses profondes. Nouvelles acquisitions dans le diagnostic mycologique et immunologique des infections mycosiques. Arch. Roum. Pathol. Exp. Microbiol. 30: 65, 1971.
37. Louria, D. B., J. K. Smith, R. G. Brayton, and M. Buse. Anti-*Candida* factors in serum and their inhibitors. I. Clinical and laboratory observations. J. Infect. Dis. 125: 102, 1972.
38. Lehner, T., H. R. Buckley, and I. G. Murray. The relationship between fluorescent, agglutinating, and precipitating antibodies to *Candida albicans* and their immunoglobulin classes. J. Clin. Pathol. 25: 344, 1972.
39. Stallybrass, F. C. *Candida* precipitins. J. Pathol. Bacteriol. 87: 89, 1964.
40. Taschdjian, C. L., P. J. Kozinn, and L. Caroline. Immune studies in candidiasis. III. Precipitating antibodies in systemic candidiasis. Sabouraudia 3: 312, 1964.
41. Chilgren, R. A., P. G. Quie, H. J. Meuwissen, and R. Hong. Chronic mucocutaneous candidiasis, deficiency of delayed hypersensitivity and selective local antibody defect. Lancet ii: 688, 1967.
42. Chilgren, R. A., P. G. Quie, H. J. Meuwissen, R. A. Good, and R. Hong. The cellular immune defect in chronic mucocutaneous candidiasis. Lancet i: 1286, 1969.
43. Hermans, P. E., J. A. Ulrich, and H. Markowitz. Chronic mucocutaneous candidiasis as a surface expression of deep-seated abnormalities. Amer. J. Med. 47: 503, 1969.
44. Pabst, H. F., and R. Swanson. Immunotherapy in candidiasis. Lancet i: 1022, 1972.
45. Smith, J. K., and D. B. Louria. Anti-*Candida* factors in serum and their inhibitors. II. Identification of a *Candida*-clumping factor and the influ-

ence of the immune response on the morphology of *Candida* and on anti-*Candida* activity of serum in rabbits. J. Infect. Dis. 125: 115, 1972.
46. Grimley, P. M., L. D. Wright, Jr., and A. E. Jennings. *Torulopsis glabrata* infection in man. Amer. J. Clin. Pathol. 43: 216, 1965.
47. Rosebury, T. Microorganisms Indigenous to Man. McGraw-Hill Book Co., New York, 1962. p. 227.
48. Gordon, M. A., J. C. Elliott, and T. W. Hawkins. Identification of *Candida albicans*, other *Candida* species and *Torulopsis glabrata* by means of immunofluorescence. Sabouraudia 5: 323, 1967.
49. Benham, R. W. Cryptococci—their identification by morphology and by serology. J. Infect. Dis. 57: 255, 1935.
50. Hasenclever, H. F., and W. O. Mitchell. Antigenic relationships of *Torulopsis glabrata* and seven species of the genus *Candida*. J. Bacteriol. 79: 677, 1960.
51. Tsuchiya, T., Y. Fukazawa, and S. Kawakita. Serological classification of the genus *Torulopsis*. Sabouraudia 1: 145, 1961.
52. Pepys, J., R. W. Riddell, K. M. Citron, Y. M. Clayton, and E. I. Short. Clinical and immunological significance of *Aspergillus fumigatus* in the sputum. Amer. Rev. Resp. Dis. 80: 167, 1959.
53. Abrahams, I., K. M. Payette, H. R. Stoffer, and F. R. Singh. Immunologic studies in human aspergillosis. Bacteriol. Proc. (Abstr.), 1970, p. 122.
54. Coleman, R. M., and L. Kaufman. Use of immunodiffusion test in the serodiagnosis of aspergillosis. Appl. Microbiol. 23: 301, 1972.
55. Proctor, A. G. Serologic methods in mycology. In C. H. Collins (ed.), Progress in Microbiological Techniques, p. 213. Plenum Press, New York, 1967.
56. English, M. P., and A. H. Henderson. Significance and interpretation of laboratory tests in pulmonary aspergillosis. J. Clin. Pathol. 20: 832, 1967.
57. Longbottom, J. L., and J. Pepys. Pulmonary aspergillosis: Diagnostic and immunological significance of antigens and C-substance in *Aspergillus fumigatus*. J. Pathol. Bacteriol. 88: 141, 1964.
58. Campbell, M. J., and Y. M. Clayton. Bronchopulmonary aspergillosis. A correlation of the clinical and laboratory findings in 272 patients investigated for bronchopulmonary aspergillosis. Amer. Rev. Resp. Dis. 89: 186, 1964.
59. Chan-Yeung, M., W. H. Chase, W. Trapp, and S. Grzybowski. Allergic bronchopulmonary aspergillosis. Clinical and pathologic study of three cases. Chest 59: 33, 1971.
60. Young, R. C., and J. E. Bennett. Invasive aspergillosis. Absence of detectable antibody response. Amer. Rev. Resp. Dis. 104: 710, 1971.

61. Walter, J. E., and R. D. Jones. Serodiagnosis of clinical cryptococcosis. Amer. Rev. Resp. Dis. 97: 275, 1968.
62. Bussard, A. Description d'une technique combinant simultanément l'électrophorèse et la précipitation immunologique dans un gel: L'électrosynérèse. Biochim. Biophys. Acta 34: 258, 1959.
63. Gocke, D. J., and C. Howe. Rapid detection of Australia antigen by counterimmunoelectrophoresis. J. Immunol. 104: 1031, 1970.
64. Prince, A. M., and K. Burke. Serum hepatitis antigen (SH): Rapid detection by high voltage immunoelectroosmophoresis. Science 169: 593, 1970.
65. Jameson, J. E. Rapid and sensitive precipitin test for the diagnosis of farmer's lung using immunoosmophoresis. J. Clin. Pathol. 21: 376, 1968.

11

Opportunistic Phycomycetes and Aspergilli in the Compromised Host

Roger Denio Baker

The presence of phycomycetes and aspergilli in the compromised host is a subject of special significance in an increasing number of cases (1). It is fitting that these two fungal types are considered together because they are the two principal fungi which become opportunistic pathogens in a compromised host, that is, a person with leukemia or cutaneous burns or one who is undergoing systemic corticosteroid therapy.

Mucormycosis in the compromised host is caused by the genera *Rhizopus*, *Mucor*, and *Absidia* of the family Mucoraceae of the phycomycetes. The term "mucormycosis" is used to designate opportunistic phycomycosis. The tropical phycomycoses are caused by other members of the phycomycetes.

I. Mucormycosis

A. Definition

Mucormycosis (opportunistic phycomycosis) is a serious, acute, infarct-producing fungal infection which develops in human hosts compromised by acidotic diabetes, leukemia, systemic corticosteroid therapy, and other predisposing conditions. Mucormycosis takes cranial, pulmonary, disseminated, gastrointestinal, and cutaneous forms.

1. *Cranial mucormycosis.* The cranial form of mucormycosis characteristically occurs in a diabetic patient in acidosis. *Rhizopus*, the usual cause of mucormycosis, enters the nose and a paranasal sinus and then grows into arteries, causing thrombosis and infarcts.

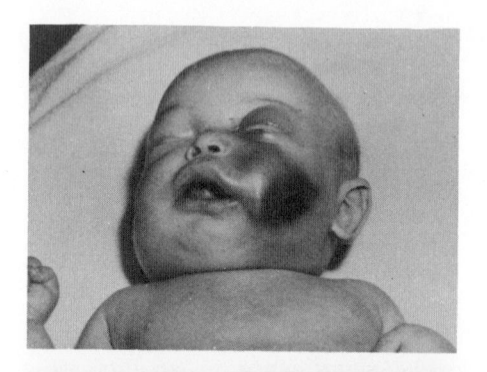

Figure 1. Infarction (gangrene) of left orbit and cheek. Case of Martin et al. (1954). Photograph reproduced by courtesy of Dr. J. M. Lukeman.

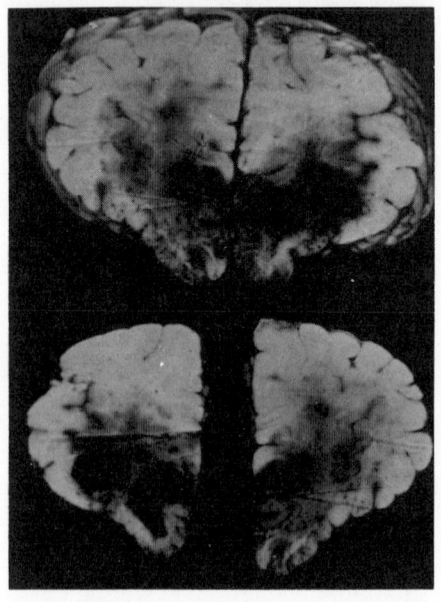

Figure 2. Cerebral mucormycosis. Bilateral hemorrhagic infarction. Reproduced by courtesy of Tinaztepe and Tinaztepe (1966).

Phycomycetes and Aspergilli

Figure 1 shows the proptosis and infarcted cheek of cranial mucormycosis. The fungus passes from the orbit or ethmoid air sinuses to the frontal lobes of the brain and causes them to become infarcted. Figure 2 shows mucormycotic hemorrhagic infarction of the frontal lobes of the brain. The fungus may cause thrombosis of an internal carotid artery, perforation of the palate, thickening of the mucous membrane of the antrum, nerve palsies of the muscles of the eye and face, and blindness of the eye on the affected side. Figure 3 shows a broad nonseptate hypha and the right-angled branching in the meninges. Death may occur in two to five days. Approximately two-thirds of the patients that develop cranial mucormycosis will die.

2. *Pulmonary and disseminated mucormycosis.* The pulmonary and disseminated forms of mucormycosis often develop in neutropenic leukemic patients who have received corticosteroid drugs. Infarction of the lung supervenes because of thrombosis of a pulmonary artery attributable to *Rhizopus*, which has come from the bronchi through the tissues. The pulmonary form of mucor-

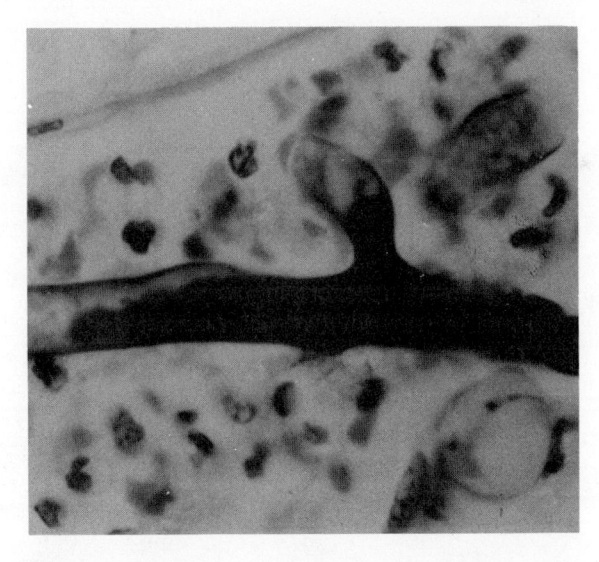

Figure 3. Hypha in meningeal mucormycosis with right-angled branching. (H & E, × 800) From Baker (2).

mycosis has had a 10% survival rate. The disseminated disease has been uniformly fatal.

3. *Gastrointestinal mucormycosis.* Gastrointestinal mucormycosis develops after the fungus enters the blood vessels locally, causing thromboses and then segmental infarcts, that is, segments of gangrene. Figure 4 shows an area of mucormycotic gangrene of the stomach.

4. *Opportunism in mucormycosis.* *Rhizopus*, an ubiquitous mold, takes on pathogenic powers and infects the compromised host, but is almost completely incapable of infecting the normal, healthy host. This has been demonstrated repeatedly in experimental animals that have been compromised by acute alloxan diabetes or by the administration of corticosteroids or nitrogen mustard, the latter to deplete the bone marrow. Under these conditions, *Rhizopus* has acted like a virulent pathogen and has spread in the animal body, producing serious lesions and sometimes death.

Mucormycosis is the very best example of fungal opportunism in the compromised host. The Mucoraceae *Rhizopus*, *Mucor*, and *Absidia* invade humans whose tissues have been altered in some not yet understood manner by diabetes, acidosis, leukemia,

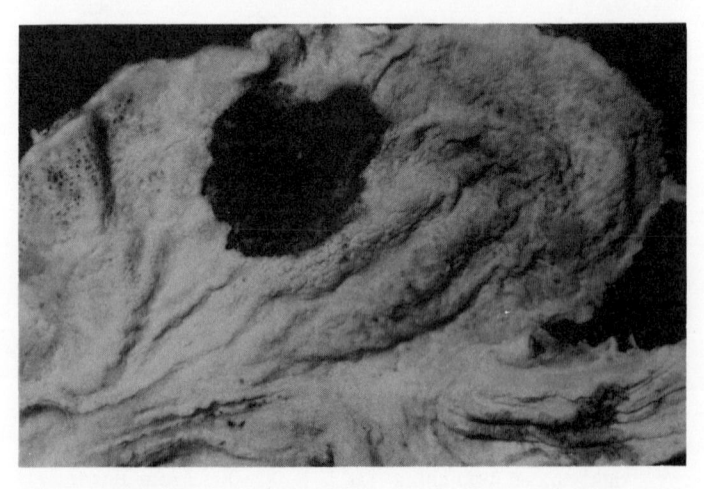

Figure 4. Gastric mucormycosis in leukemia. From Baker (2).

lymphoma, Hodgkin's disease, neutropenia, corticosteroid therapy, malnutrition, or cutaneous burns.

Normal human serum and, presumably, all normal human tissues contain an anti-*Rhizopus* factor which protects humans from infection with *Rhizopus*. This factor is diminished in some of the conditions which predispose to mucormycosis.

5. *Prognosis*. The overall prognosis in human mucormycosis is poor. However, Figure 5 shows a cutaneous mucormycotic ulcer in a diabetic patient which healed with the regulation of the diabetes. The patient has remained well except for the diabetes.

B. Diagnosis

The clinical diagnosis of the cranial form of mucormycosis is made readily by the clinician who knows about mucormycosis and who recognizes the orbital and facial features. The clinical diagnosis of the other forms of mucormycosis is difficult.

Biopsy is the best means of diagnosing mucormycosis. In hematoxylin and eosin sections, broad, nonseptate hyphae with right-angled branching are diagnostic. The Gomori methenamine silver nitrate stain shows the hyphae even better than does the hematoxylin and eosin stain.

Direct examination of wet preparations of infected tissue may give the diagnosis.

While biopsy and direct examination of wet mounts permit the diagnosis of mucormycosis, cultures are necessary to identify the

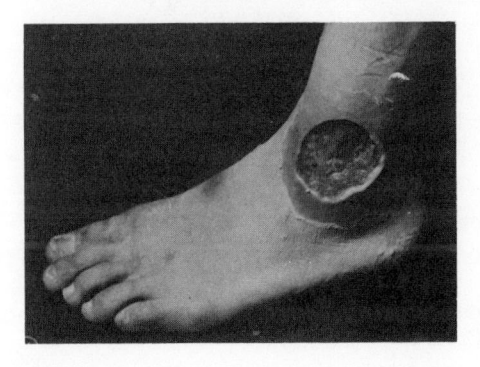

Figure 5. Cutaneous mucormycosis. Reproduced by courtesy of Josefiak et al. (1958).

genus and species. The isolation medium for *Rhizopus*, *Mucor*, and *Absidia* is Sabouraud's dextrose agar, supplemented with antibacterial antibiotics. The organism grows rapidly at room temperature, filling a Petri dish in two days. At first gray, it turns brown in four days. The pepper-grain-like sporangia can be seen with the naked eye (Fig. 6). Teased preparations may permit a differentiation between the genera mentioned, but culture mounts are really necessary. *Rhizopus* has rhizoids which are extensions of the sporangiophores (3). *Absidia* has rhizoids which come from the stolons between the points of attachment of the sporangiophores. *Mucor* possesses no rhizoids. The sporangiospores of *Rhizopus* are brownish and are much like human red blood cells in size and in character.

Positive cultures from the 255 cases of mucormycosis in the world literature up to the summer of 1968 grew *Rhizopus* 32 times, *Absidia* twice, and *Mucor* 10 times.

Rhizopus oryzae has been reported most often, followed by (in descending order of frequency): *Rhizopus arrhizus, Rhizopus nig-*

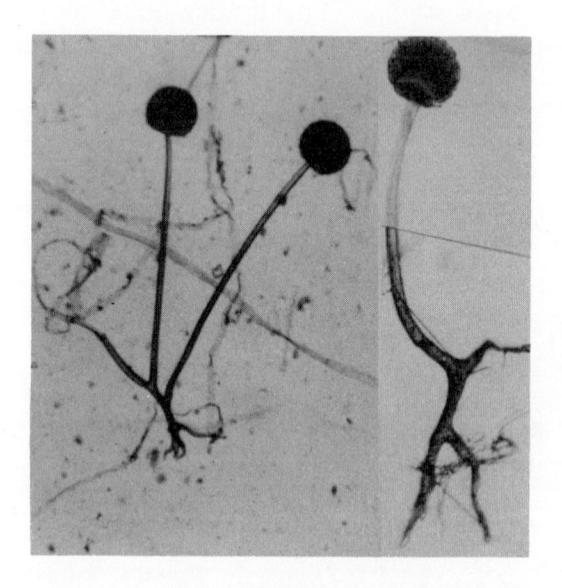

Figure 6. *Rhizopus oryzae* in a wet preparation, unstained. From Baker (1957).

ricans, *Rhizopus microsporus*, and *Rhizopus rhizopodiformis*. Speciation is based on the length and branching of the sporangiophores and the size of the sporangiospores. For example, *R. rhizopodiformis* has short sporangiophores (4). *Mucor corymbifera*, *Mucor hiemalis*, and *Mucor ramosissimus* have been cultured from cases of mucormycosis.

Absidia lichtheimi and *Absidia ramosa* have been cultured from cases of mucormycosis.

To my knowledge, serological tests have not been developed in the diagnosis of mucormycosis.

1. *Treatment.* Mucormycosis is treated by 1) improving the underlying condition; for example, by regulating diabetes in the patient, or by transfusing the leukemic patient; 2) giving amphotericin B; and 3) surgically removing infarcted tissues.

2. *Prevention.* Compromised patients might be treated in germ-free rooms. Corticosteroid drugs might be used systemically less frequently.

II. Aspergillosis

A. Definition

The excellent definition of aspergillosis given by Peña (5) cannot be improved on:

> Aspergillosis can be broadly defined as any infection or colonization of tissues or cavities by fungi of the genus *Aspergillus*. This includes proliferation in normal or dilated bronchi or caverns, a necrotizing or granulomatous pneumonitis sometimes with hematogenous dissemination, endocarditis, sinusitis, infections of the tegument, and certain cases of mycetoma pedis. In addition, the spores of the fungus may act in man as an allergen, that when inhaled, produces a hypersensitivity reaction similar to bronchial asthma.

1. *Pulmonary aspergillosis.* The lungs are the organs most frequently affected by *Aspergillus*. The pneumonia may be acute or chronic, primary or secondary. Hemoptysis may occur. However, symptoms may be absent, and the pulmonary aspergillosis may be diagnosed first after postmortem examination of the deceased

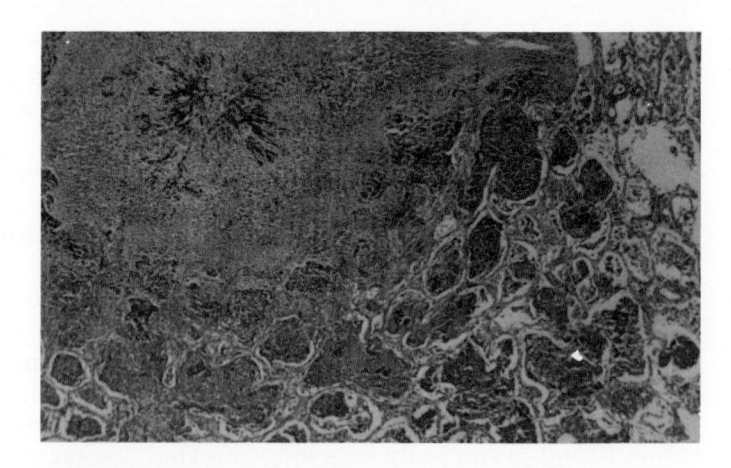

Figure 7. Pulmonary aspergillosis. (PAS, × 100) From Peña (5). Reproduced by courtesy of Dr. R. Hellstrom.

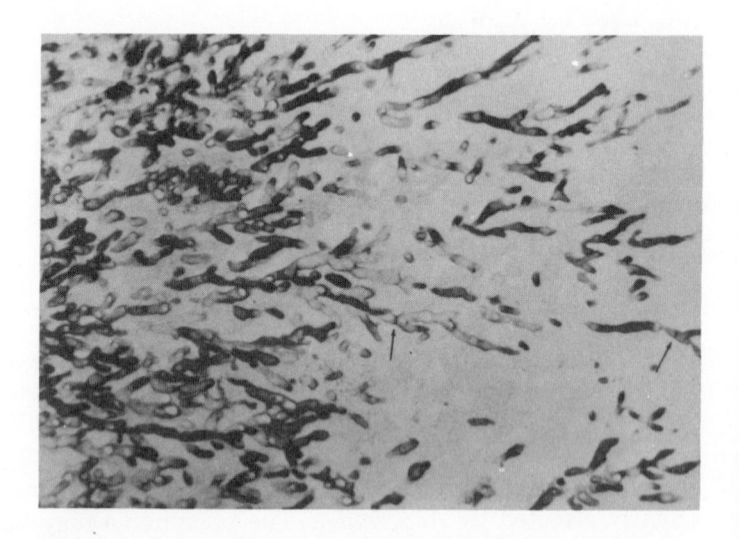

Figure 8. *Aspergillus* in tissue. The hyphae are septate (arrows) and exhibit dichotomous branching. (Gomori methenamine silver nitrate stain, × 450) From Pena (5).

patient. Figure 7 shows a colony of *Aspergillus* in the lung with surrounding pneumonia. Figure 8 shows radiating septate hyphae with the characteristic acutely angled branching. *Aspergillus fumigatus* is the species most frequently cultured.

2. *Disseminated aspergillosis.* The process may disseminate from the lungs to many organs and tissues. The frequency of extrapulmonary organ involvement in disseminated aspergillosis is, in descending order: heart, brain, kidney, liver, thyroid, spleen, intestine, and then almost any organ or tissue in the body. Figure

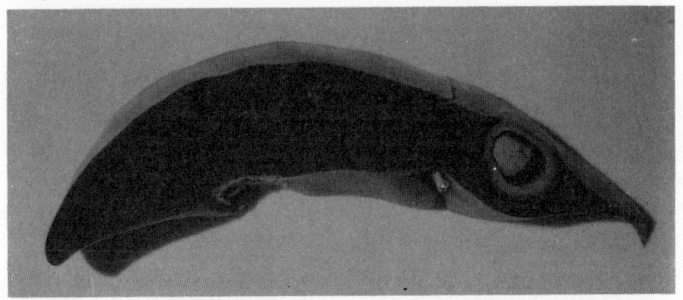

Figure 9. *Aspergillus* abscess of the liver. From Baker, R. D. Amer. J. Clin. Pathol. 37: 358, 1962.

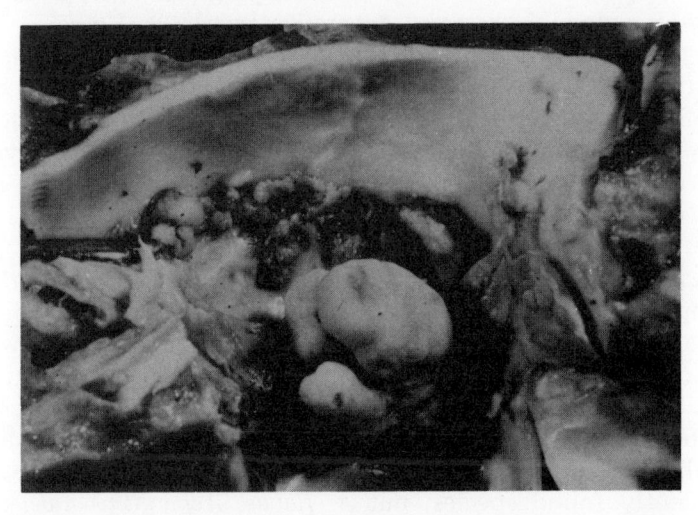

Figure 10. *Aspergillus* endocarditis. From Peña (5) (Presbyterian University Hospital, Pittsburgh, Pennsylvania).

9 shows an abscess of the liver in disseminated aspergillosis in a leukemic patient. *Aspergillus* endocarditis may develop, as shown on the aortic valve in Figure 10.

The preexisting conditions in a series of 81 cases of disseminated aspergillosis reported by Peña were as follows: leukemia, 25 cases; lymphoma, 5 cases; immunosuppressive therapy, anemia, neutropenia, or pancytopenia, 6 cases; open-heart surgery, 4 cases; and viral hepatitis, malignant tumors, tuberculosis, and prematurity with cytomegalic inclusion disease, 2 cases each. In 10 cases, there were a variety of preexisting conditions and in 11, no apparent preexisting condition existed. In 12% of the cases, therefore, *Aspergillus* appeared to be a primary pathogen rather than an opportunistic pathogen. The absence of diabetes from the list of predisposing conditions is noteworthy, in contrast to what is found in mucormycosis.

The disseminated lesions may be caseous foci, abscesses or, rarely, granulomas with giant cells. Organisms are present as in the lungs.

The species of *Aspergillus* identified in 34 cases of disseminated aspergillosis were *A. fumigatus*, 29 cases; *Aspergillus flavus*, 2 cases; *Aspergillus nidulans*, 2 cases; *Aspergillus niger*, 1 case; *Aspergillus sydowi*, 1 case; and *Aspergillus restrictus*, 1 case.

3. *Pulmonary aspergilloma (fungus ball).* Pulmonary aspergilloma is a curious condition. A fungus ball is discovered by X-ray, usually in an upper lobe. The aspergilloma apparently develops in a preexisting, fibrotic, tuberculous cavity, bronchiectatic cyst, or cyst of uncertain origin. Hemoptysis is the most frequent symptom in pulmonary aspergilloma. *A. fumigatus* is the fungus most frequently found in pulmonary aspergilloma.

It is questionable whether we should consider the *Aspergillus* as an opportunistic pathogen in these instances of fungus ball. It is more like a saprophytic growth in a cavity in a person who is immunologically sound.

4. *Aspergillosis of the eye.* *Aspergillus* may produce ulceration of the cornea of the eye and may even invade the eyeball, but usually, there is preceding trauma. *A. fumigatus* is the most frequently found species, but *A. flavus*, *Aspergillus niveus*, and *Aspergillus versicolor* also have been found.

5. *Aspergillosis of the paranasal sinuses.* Aspergillosis of the

nose and paranasal sinuses affects women more frequently than men in a ratio of 5 to 1. The reason for this difference in frequency is not yet understood. The antrum is most often involved. Very rarely does the process extend to the brain. The orbitofacial-cerebral complex of mucormycosis apparently does not occur, and the process is suppurative or granulomatous rather than ischemic in nature. Apparently, the *Aspergillus* is a primary pathogen in these cases.

6. *Otomycosis. Aspergillus* thrives in cerumen and cellular debris that accumulates in the external ear; this is spoken of as "otomycosis." This is often a saprophytic growth in a moist, undisturbed environment; but sometimes, an eczematoid inflammation develops.

B. Diagnosis

For the laboratory diagnosis of aspergillosis, place pus or sputum, with or without potassium hydroxide, on slides, flatten under cover slips, and look for hyphal fragments (6). In cavitary

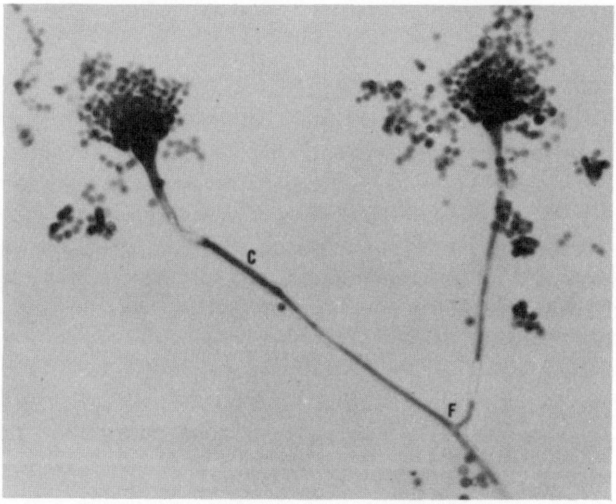

Figure 11. *Aspergillus fumigatus.* Slide culture. (Lactophenol cotton blue stain, × 450)

aspergillosis, hyphal fragments are usually numerous. There may be conidiophores in the sputum. The conidiophores of *A. fumigatus* are distinctive, so that the fungus can be identified with as much certainty as from a culture.

For culturing *Aspergillus*, spread pus or blood-tinged sputum over the surface of Sabouraud's dextrose agar supplemented with antibacterial antibiotics. Incubate at room temperature up to 45°C. Temperatures of 37°C and above are favorable for *A. fumigatus* and will inhibit growth of many fungal contaminants. Conidiophores are often present in cultures after 48 hr of incubation. Young cultures are preferable for identification. Figure 11 shows the conidiophores and fruiting heads of *Aspergillus*.

III. Mechanisms of Opportunism

In comparison, mucoraceous infections are more frequently opportunistic than are the aspergillic infections. Also, diabetic acidosis is more important in predisposing to mucormycosis than to aspergillosis.

A. Neutropenia

Leukemia, treatment with corticosteroid drugs, and cutaneous burns are predisposing conditions to both infections. I believe that the neutropenia of leukemia and the antiinflammatory effect of the corticosteroids are the factors which favor both mycoses. The corticosteroid drugs decrease the intensity of the inflammatory reaction, the number of the polys locally, and the quantity of the hydrolyzing enzymes released from lysosomes of the polys. Failure of phagocytosis cannot be a factor because the large fungus organisms are not phagocytized by polys. Very rarely are hyphae of *Rhizopus* found in giant cells.

B. Immunoglobulin Deficiency

In some of the leukemias, deficiencies in immunoglobulins have been demonstrated. These deficiencies may favor infection with the two molds under consideration. However, in the majority of cases of mucormycosis and aspergillosis, the essential predisposing mechanisms have not yet been demonstrated.

Acknowledgment

The eleven illustrations are reproduced from Baker's *Human Infection with Fungi, Actinomycetes, and Algae*, Springer-Verlag, Inc., New York, Heidelberg, Berlin, 1971, with the publisher's permission and through his courtesy.

Literature Cited

1. Remington, J. S. The compromised host. Hospital Practice 7: 59, 1972.
2. Baker, R. D. Mucormycosis (opportunistic phycomycosis). *In* R. D. Baker (ed.), Human Infection with Fungi, Actinomycetes, and Algae, p. 832. Springer-Verlag, New York, Heidelberg, Berlin, 1971.
3. Baker, R. D. The phycomycoses. Ann. N. Y. Acad. Sci. 74: 592, 1970.
4. Baker, R. D., J. H. Seabury, and J. D. Schneidau, Jr. Subcutaneous and cutaneous mucormycosis and subcutaneous phycomycosis. Lab. Invest. 11: 1091, 1962.
5. Peña, C. E. Aspergillosis. *In* R. D. Baker (ed.), Human Infection with Fungi, Actinomycetes, and Algae, p. 762. Springer-Verlag, New York, Heidelberg, Berlin, 1971.
6. Emmons, C. W., C. H. Binford, and J. P. Utz. Medical Mycology. 2nd Ed. Lea & Febiger, Philadelphia, 1970.

12

Nocardia Species as Opportunists and Current Methods for Their Identification

Lucille K. Georg

I. *Nocardia* Species as Opportunists

Nocardia asteroides, *Nocardia brasiliensis*, and *Nocardia caviae*, three well-characterized species of the genus *Nocardia*, are primary pathogens. All of these organisms may produce severe, even fatal, disease in apparently normal hosts. In a review of reports of nocardiosis from the U. S. Armed Forces Institute of Pathology, Cross and Binford (1) stated that *N. asteroides* appeared to be solely responsible for the illness or death of the patients in over half of 44 recorded cases. Similarly, Goodman and Koenig (2), in a study of 15 patients with *N. asteroides* infections, determined that nine had no apparent underlying disease. However, as will be discussed below, *N. asteroides* frequently also produces disease as an opportunist.

On the other hand, Gonzalez-Ochoa (3), who has observed hundreds of persons with *N. brasiliensis* infections in Mexico, states that *N. brasiliensis* should be considered only as a primary pathogen, since mycetoma, the most common form of infection caused by this organism, develops in active laborers who are particularly exposed. He also reports that the disease practically always is observed in persons who do not show any evidence of concurrent chronic disease. Berd (4) has recently reviewed 26 case histories of *N. brasiliensis* infections that have occurred in the United States. The most common form encountered was an abscess involving the skin and subcutaneous tissues. If left untreated, such infections might develop into mycetomas. Disseminated infections caused by *N. brasiliensis* are rare, and usually result from metasases from cutaneous and subcutaneous lesions. At present, there appears to be little evidence that nocardiosis caused by *N. brasiliensis* is an opportunistic disease, except for the localized tissue trauma that occurs when the organism is inoculated accidentally into the epidermal tissues.

Only five human cases of *N. caviae* infections have been recorded, and all five of these were mycetomas (5). However, a few systemic infections have been seen in animals (6–8). With only these few cases described, it is not possible to form any opinion as to whether *N. caviae* may be considered an opportunist. Since pathogenicity studies (9, 10) have shown that the virulence of *N. caviae* in mice is equal to that of *N. asteroides*, it may well be considered a primary pathogen.

However, considerable evidence has accumulated which indicates that *N. asteroides* frequently produces clinical disease as an opportunist. *N. asteroides* is seen quite commonly as a secondary invader in patients with chronic, debilitating, primary diseases, particularly pulmonary diseases such as tuberculosis, pulmonary alveolar proteinosis, silicosis, and bronchiectasis (2, 11–14). Tissue damage from such chronic illnesses, preexisting pulmonary cavities, the prolonged use of corticosteroids, or hyperadrenal corticoidism (Cushing's syndrome) apparently play a role in allowing invasion by this organism. The specific primary disease entities with which *N. asteroides* is most commonly associated are listed as follows, in order of their importance on the basis of the number of reports found in the literature: 1) leukemia and lymphoma; 2) pulmonary alveolar proteinosis; 3) tuberculosis; 4) Hodgkin's disease; 5) emphysema and bronchiectasis; 6) Cushing's syndrome; 7) dysproteinemias; 8) solid neoplasms; and 9) nephrotic syndrome, including renal transplant recipients.

Nocardiosis caused by *N. asteroides* also plays an important role in complicating neoplastic diseases such as Hodgkin's disease and various types of leukemias and lymphomas, as well as sarcomas and carcinomas. Young et al. (15) recently reviewed 13 cases of *N. asteroides* infections complicating neoplastic disease. In all of these, the patients had been receiving radiation or chemotherapy including cytotoxic drugs. Clinical manifestations included bronchopneumonia, lobar pneumonia, and necrotizing pneumonia with abscesses in other parts of the body, particularly the brain.

However, in a second group of persons suspected of having neoplastic disease, Young et al. (15) described seven cases in which the isolation of *N. asteroides* was "of uncertain significance." In this group of seven, cultures were taken from sputum to evaluate fever or symptoms of the upper respiratory tract. Two patients did have neoplastic disease, one had glomerulonephritis, and a fourth had chronic pancreatitis. The remaining three patients eventually were shown to be free of any underlying disease. None in this group was being treated with corticosteroids. Although *N. asteroides* was isolated from all the patients in this group (in some cases, multiple cultures were obtained while symptoms continued), there was no conclusive laboratory evidence of infection, and the symptoms disappeared without treatment.

All three of the *Nocardia* species, *N. asteroides*, *N. brasiliensis*, and *N. caviae*, have been found to exist as saprophytes in nature. Numerous soil isolations have been recorded from various parts of the world (9, 16). *N. asteroides* also has been isolated from normal skin (17). There is little question that many nocardial infections result from the contamination of wounds by soil particles containing mycelial elements of the etiological agents (3, 18). Cattle frequently develop mastitis when soil-contaminated canulas are used in the treatment of mammary infections (19).

Actinomycetes that exist in the environment, of course, enter the mouth and respiratory passages as airborne particles. The common involvement of the upper respiratory tract and the pulmonary areas with *N. asteroides* infections suggests that systemic nocardiosis usually is caused by inhalation of the organism.

The frequency with which *N. asteroides* is isolated from bronchial washings and sputum specimens, however, often in the absence of demonstrable pulmonary lesions, as shown either by X-Ray or tissue biopsy, makes the diagnosis of pulmonary nocardiosis very difficult. It has led some to speculate either that *N.*

asteroides may exist as a commensal in the mouth and respiratory passages (20) or that it may cause mild infections that do not produce objective pulmonary evidence (15).

The fact that the most frequent isolations of *N. asteroides* from clinical materials are from sputum specimens submitted for "acid-fast studies" suggests the organism's frequent association with pulmonary tuberculosis or clinically similar diseases. Another explanation for this frequency of isolation is the similarity in clinical presentation of tuberculosis and nocardiosis. On the other hand, the apparent association of the two diseases may, in some cases, reflect mistakes in diagnosis.

Table 1 is a summary of data covering an 8.5-year period from the Alabama State Department of Health, 1957–1960 (20), and from the South Carolina State Board of Health, 1967–1972, on the prevalence of *N. asteroides* in sputum specimens submitted for acid-fast studies.

In the Alabama study, sputum specimens taken from 134 patients were treated with 4% NaOH and mechanically shaken; 175 isolations of *N. asteroides* were made from the specimens. From 122 individuals, single isolations were made, and from 12 various numbers of isolations were made, up to 21 from one individual.

In the South Carolina study, where N-acetylcysteine concentration procedures were used, 174 isolations of *N. asteroides* were made from sputum specimens from 140 patients over a five-year period. From 111 individuals, single isolations were obtained, and from 29, multiple isolations were made, up to 10 from one person.*

In both series, the percentage of *N. asteroides* isolations, about 0.23% was remarkably constant. A number of the isolations were made from patients with histories of tuberculosis. In three instances, *N. asteroides* was isolated concurrently with *Mycobacterium tuberculosis*. In more than 10 instances, *N. asteroides* was isolated together with "atypical mycobacteria."

In spite of what appears to be a large number of isolations of *N. asteroides*, the incidence, only about 0.2%, precludes the possibil-

---

* Data from the South Carolina Board of Health have been furnished kindly by Dr. Arthur DiSalvo, Chief, and Miss Gene N. Lindler, Supervisor, Mycobacteriology Section, Bureau of Laboratories.

Table 1. Prevalence of *N. asteroides* in sputa submitted for acid-fast studies

Source of study	Total no. of specimens	*N. asteroides* isolations	*N. asteroides* + atypical mycobacteria	*N. asteroides* + *M. tuberculosis*	*N. asteroides* from patients with tuberculosis history	*M. tuberculosis* isolated (*N. asteroides* not isolated)
Alabama State Dept. of Health July, 1957–Aug., 1960 (2.5 years)	85,435	175 (0.2%)	Frequently both isolated*	2	15†	10,197 (12%)
South Carolina State Bd. of Health July, 1967–June, 1972 (5 years)	56,998	174 (0.31%)	10	1	29	3,032 (5.3%)
Total	142,433	349 (0.24%)		3	44	13,229 (8.6%)

* Number of acid-fast chromogens isolated with *N. asteroides* was not recorded. However, it was stated that "they were frequently concurrently present" (20).

† Fifty-two of the patients from whom *N. asteroides* was isolated either were suspected of having tuberculosis or were under treatment for that disease. In two, *M. tuberculosis* was isolated along with *N. asteroides*. In 37 patients, tuberculosis was ruled out. In 13, data were insufficient.

ity that the microorganism is a "normal inhabitant" of the human mouth or respiratory tract, as is the case with *Candida albicans*. Unfortunately, adequate cultural studies of the normal mouth and pharynx, that is, in individuals who do not have clinical evidence of pulmonary disease and are not producing sputum, have not been made.

Saltzman et al. (12) have emphasized the need for considering such isolations as important, and have demonstrated the astonishing effectiveness of specific therapy. In the review by Young et al. (15) of nocardial infections that complicate neoplastic disease, the authors stress the need for multiple cultural studies when a superimposed infection is suspected in patients with neoplastic disease. In their experience with several patients who were being maintained on anticancer therapy, Young et al. (15) noted excellent responses to sulfonamides; the superimposed pulmonary disease was resolved, although the underlying disease usually was fatal.

Adequate isolation techniques and identification of the isolates by a battery of morphological, physiological, and biochemical tests are very important in choosing the proper therapy for such patients.

Berd (21) has recently evaluated current methods and has devised flow charts to facilitate the laboratory identification of the *Nocardia* species. Section III of this chapter contains formulas of the media used and step-by-step procedures of techniques.

II. Current Methods for the Isolation and Identification of *Nocardia* Species from Clinical Materials

The following methods, based on experience as well as on recent evaluations of new methods, are used currently by the Mycology Branch of the Center for Disease Control in Atlanta, Ga. Exact formulations of media and procedural steps are included in Section III of this chapter.

Nocardia Species

A. *Direct Examination of Clinical Materials*

Pus, sputum, bronchial washings, spinal fluid, and other clinical materials should be collected in sterile containers and taken to the laboratory as quickly as possible. Pus should be examined for granules (compact colonies of the organism surrounded by "tissue-reaction material"). Granules usually are not present in material from persons with systemic nocardiosis. However, granules are characteristic of nocardial mycetomas, particularly infections caused by *N. brasiliensis*.

Smears of the fresh materials (centrifuged sediment, in the case of spinal fluids or urine, when the volume is sufficient), as well as of concentrates of sputum, bronchial, or gastric washings should be made (see Section III-A for preparation methods). Smears are stained by both Gram and acid-fast methods. For the "modified Kinyoun acid-fast stain" that is appropriate for these partially acid-fast organisms, see Section III-B. Smears are examined under oil immersion for Gram-positive, partially acid-fast, mycelial elements.

In stained smears from clinical materials, the *Nocardia* species appear as bacillary or filamentous, occasionally branched forms measuring 1 μ or less in diameter. Coccoid forms also are seen frequently. It is important to search for filamentous, branched forms, since bacillary or coccobacillary forms may be mistaken for mycobacteria. Coccoid forms may be the spores of *Streptomyces* species that occasionally retain the acid-fast stain. The forms most characteristic of *Nocardia* species are very delicate filaments, occasionally branched and usually showing beading along their length. In fresh clinical materials, the entire filament may retain the acid-fast stain, but frequently, only the fine granulations along the length of the filament will stain red.

Although the demonstration of partially acid-fast forms, as described above, is presumptive evidence of nocardial infection, cultural studies always should be undertaken for confirmation. Furthermore, the organisms frequently are missed in such examinations. Young et al. (15) reported that *N. asteroides* was recovered by cultures from 22% of 42 specimens in which acid-fast organisms were not seen on direct smear. The reverse condition is also occasionally true, i.e., the organism may be seen by direct examination, yet not grown in culture.

B. Isolation from Clinical Materials

1. *Routine culture.* Clinical materials should be cultured whether or not organisms which suggest *Nocardia* species are observed in stained smears. Inoculated media should be held for three weeks before being considered negative for *Nocardia* species. It is a well-recognized experience that *Nocardia* species isolations frequently are missed in the routine diagnostic laboratory, where cultures are maintained only for three to four days.

Most isolates grow well on Sabouraud dextrose agar at room temperature with or without the addition of chloramphenicol (0.05 mg per ml) and cycloheximide (0.5 mg per ml). Although *N. asteroides* shows some sensitivity to chloramphenicol in vitro, it is an advantage to use media with and without this antibiotic for primary isolation purposes. In many instances, although the growth may be partially inhibited by chloramphenicol, it may be only on such antibiotic-containing media that the *Nocardia* species are isolated. This results from the fact that bacteria are inhibited frequently by chloramphenicol to a greater degree than the *Nocardia* species. However, if a *Nocardia* species is sought specifically, media with other antibacterial antibiotics, such as penicillin (20 units per ml), may be more appropriate. It should be noted, however, that some isolates of *N. asteroides* may be sensitive to penicillin. The use of cycloheximide aids isolation by inhibiting the development of saprophytic molds.

Recent experience has shown that some isolates of the *Nocardia* species require media that are more nutritious than Sabouraud dextrose agar. In addition, many isolates grow much more rapidly at 35–37°C than at room temperature. For these reasons, it is recommended that streaking on brain heart infusion agar with and without antibiotics* and incubation at 35–37°C be included in routine cultural procedures. Heart infusion blood agar plates with

---

* Both Sabouraud dextrose agar and brain heart infusion agar with chloramphenicol and cycloheximide, in the amounts recommended above, are available commercially.

added penicillin are recommended also. It is important to point out that the nocardias grow well in thioglycolate broth. They also develop very slowly on plates incubated in an anaerobe jar; however, when removed from the jar, they grow quickly and develop characteristic morphology.

2. *Use of concentration procedures.* The isolation of *Nocardia* species, as well as the fungi that cause systemic diseases, may be greatly facilitated by the use of concentration procedures. Details of such a procedure that involves the use of preliminary digestion, concentration by centrifugation, and treatment with antibiotics are given in Section III-A.

It is well recognized that most of the procedures routinely used in the Mycobacteriology Laboratory allow isolation of *Nocardia* species from sputum (20, 22). In a recent evaluation of such procedures by Reep and Kaplan (23, 24), it was shown that fungi differed in their ability to survive the currently used digestion-decontamination procedures. *N. asteroides* was found to be relatively resistant to the action of *N*-acetyl-l-cysteine-sodium hydroxide and dithiothreitol-sodium hydroxide procedures. This actinomycete was recovered from more than 75% of the specimens treated by these two procedures. The use of these reagents without NaOH, however, allowed 100% recovery rates. Results with the trisodium phosphate-zephiran procedure were not favorable for the recovery of the *Nocardia* species. These authors (23, 24) also pointed out that the recovery rate of *N. asteroides* was greatly reduced when cultures were attempted on chloramphenicol-containing media, as opposed to similar media without chloramphenicol.

Since we know from practical experience as well as from experimental studies that *Nocardia* species usually survive the commonly used concentration procedures, culture tubes inoculated for the isolation of mycobacteria should be examined carefully for *Nocardia* species. These organisms grow well on media such as Lowenstein-Jensen or 7H10 that have been incubated at 37°C.

When *N. asteroides* is present, its growth is usually apparent on Lowenstein-Jensen slants in five to six days. However, in some instances, the growth is so scanty that after two weeks, the time when the majority of cultures are examined routinely for mycobacteria, nocardial growth appears only as a discoloration of the medium. As the colonies develop, the colonial coloration is quite variable. Most are a light, tannish orange and show a moist, skin-like surface. They have neither the clear orange coloration of the rapidly growing, chromogenic, atypical mycobacteria nor the chalk-white or powdery surface growth as seen on *Nocardia* cultures grown on dry-surfaced media, such as Sabouraud dextrose agar slants with nonadsorbent cotton plugs. All cultures should be held at least three weeks before they are considered negative for *Nocardia* species.

C. Routine Methods for the Identification of Nocardia *Species in Culture*

Methods for the identification of *Nocardia* species include not only the demonstration of species differences but also the separation of these organisms from the morphologically similar members of the genera *Actinomadura* and *Streptomyces.* Certain species of these later genera, such as *Actinomadura madurae, Actinomadura pelletierii* and *Streptomyces somaliensis,* are also clinically important and should be identified specifically. This is particularly true when isolation has been made from localized, suppurating lesions or obvious mycetomas.

Berd (21) recently reviewed and evaluated current methods for the laboratory identification of *Nocardia* species and other clinically important aerobic actinomycetes. Practical methods as well as special procedures for problem cultures will be reviewed here. (Technical details and media formulas will be found in Section III.) Detailed flow charts and test results obtained for the various species may be found in Berd's publications (4, 21, 25), as well as in those of Gordon and her associates (6, 26-30) and of Lechevalier and her associates (31, 32).

1. *Selection of a pure culture.* Isolates suspected of being *Nocardia* species are streaked on brain heart infusion agar plates to determine their purity before they are studied further. If bacterial contamination is noted or if two colony types are seen, individual colonies are picked or the growth is treated with appropriate antibiotics until it is free of contamination.

2. *Gross morphology.* Gross morphology on a moist, enriched medium, such as Lowenstein-Jensen agar incubated at 37°C, has been described above. More characteristic morphology, as usually described for the *Nocardia* species, is observed after two to three weeks of growth on Sabouraud dextrose agar in cotton-plugged tubes that have been incubated at room temperature. Colonies of all the *Nocardia* species, as well as those of the *Actinomadura* and *Streptomyces* species, are basically similar. They are characteristically heaped and folded. They may have a moist, glabrous surface or be covered with a powdery or short, downy, aerial mycelium. In addition, they may be white, cream to tan, or shades of yellow to reddish orange. When aerial mycelium is present, the surface is often chalky white. Colonies that remain moist or glabrous frequently are contaminated by bacteria. Many isolates produce a browning of the medium (tyrosinase reaction).

3. *Microscopic morphology.* Microscopic morphology is determined chiefly by the use of slide cultures. Potato dextrose agar or cornmeal agar are usually satisfactory. Berd (21) preferred tap water agar (20 g of crude agar in 1000 ml of tap water) for the study of sporulation for some isolates. Examination of microcolonies on agar plates may be helpful, particularly when aerial mycelium is not demonstrated by the slide culture method. Slide cultures should be retained and examined for two to four weeks. Agar plates may be held for up to eight weeks. It is important to be able to recognize true aerial branched mycelium as produced by the *Nocardia* and *Streptomyces* species and species of *Actinomadura* in order to separate them from organisms such as *Mycobacterium fortuitum* or members of the "rhodochrous group." This is best accomplished on slide cultures examined for growth that extends from the agar block onto the glass. True aerial mycelium extends away from the agar and, in most isolates, shows filaments with branching produced at right angles. However, false "branched filaments" also may extend onto the glass and must be differentiated morphologically (33).

Production of spores in some isolates may not be apparent until after three to four weeks of incubation. Slide cultures should be examined weekly to determine the type of sporulation produced. Members of the genera *Nocardia*, *Actinomadura*, or *Streptomyces* produce no spores; or, if spores are produced, it is in delicate chains on the aerial mycelium or on the vegetative mycelium (in the agar). This type of sporulation distinguishes members of these genera from *Microbispora* and *Dermatophilus* species, which have distinctive sporulation patterns, and the genus *Micromonospora*, which produces minute, singly borne spores only in the submerged growth (34).

Acid-fast stains of cultures are made by the modified Kinyoun's cold stain (Section III-B). In general, acid fastness is more easily demonstrated in cultures when the smear is made from fresh growth on media rich in proteins, such as casein agar, Lowenstein-Jensen medium, or blood agar, than from Sabouraud dextrose agar. It is very important that control smears from a known *Streptomyces* species (acid-fast-negative) culture and a *N. asteroides* (acid-fast-positive) culture be stained with every group of unknowns. However, failure to demonstrate acid fastness does not rule out a *Nocardia* species, since it is not possible to demonstrate this with all isolates.

4. *Physiological tests.* The basic tests recommended for the identification of the *Nocardia* species include 1) decomposition of a number of substrates, 2) ability to grow in dilute (0.4%) gelatin, 3) resistance to lysozyme, 4) ability to produce acid from carbohydrates, 5) ability to grow at 10°C, and 6) whole-cell hydrolysate analyses by paper chromatography that includes diaminopimelic acid (DAP) determinations as well as analysis for monosaccharides. (Details of most of these procedures are given in Section III. For all physiological tests, cultures are incubated at room temperature, unless better growth is obtained at 35–37°C.

Fortunately, not all these tests are necessary for every *Nocardia*-like isolate that appears in the diagnostic laboratory. Figure 1 shows a schema that allows the identification of the majority of the clinically important isolates given in the abbreviated flow-chart of Berd (21). If results do not fit patterns as indicated or if further tests are needed, these cultures should be selected for further studies. If such additional tests cannot be performed because of lack of time, personnel, or adequate facilities, these cultures should be referred to a special research laboratory.

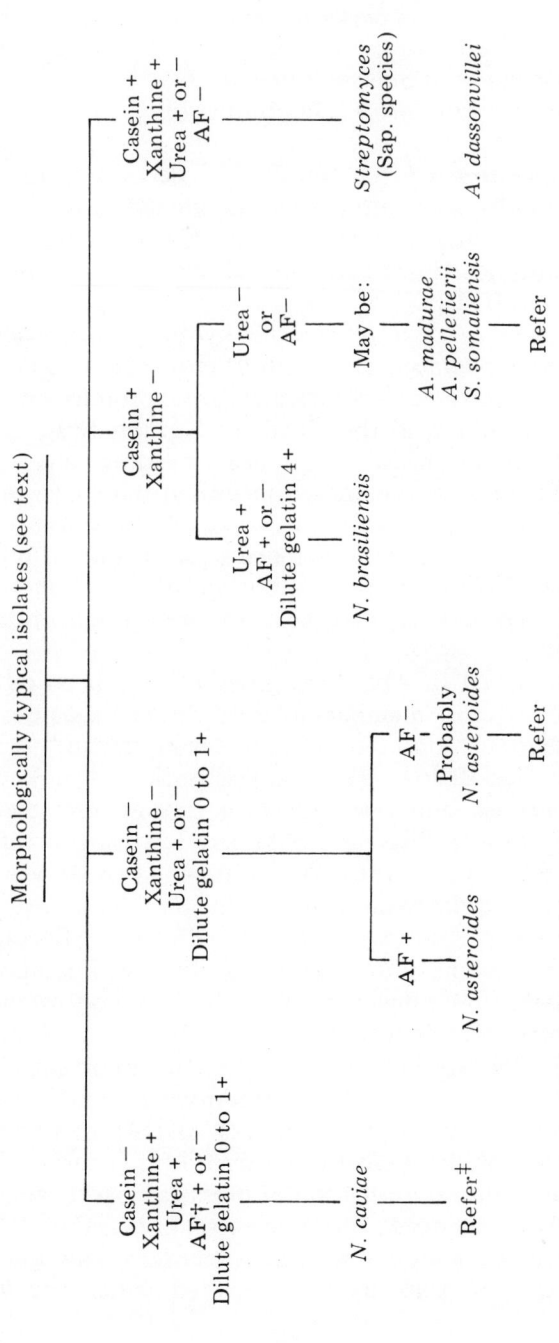

```
                                                              Casein +
                                                              Xanthine +
                                                              Urea + or −
                                                              AF −
                                                                  │
                                                          Streptomyces
                                                          (Sap. species)
                                                          A. dassonvillei
```

Morphologically typical isolates (see text)

```
Casein −              Casein −                Casein +                   Casein +
Xanthine +            Xanthine −              Xanthine −                 Xanthine +
Urea +                Urea + or −                                        Urea + or −
AF† + or −            Dilute gelatin 0 to 1+                             AF −
Dilute gelatin 0 to 1+
                      AF +      AF −          Urea +          Urea −
                                              AF + or −       or
                                              Dilute gelatin 4+   AF−

N. caviae             N. asteroides  Probably                  May be:
                                     N. asteroides
                                                  N. brasiliensis    A. madurae
Refer‡                         Refer                                 A. pelletierii
                                                                     S. somaliensis

                                                                        Refer
```

Figure 1. Simplified flow chart for the identification of *Nocardia*-like species.*

* Adapted from Ref. 21.
† AF, acid-fast or partially acid-fast.
‡ Refer for further tests for confirmation, or to other speciation if necessary.

Lucille K. Georg

D. Discussion of Special Procedures for Generic and Species Determinations

1. *Decomposition of substrates.* The decomposition of casein and xanthine is used routinely in the identification of *Nocardia* species. Other substrates that are particularly useful are tyrosine and hypoxanthine. (Formulas, procedures, and specific uses are given in Section III-C, D.)

2. *Production of acid from carbohydrates.* Organisms of the genera *Nocardia*, *Actinomadura*, and *Streptomyces* do not ferment sugars, but do utilize certain sugars with the production of acid. A special basal medium, as described by Gordon (30), is required (Section III-G). Sugar utilization patterns now have been well established for most of the known species of the above genera (28, 29, 35).

3. *Lysozyme resistance.* Resistance to the action of lysozyme is characteristic of *Nocardia* species, but not of the *Actinomadura* or *Streptomyces* species. It is variable for the "rhodochrous group" (Section III-H).

4. *Growth at 10°C.* Ability to grow at 10°C is an outstanding characteristic of most members of the "rhodochrous group." For further characterization of the "rhodochrous group," see Gordon (28, 29) and Goodfellow, Fleming, and Sackin (36). Some *Nocardia*, *Streptomyces*, and *Actinomadura* species also grow at this temperature. Best results are obtained by using a refrigerated water bath set at 10°C, with control tubes at room temperature.

5. *Whole-cell hydrolysate analyses for diaminopimelic acid and monosaccharides.* Studies concerned with cell-wall constituents have given important information on the basic composition of various bacteria and fungi (34, 37, 38). In many instances, they have confirmed generic and species separations and relationships. Some of the findings have, in fact, led to important changes in classification. For the aerobic actinomycetes under discussion, information on the presence of absence of DAP and whether it is in the L-isomer or the meso-form is useful for generic delineation. Also of value is the determination of monosaccharide constituents. In general, for the aerobic actinomycetes, organisms of the genera *Actinomadura*, *Dermatophilus*, and *Nocardia* contain meso-DAP. This is also true of members of the related genus *Mycobacterium*

and some corynebacteria. LL-DAP is characteristic of the genus *Streptomyces*. It also occurs in the microaerophilic genus *Arachnia*.

Lechevalier and Lechevalier (34) have shown that those actinomycetes that contain meso-DAP may be further separated on the basis of the monosaccharides found in whole-cell preparations. For example, *Nocardia* as well as *Mycobacterium* species and some corynebacteria show galactose and arabinose, but no xylose. Some members of the genus *Actinomadura* that are mycetoma agents, namely, *A. madurae* and *A. pelletierii*, show a specific sugar madurose, 3-O-methyl-D-galactose (32), but no arabinose or xylose. On the other hand, *Streptomyces* species and *Actinomadura dassonvillei* show no sugars of diagnostic significance. It should be noted that glucose, mannose, ribose, and rhamnose are commonly present in all these genera.

Methods for the preliminary preparation of cultures and the paper chromatographic determination of these cell-wall constituents, as adapted from Lechevalier and Lechevalier (34), Becker et al. (38), and Hoare and Work (39), are described in Section III-I.

6. *Determination of lipids.* The separation of *Nocardia* species from *Mycobacterium* or *Corynebacterium* species usually is not a problem if well-developed aerial mycelium can be demonstrated. However, difficulties arise when glabrous, waxy, or moist colonies are encountered. In such cases, the study of whole-cell hydrolysates for DAP and monosaccharides is not adequate, since members of these genera all show the same cell-wall pattern, i.e., meso-DAP in combination with arabinose and galactose.

These genera can be separated, however, on the basis of cellular lipids. Lechevalier, Horan, and Lechevalier (40) have found that one of the characteristic lipids of the *Nocardia* species, the so-called "nocardomycolic acid," has a skeleton of 50 carbon atoms. When pyrolyzed, this lipid breaks down into a series of fatty acids with shorter carbon chains. The most abundant of these fatty acids are myristic acid (C_{14}), palmitic acid (C_{16}), and stearic acid (C_{18}). *Mycobacterium* species contain lipids, "mycolic acids," that have skeletons of about 80 carbons, and *Corynebacterium* species contain lipids, "corynemycolic acids," of only about 32 carbons. The lipid constituents of these organisms may be demonstrated by gas pyrolysis methods (40).

Recently, more practical methods for separation on the basis of characteristic lipids have been described by Kanetsuna and Bartoli (41) and by Mordarska, Mordarski, and Goodfellow (42). In the former publication, a simple and rapid chemical test was described. The procedure involved the saponification of cells with KOH in methanol and benzene (1:1, v/v) at 37°C, followed by extraction with ether, and then precipitation of the ethereal solution with ethanol. Mycobacteria produced large amounts of white precipitate (about 10 mg per g of wet whole bacteria) with a melting point between 45 and 70°C, whereas the nocardias gave no precipitate, or very small amounts (less than 2 mg per g of whole bacteria), which did not melt below 150°C or which for a few isolates melted near 80°C.

In the procedure described by Mordarska et al. (42), a specific lipid for *Nocardia* species, which they designate as LCN-A (Lipid Characteristic of *Nocardia*), may be demonstrated by thin-layer chromatography.

A combination of these two procedures may serve well as a practical method for the diagnostic laboratory when the distinction between *Nocardia*, *Mycobacteria*, and certain *Corynebacterium* species is necessary.

III. Appendix

A. Preparation of Sputum or Bronchial Washings for the Isolation of Nocardia Species

After direct inoculation of any granules or purulent portions, the remaining specimen may be digested, concentrated, and treated with antibiotics.

1. Place equal volumes of digestant (*N*-acetylcysteine or dithiothreitol without NaOH) and specimen in a 50-ml, graduated, screw-capped centrifuge tube.
2. Place in a vortex-type mixer for 5–10 sec.
3. Bring to a volume of 50 ml with phosphate-buffered saline.
4. Centrifuge at 2100 rpm for 15 min.

5. Decant supernatant.
6. Add penicillin* to give a final concentration of 20 units per ml.

B. *Modified Kinyoun Acid-Fast Stain*

This stain is used for clinical materials suspected of containing *Nocardia* species and also for study of cultures suspected of being *Nocardia* species.

1. Composition of Kinyoun carbol fuchsin.
   a. Basic fuchsin   4.0 g
   b. Phenol crystals   8.0 g
   c. Alcohol (95%)   20.0 ml
   d. Water (distilled)   100.0 ml

2. *Staining procedure.*
   a. Apply to heat-fixed smears:†
      1) Kinyoun carbol fuchsin—5 min (room temperature—do not heat)
      2) H_2O rinse
      3) 50% ethyl alcohol rinse (flood and pour off until excess red dye is removed)
      4) H_2O rinse
      5) 1% aqueous H_2SO_4 rinse—3 min
      6) 1% aqueous methylene blue—1 min
      7) H_2O rinse
   b. Blot dry and examine under oil immersion

---

* If other pathogenic fungi that are not sensitive to chloramphenicol are sought, a portion of the sediment may be treated with this antibiotic to give a final concentration of 0.05 mg per ml.

† Control smears of *N. asteroides* (mycelium partially acid-fast) and *Streptomyces* species (mycelium not acid-fast) should be run with each group of unknown smears.

C. Casein Decomposition

Prepare and autoclave separately: 10 g of skim milk (dehydrated) in 100 ml of distilled water and 2 g of agar in 100 ml of distilled water. Cool to 45°C, mix the two solutions, and pour into four-compartment Petri dishes (25 ml in a 15- × 100-mm dish).

Inoculate sectors with unknown cultures; streak a large amount of inoculum on the agar surface. If possible, select plates with the same agar thickness, and inoculate unknowns and one positive and negative control culture at the same time. Examine plates at 7 and 21 days for clearing of the casein underneath and around the growth.

Important casein-positive species are indicated on the flow chart. Some isolates of *N. brasiliensis* hydrolyze casein very slowly.

A. dassonvillei, a saprophytic species recently described by Gordon (43), also hydrolyzes casein.

D. Xanthine, Hypoxanthine, and Tyrosine Decomposition

Suspend 0.4 g of xanthine, 0.5 g of hypoxanthine, or 0.5 g of tyrosine in individual, 10-ml aliquots of distilled water and autoclave. Mix each sterile suspension with 100 ml of melted or freshly sterilized nutrient agar (peptone, 5 g; beef extract, 3 g; agar, 15 g; distilled water, 1000 ml, at pH 7.0). Cool the mixtures to about 50°C and pour into four-compartment dishes like those used for casein decomposition. It is important to swirl the flasks while pouring to keep the crystals evenly distributed. Inoculate the sectors heavily and examine them weekly for clearing of granules underneath and around the inoculum. Positive and negative controls should be inoculated and read at the same intervals.

Important xanthine-positive species are indicated on the flow chart. *A. dassonvillei* also may hydrolyze xanthine.

Hypoxanthine-positive species are *N. caviae*, *A. dassonvillei*, and some *Streptomyces* species. *N. brasiliensis* is variable in its ability to hydrolyze hypoxanthine.

Tyrosine-positive species are *N. brasiliensis*, *A. dassonvillei*, and some *Streptomyces* species, including *S. somaliensis*.

E. Urea Decomposition

From actively growing cultures, heavily inoculate 3-ml aliquots of sterile urease test medium (BBL Division of BioQuest, Cockeysville, Md.)* at pH 6.8 in cotton-stoppered tubes. Check the tubes at weekly intervals for four weeks for development of an alkaline reaction. An uninoculated tube should be incubated with the tests for color comparison.

Urease-positive species are indicated on the flow chart.

F. Ability to Grow in Dilute (0.4% Gelatin)

Adjust dilute gelatin (4 g of gelatin in 1000 ml of distilled water) to pH 7.0, distribute into tubes in 5-ml amounts, and autoclave. Inoculate the tubes with a very small fragment of growth from unknown cultures. Examine for quality and type of growth after three to four weeks. The following growth patterns are obtained:

1. *N. asteroides:* no growth or very small amount of thin, flaky growth; pH, acid or unchanged.
2. *N. brasiliensis:* good growth (3–4+, in amount, as compared to above), usually with firm, spherical, compact colonies; pH, usually alkaline.
3. *N. caviae:* fair growth (1–2+) with small, but usually discrete colonies.
4. *Streptomyces* species: growth (1+) usually thin and stringy.

If it is difficult to read tests grossly on the basis of the amount of growth or pH change, the presence of free amino acids should be determined by the ninhydrin reaction in order to demonstrate utilization of the gelatin. *N. brasiliensis* species break down gelatin into amino acids. *N. asteroides* and most other *Nocardia* species do not (44).

---

* Use of trade names is for identification only and does not constitute endorsement by the U. S. Public Health Service or by the U. S. Department of Health, Education, and Welfare.

G. Production of Acid from Carbohydrates

Use basal medium recommended by Gordon (30): $(NH_4)_2PO_4$, 1 g; KCl, 0.02 g; $MgSO_4 \cdot 7H_2O$, 0.2 g; agar, 15 g; distilled water, 1000 ml. Add 15 ml of 0.04% solution of bromcresol purple to each liter. Adjust the pH to 7.0. Place 5-ml aliquots in cotton-plugged tubes and sterilize the medium. Maintain the tubes in a 50–55°C water bath, and add 0.5-ml aliquots of Seitz-filtered 10% carbohydrate solutions to the basal medium in each tube. Rotate and slant the tubes. To perform the test, inoculate the slants with several drops of an actively growing broth culture suspension with a capillary pipet and incubate the slants for four weeks. An acid reaction, indicated by a yellow color, is considered positive. The following carbohydrates appear to be useful: adonitol, arabinose, dulcitol, fructose, galactose, glucose, glycerol, inositol, lactose, maltose, mannitol, mannose, rhamnose, salicin, sorbitol, starch, sucrose, trehalose, and xylose.

Production of acid from sugars for identification of the aerobic actinomycetes has been reviewed by Berd (21).

See also the work of Gordon and co-workers (27–30) and of Goodfellow (35).

H. Lysozyme Resistance

Mix 95 ml of sterile glycerol broth (peptone, 5 g; glycerol, 70 ml; distilled water, 1000 ml) with 5 ml of lysozyme solution [100 mg of lysozyme (Difco Bactolysozyme; Difco Laboratories, Detroit, Mich.) in 100 ml of 0.01 N HCl, sterilized by Seitz filtration], and dispense into test tubes. Inoculate these tubes and controls containing glycerol broth without lysozyme with one drop of culture suspension. Make weekly readings for four weeks. The result is considered positive if good growth is obtained in both tubes, and negative if growth is good in the control tube but poor or absent in lysozyme.

Nocardia species generally are resistant to lysozyme; *Actinomadura* and *Streptomyces* species are not.

I. Whole-Cell Hydrolysate Analyses

Grow the cultures in Trypticase soy broth in flasks on a rotary shaker for a period of time varying from three days to two weeks, and then kill them with 1% (w/v) formalin. Harvest the cultures by centrifugation, wash them once in distilled water and then in 95% alcohol, and thoroughly dry them in small Petri dishes in a 45°C oven. To facilitate weighing, some of the dried preparations may be ground with a mortar and pestle before hydrolysis.

1. *DAP analysis.* The method of Becker et al. (38) is used for this analysis. Place 10 mg of dried cells in a 5-ml ampule, and then add 1 ml of 6-*N*-hydrochloric acid. Seal the ampule and put it in an oven at 100°C for 18 hr. Cool the ampule, and then filter the hydrolysate with 4.25-cm filter paper attached to a 20-ml beaker with a paper clip. Wash the material on the paper with three or four drops of distilled water. Dry the liquid hydrolysate on a steam bath. To make sure that all hydrochloric acid is removed, add and evaporate 1 ml of water twice. Reconstitute the hydrolysate with 0.3 ml of distilled water, and spot 10 μl onto Whatman No. 1 chromatography paper. As a standard, spot 10 μl of 0.01 M DL-diaminopimelic acid (Sigma Chemical Co., St. Louis, Mo.), which contains both the meso- and L-isomers. To perform descending chromatography, use methanol-water-10 N hydrochloric acid-pyridine (80:17.5:2.5:10, by volume) for 16–18 hr. After the paper is dried, dip it into 0.2% acetonic ninhydrin and heat it in an oven at 100°C for 2 min to reveal the spots. DAP spots are olive green which fade to yellow; the L-isomer moves several centimeters ahead of the meso-isomer. Other amino acid spots are purple; this color rapidly fades and these spots move ahead of the DAP spots.

2. *Monosaccharide analysis.* This is performed according to the method of Lechevalier and Lechevalier (34) with minor modifications by Berd (21). Place 100 mg of dried cells in an ampule with 2 ml of 1.0 N sulfuric acid. Seal the ampule and put it into boiling water for 2 hr. Then transfer the contents to a centrifuge tube and add saturated barium hydroxide dropwise until the pH is 5.0–5.5; determine this with short-range pH paper and then check with a pH meter. Centrifuge the mixture and filter the supernatant into 50-ml beakers to which have been added 2 ml of chloroform as an

anticontaminant. The material is evaporated to dryness in a 45°C oven overnight and reconstituted with 0.3 ml of distilled water. Spot 30 µl of the hydrolysate onto Whatman No. 1 paper. As a reference standard, spot 10 µl of a mixture of sugars (arabinose, galactose, glucose, mannose, rhamnose, ribose, and xylose), each in a 1% concentration. Spot a hydrolysate of a known culture of *A. madurae* or *A. pelletieri* as a reference standard for madurose.* Perform descending chromatography with the organic (top) phase of a mixture of *n*-butanol-water-pyridine-toluene (5:3:3:4, by volume) as the solvent. Develop the paper for 48–54 hr and then dry. Reveal the spots by spraying with acid aniline phthalate (3.25 g of phthalic acid dissolved in 100 ml of water-saturated butanol plus 2 ml of aniline) and heating in an oven at 110°C for 3 min.

Hexoses (galactose, glucose, mannose, and rhamnose) produce brown spots, and pentoses (arabinose, ribose, and xylose) produce reddish spots. Because of differences in rate of migration, the spots will be aligned in the following sequence: galactose, glucose, mannose, arabinose, xylose, ribose, and rhamnose (usually off the sheet). Madurose moves at about the same distance as xylose, but is easily identifiable because it produces a brown spot.

3. *Grouping of aerobic actinomycetes on the basis of cell-wall studies.* On the basis of cell-wall studies such as those described above, the *Nocardia* species and some morphologically similar genera can be separated into groups:

a. Group I. Meso-DAP + arabinose and galactose
  1) *N. asteroides*
  2) *N. brasiliensis*
  3) *N. caviae*
  4) Also *Mycobacterium* species, the "rhodochrous group," and most species of *Corynebacterium*
b. Group II. Meso-DAP + madurose
  1) *A. madurae*
  2) *A. pelletierii*
c. Group III. Meso-DAP, but no diagnostic sugars: *A. dassonvillei*

---

* Madurose was originally so named because it was found in *A. madurae*; it recently has been identified as 3-*O*-methyl-D-galactose (32).

d. Group IV. LL-DAP, but no diagnostic sugars
   1) *Streptomyces* species
   2) *Arachnia propionica*
e. Group V. No DAP and no diagnostic sugars: *Actinomyces* species

Literature Cited

1. Cross, R. M., and C. H. Binford. Infections by fungi that are commonly primary pathogens. Is *Nocardia asteroides* an opportunist? Lab. Invest. 11:1103, 1962.
2. Goodman, J. S., and M. G. Koenig. *Nocardia* infections in a general hospital. Ann. N. Y. Acad. Sci. 174: 552, 1970.
3. Gonzalez-Ochoa, A. Mycetomas caused by *Nocardia brasiliensis*, with a note on the isolation of the causative organism from soil. Lab. Invest. 11: 1118, 1962.
4. Berd, D. *Nocardia brasiliensis* infection in the United States. A report of nine cases and a review of the literature. Amer. J. Clin. Pathol. Aug. 1973.
5. Mariat, F. Étude comparative de souches de *Nocardia* isolées de mycetomes. Ann. Inst. Pasteur 109: 90, 1965.
6. Gordon, R. E., and J. M. Mihm. Identification of *Nocardia caviae* (Erikson) nov. comb. Ann. N. Y. Acad. Sci. 98: 628, 1962.
7. Kinch, D. A. A rapidly fatal infection caused by *Nocardia caviae* in a dog. J. Pathol. Bacteriol. 95: 540, 1968.
8. Pier, A. C., A. K. Takayama, and A. Y. Miyarhara. Cetean nocardiosis. J. Wildl. Dis. 6: 112, 1970.
9. Kurup, P. V., and R. S. Sandhu. Isolation of *Nocardia caviae* from soil and its pathogenicity for laboratory animals. J. Bacteriol. 90: 822, 1965.
10. Smith, I. M., and A. H. S. Hayward. *Nocardia caviae* and *Nocardia asteroides:* Comparative bacteriological and mouse pathogenicity studies. J. Comp. Pathol. 81: 79, 1971.
11. Murray, J. F., S. M. Finegold, S. Froman, and D. W. Will. The changing spectrum of nocardiosis. A review and presentation of nine cases. Amer. Rev. Resp. Dis. 83: 315, 1961.
12. Saltzman, H. A., E. W. Chick, and N. F. Conant. Nocardiosis as a complication of other diseases. Lab. Invest. 11: 1110, 1962.
13. Carlsen, E. T., R. B. Hill, and D. T. Rowlands, Jr. Nocardiosis and pulmonary alveolar proteinosis. Ann. Intern. Med. 60: 275, 1964.

14. Andriole, V. T., M. Ballas, and G. L. Wilson. The association of nocardiosis and pulmonary alveolar proteinosis. Ann. Intern. Med. 60: 266, 1964.
15. Young, L. S., D. Armstrong, A. Blevins, and P. Lieberman. *Nocardia asteroides* infection complicating neoplastic disease. Amer. J. Med. 50: 356, 1971.
16. Kumar, R., and L. N. Mohapatra. Studies on aerobic actinomycetes isolated from soil. I. Isolation and identification of strains. Sabouraudia 6: 140, 1968.
17. Stropnik, Z. Isolation of *Nocardia asteroides* from human skin. Sabouraudia 4: 41, 1965.
18. Whyte, H. J., and W. Kaplan. Nocardial mycetoma resembling granuloma faciale. Arch. Dermatol. 100: 720, 1969.
19. Pier, A. C., E. H. Willers, and M. J. Mejia. *Nocardia asteroides* as a mammary pathogen of cattle. II. The sources of nocardial infection and experimental reproduction of the disease. Amer. J. Vet. Res. 22: 698, 1961.
20. Hosty, T. S., C. McDurmont, L. Ajello, L. K. Georg, G. L. Brumfield, and A. A. Calix. Prevalence of *Nocardia asteroides* in sputa examined by a tuberculosis diagnostic laboratory. J. Lab. Clin. Med. 58: 107, 1961.
21. Berd, D. The laboratory identification of clinically important aerobic actinomycetes. Appl. Microbiol. 25: 665, 1973.
22. Ajello, L., V. Q. Grant, and A. B. Gutske. The effect of tubercle bacillus concentration procedures on fungi causing pulmonary mycoses. J. Lab. Clin. Med. 38: 486, 1951.
23. Reep, B. R., and W. Kaplan. The effect of newer tubercle digestion and decontamination procedures on fungi causing pulmonary diseases. Mycopathol. Mycol. Appl. 41: 167, 1971.
24. Reep, B. R., and W. Kaplan. The use of N-acetyl-l-cysteine and dithiothreitol to process sputa for mycological and fluorescent antibody examinations. Health Lab. Sci. 9: 118, 1972.
25. Berd, D. *Nocardia asteroides:* A taxonomic study with clinical correlations. (In preparation)
26. Gordon, R. E., and M. M. Smith. Proposed group of characters for the separation of *Streptomyces* and *Nocardia*. J. Bacteriol. 69: 147, 1955.
27. Gordon, R. E., and J. M. Mihm. A comparison of *Nocardia asteroides* and *Nocardia brasiliensis*. J. Gen. Microbiol. 20: 129, 1959.
28. Gordon, R. E. Some strains in search of a genus—*Corynebacterium, Mycobacterium, Nocardia* or what? J. Gen. Microbiol. 43: 329, 1966.
29. Gordon, R. E. Some criteria for the recognition of *Nocardia madurae* (Vincent) Blanchard. J. Gen. Microbiol. 45: 355, 1966.
30. Gordon, R. E. The taxonomy of soil bacteria. *In* T. R. G. Gray and D. Parkinson (eds.), The Ecology of Soil Bacteria, p. 305. Liverpool University Press, Liverpool, England, 1967.

31. Lechevalier, M. P. Identification of aerobic actinomycetes of clinical importance. J. Lab. Clin. Med. 71: 934, 1968.
32. Lechevalier, M. P., and N. N. Gerber. The identity of madurose with 3-O-D-galactose. Carbohydrate Res. 13: 451, 1970.
33. George, L. K., L. Ajello, C. McDurmont, and T. S. Hosty. The identification of *Nocardia asteroides* and *Nocardia brasiliensis*. Amer. Rev. Resp. Dis. 84: 337, 1961.
34. Lechevalier, M. P., and H. Lechevalier. Chemical composition as a criterion in the classification of aerobic actinomycetes. Internatl. J. Syst. Bacteriol. 20: 435, 1970.
35. Goodfellow, M. Numerical taxonomy of some nocardioform bacteria. J. Gen. Microbiol. 69: 33, 1971.
36. Goodfellow, M., A. Fleming, and M. J. Sackin. Numerical classification of *"Mycobacterium" rhodochrous* and Runyon's Group IV Mycobacteria. Internatl. J. Syst. Bacteriol. 22: 81, 1972.
37. Cummins, C. S. Chemical composition and antigenic structure of cell walls of *Corynebacterium, Mycobacterium, Nocardia, Actinomyces,* and *Arthrobacter*. J. Gen. Microbiol. 28: 35, 1962.
38. Becker, B., M. P. Lechevalier, and H. A. Lechevalier. Chemical composition of cell wall preparations from strains of various form-genera of aerobic Actinomycetes. Appl. Microbiol. 13: 236, 1965.
39. Hoare, D. S., and E. Work. The stereoisomers of $\alpha\epsilon$-diaminopimelic acid. Their distribution in the bacterial order Actinomycetales and in certain Eubacteriales. Biochem. J. 65: 441, 1957.
40. Lechevalier, M. P., A. C. Horan, and H. Lechevalier. Lipid composition in the classification of nocardiae and mycobacteria. J. Bacteriol. 105: 313, 1971.
41. Kanetsuna, F., and A. Bartoli. A simple chemical method to differentiate *Mycobacterium* from *Nocardia*. J. Gen. Microbiol. 70: 209, 1972.
42. Mordarska, H., M. Mordarski, and M. Goodfellow. Chemotaxonomic characters and classification of some nocardioform bacteria. J. Gen. Microbiol. 71: 77, 1972.
43. Gordon, R. E., and A. C. Horan. *Nocardia dassonvillei*, a macroscopic replica of *Streptomyces griseus*. J. Gen. Microbiol. 50: 235, 1968.
44. Bojalil, L. F., and J. Cerbon. Schema for the differentiation of *Nocardia asteroides* and *Nocardia brasiliensis*. J. Bacteriol. 78: 852, 1959.

13

Toxoplasmosis and Pneumocystosis: Clinical and Laboratory Aspects in Immunocompetent and Compromised Hosts

J. K. Frenkel

I. Introduction

Toxoplasmosis and pneumocystosis are asymptomatic infections in most adults, but both can give rise to disease in patients who are generally or locally "compromised" or immunosuppressed. Although toxoplasmosis may occur in clinical form in patients who are immunologically competent, clinically apparent pneumocystosis appears to occur only in patients whose immunological mechanisms are compromised. However, local factors are also apparent. Focal toxoplasmosis occurs most often in brain and eye, where the expression of cellular and antibody immunity normally is impaired. In addition, the growth of *Pneumocystis* generally is confined to the alveoli, probably because the organisms are phagocytized in solid tissues.

Original research by the author reported herein was supported by Research Grants AI-07489 and AI-07810 of the National Institute of Allergy and Infectious Diseases, U. S. Public Health Service, Bethesda, Md.

It may be well to reexamine our central theme briefly. Probably all potential microbes are opportunistic, limited only by their requirements for substrates and by host defenses. What we are interested in is 1) which microbes invade only, or mostly, under conditions of immune deficiency, and 2) what are the conditions of immunodeficiency during which they invade. Immune deficiency may be generalized, and we speak of "the compromised host." Corticosteroids, cyclophosphamide, and certain other treatments interfering with immunocompetent lymphoid cells are more important than the underlying diseases in the production of symptomatic toxoplasmosis and pneumocystosis. Immunosuppression directed against the rejection of an organ transplant also impairs host immunity to the infections discussed. Immune deficiency also may be localized, as in the adrenal gland, where corticosteroids are elaborated, or in the brain and eyes, where cellular and antibody factors do not penetrate well. Particularly with toxoplasmosis, brain and eye involvement are important, and especially so when patients are additionally immunosuppressed by the treatments mentioned. The expression of immunity sometimes is interfered with, as when there is neutropenia, macrophage dysfunction, complement deficiency, or epithelial defects. Some of these may play a role in some patients with pneumocystosis.

II. Toxoplasmosis

Toxoplasma, an obligate intracellular sporozoan (protozoa), infects humans and a wide variety of mammals and birds. Felines, especially domestic and feral cats, are the complete (final, definitive) hosts, in which the entire cycle, including the enteroepithelial proliferative and sexual cycles, leading to the formation of oocysts, take place. The *Isopora*-type oocysts, measuring $10 \times 12 \mu$, are shed in the feces and sporulate in one to five days, when they become infectious (Fig. 1; Refs. 1 and 2). Man, nonfeline mammals, and birds are incomplete (intermediate) hosts, in which only the extraintestinal, or "tissue stages," are found. During the acute infection, these are principally the "tachyzoites"* (rapidly multi-

---

* These are new terms to designate better the various stages of *Toxoplasma* (3).

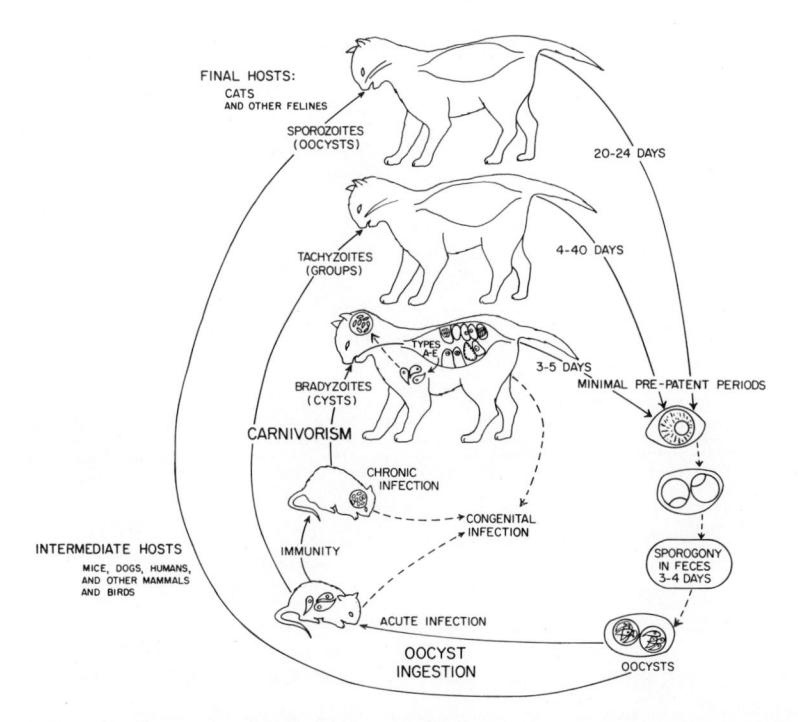

Figure 1. Life cycle of *Toxoplasma*. Three cats are used to indicate prepatent periods to oocyst appearance with the three infectious stages of *Toxoplasma*. After the ingestion of bradyzoites from cysts, the minimal prepatent period is three to five days. After the ingestion of groups of tachyzoites from the acute infection, the prepatent period is variable from three to 40 days. After the ingestion of sporozoites from oocysts, the minimal prepatent period is 20–24 days. Details of the cyst-induced intestinal cycle have been described (139), but the others are not yet known. Cats are "complete hosts" in the sense that in addition to the intestinal cycle, an extraintestinal or tissue cycle is present. Mice are shown to represent the many "incomplete hosts," both mammals and birds, in which only the extraintestinal or tissue cycle of *Toxoplasma* is found. Congenital infection has been observed during the acute infection in humans and during the chronic infection in mice.

plying forms, trophozoites) forming "groups"* of organisms, and during the chronic infection, there are "bradyzoites"* (slowly multiplying forms) forming cysts (Fig. 2). Transmission to humans is by ingestion of the oocysts from contact with cats or with soil

J. K. Frenkel

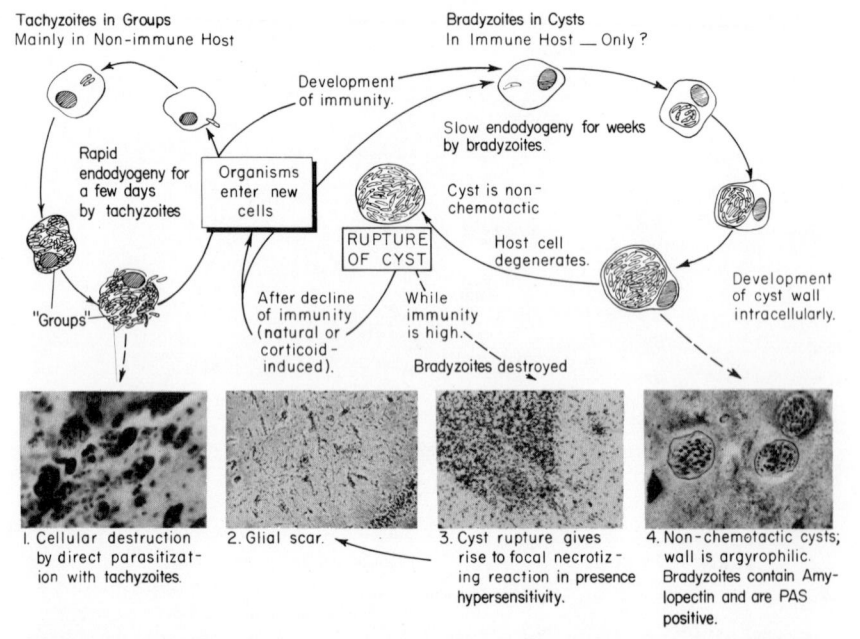

Figure 2. Extraintestinal or tissue cycle of *Toxoplasma* and histological reaction.

contaminated by cat feces, by ingestion of cysts in raw and undercooked meat, and, rarely, transplacentally or by blood transfusion [reviewed by Frenkel (3)] (Fig. 3).

A. Infection and Disease

Most *Toxoplasma* infections in man are asymptomatic, and only a few give rise to disease. Toxoplasmosis as an infection can be classified as:

1. *Acute:* a primary infection principally with tachyzoites in the immunologically virgin host. This infection usually is self-limited if the host is immunocompetent. It may be progressive in the compromised host.
2. *Subacute:* an attenuated but prolonged infection in newborns infected in utero. The passive immunization with maternal

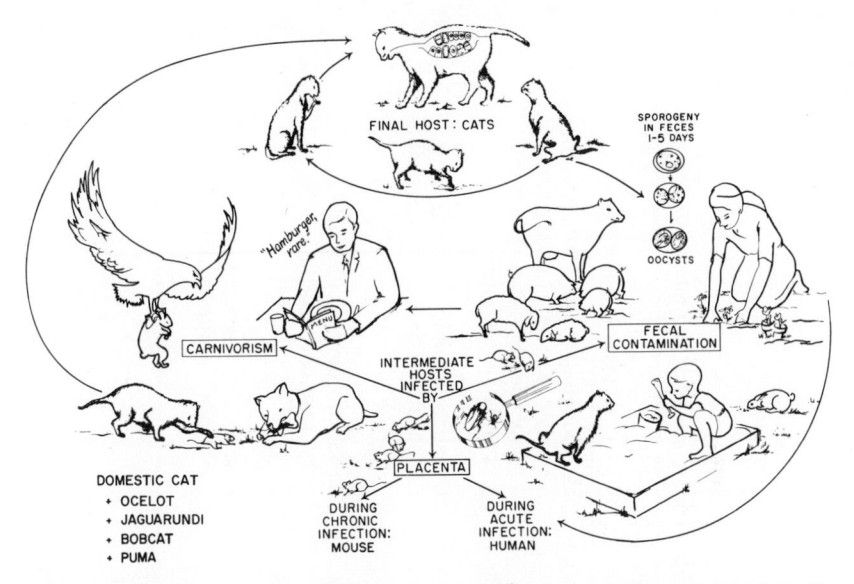

Figure 3. Postulated transmission of toxoplasmosis. Oocysts are shed in the feces of cats and after sporulation are infectious to a great variety of hosts by fecal contamination (right), probably directly and via transport hosts, such as flies and cockroaches. Carnivorism is another important means of transmission (left). Cats probably contract infection more often by carnivorism than by the ingestion of oocysts. Transplacental transmission also is indicated (bottom) (by permission of The Williams & Wilkins Co.; from Ref. 6).

antibody accounts for the attenuation, and the limited immune potential of the newborn accounts for the prolonged illness.

3. *Chronic:* since the cysts of *Toxoplasma* persist for an indefinite period of time, sometimes for the lifetime of the host, chronic infection may be latent and inactive, or there may be symptoms from cyst rupture. While immunity is being acquired slowly in the brain, there may be some proliferation of *Toxoplasma*, and, with immunosuppression, there may be reactivation of toxoplasmosis.

The symptoms of the various stages of *Toxoplasma* can be related to the stages of infection, as shown in Table 1.

Table 1. Correlation of biological parameters with disease manifestations of toxoplasmosis

Stage of *Toxoplasma* infection	Forms of *Toxoplasma*	Antibody titer (dye test)	Disease manifestations
Acute	Trophozoites	Rising or high	Maculopapular rash, fever; pneumonia; transmission to fetus; hepatitis; lymphadenopathy myocarditis, myositis; encephalitis
Subacute	Trophozoites and a few cysts	High	Hepatitis; hemolytic anemia; myocarditis, myositis; encephalitis; retinochoroiditis
Chronic	Cysts and a few trophozoites	Stable high or low	Retinochoroiditis; encephalitis; myocarditis, myositis
Relapse	Trophozoites and a few cysts	Variable	Encephalitis; myocarditis, myositis; retinochoroiditis

I will discuss mainly the acute and chronic infections in this chapter, with emphasis on the symptomatic disease, as these infections appear in the immunocompetent and compromised host. Subacute infection as defined here occurs only in the newborn, and its symptomatology and diagnosis are reviewed elsewhere (4–8).

B. Acute Toxoplasmosis

The vast majority of acute *Toxoplasma* infections are not recognized, either because they are asymptomatic or because they are accompanied by such nonspecific and vague symptoms as rash, fever, headache, anorexia, and myalgia. However, occasionally, acute, febrile toxoplasmosis is diagnosed with such localizing signs as: pneumonia (9, 10), myocarditis, and, rarely, meningoencephalitis (11, 12), hepatitis (13), and a maculopapular rash (9, 14). In general, the lesions and symptomatology result from a proliferation of *Toxoplasma* tachyzoites which destroy individual cells. Lymphadenitis may occur proximally to the portal of entry and then coincides with the febrile response after the accidental inoculation of a finger. A generalized lymphadenopathy persisting for several weeks or months may occur with clinical improvement, with sections showing lymphoreticular hyperplasia, which can be interpreted as a reaction of immunity.

Rarely in primary toxoplasmosis have retinochoroiditis (15), myositis (11), or hemolytic anemia (16) been observed.

When primary infection occurs in a compromised host, dissemination of the organisms and lesions is much more widespread. Symptoms of pneumonia, hepatitis, and rash are followed commonly by encephalitis. One such patient died with lesions in heart, pancreas, brain, bone marrow, lymph nodes, and elsewhere (17, 18).

Physical examination. The rash is maculopapular, covering most of the body but sparing the palms of the hands and soles of the feet, and the lesions may coalesce and appear purpuric. Jaundice also may be present. Pharyngitis has been reported without purulent exudate. The lymph nodes may be enlarged and tender, and they generally are discrete and freely movable. There may be signs of pulmonary consolidation with fine rales. The radiographic findings are generalized, since pneumonia depends on hematogenous dissemination. Myocarditis and pericarditis may be accompanied by a friction rub. In the abdomen, hepatomegaly, splenomegaly, or both occur in acute toxoplasmosis, and a tenderness of the abdominal lymph nodes may be elicited. There may be headache, convulsions, and other signs of meningoencephalitis.

C. Chronic Toxoplasmosis

1. *Cysts.* Toward the end of the period of acute toxoplasmosis, when lesions have been produced by proliferation of tachyzoites leading to destruction of parasitized cells, cysts of *Toxoplasma* make their appearance, especially in brain, retina, myocardium, and skeletal muscle. These cysts contain ten to hundreds or thousands of tightly packed bradyzoites. The cysts persist in the tissues for months to years and may be regarded as "resting stages," which are waiting to continue their biological cycle until ingested by a cat, in which they develop toward the oocyst stage (Fig. 1), or until ingested by a nonfeline carnivore, in which they develop into tachyzoites.

In most humans and other mammals, the long persistence of cysts is of no serious consequence. When a cyst ruptures, most liberated bradyzoites usually are destroyed by immune processes (Fig. 2). However, in the presence of hypersensitivity, an area of host tissue, many times the cyst diameter, also may be destroyed. When large numbers of cysts degenerate, this may become symptomatic in brain, heart, and skeletal muscle (11, 19). Even the rupture of a single cyst may be symptomatic in the retina, where function is highly concentrated in a small area (20). Thus, the most important clinical manifestation of chronic toxoplasmosis is retinochoroiditis. The second most important problem is a relapse of toxoplasmosis in the immunosuppressed host, where the bradyzoites liberated by cyst rupture are not destroyed, but multiply as tachyzoites mainly in the retina and in the brain.

2. *Retinochoroiditis.* Two types of retinal lesions have been observed, related to 1) cyst rupture and 2) tachyzoites. Although in the majority of humans we can only infer which of these types

of organisms is present, on the basis of observations of animals with toxoplasmosis and besnoitiosis, it appears that the suddenly appearing lesions with intense inflammation are caused by cyst rupture, and that the more chronic lesions, which smolder for many months, are caused by low-grade proliferation of tachyzoites in this area of reduced immune potential (7, 20, 21).

The presumably cyst-rupture-related lesion is of sudden onset, is circumscribed focally in the retina, accompanied by vitreous exudate, and generally heals within two months. Since the lesion ordinarily is self-limited, no treatment may be necessary. However, it is uncertain whether all bradyzoites are indeed killed by immunity; and, since corticosteroids often are used to diminish the hypersensitive inflammatory reaction, it is even less certain whether immunity remains adequate.

The presumably tachyzoite-related lesion is slowly progressive, marked by reactivations and remissions over a period of several months, and generally is poorly visualized because of the amount of vitreous exudate. Proliferation of *Toxoplasma* can be explained by the inherent immunodeficiency of the retina, similar to that of the brain. Before chemotherapy with sulfadiazine-pyrimethamine was available, these lesions tended to produce progressive visual loss. When such blind eyes became painful because of glaucoma, they often were enucleated (22, 23). On histological sections, tachyzoites are found in the retina, with an intense granulomatous inflammatory reaction in the choroid, which was formerly mistakenly attributed to tuberculosis or syphilis. Nowadays, I suspect that such lesions are often the result of treatment with corticosteroids unaccompanied by the essential *Toxoplasma*-static sulfadiazine-pyrimethamine combination. An illustrative case has been published by Hoeprich (24), which should be a warning of the disastrous effects of immunosuppression by corticosteroids (7).

3. *Encephalitis.* Toxoplasmic encephalitis either is a sequel of acute infection and related to the delay by which immunity is acquired in the central nervous system or it represents a relapse of chronic infection, often iatrogenous in origin.

An acute, febrile disease with generalized visceral symptoms may precede signs and symptoms of encephalitis (9, 11, 12), or symptoms of encephalitis may be the only ones, accompanied by fever (25–27). Focally limited toxoplasmic relapse in the brain also has been observed and first suggested in space-consuming neoplastic lesion (28, 29).

Patients with untreated lymphoreticular disease also may develop acute toxoplasmosis with encephalitis (30, 31).

Chronic, progressive encephalitis caused by relapsing toxoplasmosis was first observed by Arias-Stella (J. Arias-Stella, personal communication, 1956) in a patient with Hodgkin's disease, who was treated daily with 100—200 mg of cortisone, with nitrogen mustard, and with radiation (32). The lesions consist of large, necrotic foci with numerous *Toxoplasma* tachyzoites. *Toxoplasma* cysts also were present near the lesion and in uninvolved brain. Proliferative toxoplasmosis was restricted to the brain, although the patient also had cytomegalovirus pneumonia. Since then, numerous other patients with a similar syndrome have been observed (31, 33, 34) (Figs. 8 and 9).

Clinical signs and symptoms consist of headache, drowsiness, and disorientation, with focal palsies to hemiparesis, reflex changes, convulsions, and coma. The location of lesions is variable. Spinal fluid pleocytosis and protein elevation usually are present, although they may be depressed in patients treated with antiinflammatory drugs. The initial clinical diagnoses included brain tumor or metastasis, alcoholic psychosis, meningeal leukemia, cerebral abscess, hypertensive encephalopathy, and others.

D. Laboratory Diagnosis

Diagnosis ideally depends on isolation of *Toxoplasma* from tissues containing the lesions. Biopsy material and body fluids are useful. Histological identification is fairly safe if morphologically similar organisms can be differentiated. Serological tests offer useful but indirect information which requires skill in interpretation. Inasmuch as *Toxoplasma* antibody is common in most human populations, a positive serological test merely indicates past and persistent infection, but not necessarily a relationship with the disease in question. The indirect fluorescent antibody test (IFAT) and the Sabin and Feldman dye test are most useful to aid in diagnosis.

1. *Indirect fluorescent antibody test.* With the availability of a

microscope and a UV light source, only the *Toxoplasma* antigen and the fluorescein-conjugated antispecies serum are required to carry out the serological diagnosis of toxoplasmosis. Antigen may be obtained either as formalinized suspensions (35), lyophilized (36), or as direct smears of *Toxoplasma* from mouse peritoneal exudate or cell culture. In our studies, we fix the slides with 5% trichloroacetic acid, wash them, and store them at −20°C. The fluorescent antispecies globulin must be free from *Toxoplasma* antibody; it should not stain *Toxoplasma* without added specific antiserum. The procedures have been described by Walton et al. (35) and by Suggs, Walls, and Kagan (37), and general aspects of IFAT have been discussed by Goldman (38). Titers and interpretation are similar to those of the dye test (below) (Table 2).

A variant testing for the presence of IgM antibody, the IgM-IFAT, has been applied to identify patients with early acquired infection, especially newborns, differentiating them from uninfected newborns carrying passively transferred maternal IgG *Toxoplasma* antibody (39). IgM usually is not transferred transplacentally. Specific antibody in this class of immunoglobulins indicates active infection. However, not all patients develop this type of antibody globulin, and it may persist for only a few weeks.

The IFAT can be applied to tissue sections in order to detect small numbers of *Toxoplasma*. The test, using anti-*Toxoplasma* serum, reportedly is useful even in formalin-fixed, paraffin-embedded tissues (40), although only the alcohol-acetic fixation of Carver and Goldman (41) has given satisfactory results in our tests. Specificity of staining should be controlled with *Toxoplasma*-absorbed antiserum, which should no longer stain the structures in question in tissue (41). The identification of *Toxoplasma* also can be confirmed by noting the location of the fluorescent groups, removing the glycerol mounting medium, and staining the slide with hematoxylin or Giemsa. These stains will demonstrate the nuclei of *Toxoplasma*, while the cytoplasm generally has been lysed (J. K. Frenkel, unpublished observations).

2. *Dye test.* This test depends on lysis of living *Toxoplasma* after exposure to antibody by a complement-like "accessory factor" present in normal human serum. Lysis can be visualized directly by phase microscopy (42) or by the addition of alkaline methylene blue as indicator (42a). Any standard *Toxoplasma*

Table 2. Guide to the interpretation of serological tests for toxoplasmosis (dye test or indirect fluorescent-antibody test)[a]

Clinical problem	Titer				
	0	1:2–1:16[b]	1:32–1:128[b]	1:256–1:512[b]	1:1024+
None (Asymptomatic)	Susceptible to infection	Remote infection, probably immune	Remote infection, probably immune	Remote infection, probably immune	Recent infection(?)
Pregnancy	Susceptible to infection	Remote infection, probably immune	Remote infection, probably immune	Remote infection, probably immune	Need to check newborn baby for infection
Newborn, asymptomatic or with jaundice[f]	Incompatible[c]	Incompatible	Unlikely[d,f] (can be found in patients treated for toxoplasmosis)	Unlikely[f]	Possible[e,f]
Newborn with encephalitis	Incompatible	Incompatible	Incompatible	Unlikely	Likely if titer is stable or rises
Lymphadenopathy	Incompatible	Incompatible	Incompatible	Unlikely	Possible
Fever with pneumonia, myocarditis, or hepatitis	Incompatible	Incompatible	Unlikely	Unlikely	Possible
Retinochoroiditis	Incompatible	Possible	Possible	Possible	Possible

Encephalitis	Incompatible	Incompatible	Unlikely	Unlikely	Possible
Encephalitis in patient who is immunosuppressed[g]	Incompatible	Unlikely[g]	Unlikely[g]	Possible[g]	Possible[g]

[a] The titers listed are based on experience in the author's laboratory. Depending on the amount of accessory factor used, whether plasma or serum, and the number of organisms employed in the test, these titers may be two- to four-fold higher.

[b] At least two serological specimens taken a week or, preferably, two weeks apart are necessary to differentiate low titers, whether rising during the early acute infection, or stable and related to chronic infection. If the toxoplasmin skin test is positive, the low titer indicates chronic infection.

[c] Incompatible: with such a titer, toxoplasmosis should not be diagnosed.

[d] Unlikely: the lowest titers found in typical form of the syndrome.

[e] Possible: characteristic titer, but not necessarily related to signs and symptoms. If possible, try to obtain additional evidence from isolation of *Toxoplasma* and from consistent histological lesions.

[f] More than 99% of newborns with antibody are not infected.

[g] Antibodies could have been transfused.

strain, yielding about a million organisms per ml in mouse peritoneal exudate or in cell culture, can be used (43, 44). "Accessory factor" is obtained from human serum, or better, from citrated plasma (45) devoid of *Toxoplasma* antibody. We sample freshly drawn, blood-bank blood in citrate-dextrose solution for its suitability. We then separate the plasma and freeze it at −70°C (or −20°C) within 6 hr, usually in 5- or 10-ml amounts, as necessary for a one-day test. In other laboratories, all sera are frozen if they are received within a few hours after drawing; pools of accessory factor are prepared from the sera found to be without *Toxoplasma* antibody. Portions of patient sera to be tested are inactivated at 56°C for 30 min. The test procedures have been outlined (43). Standardization procedures have been worked out by Desmonts (45a), but have not yet been published in detail. A micromodification requiring less serum and accessory factor but an inverted microscope also has been described (46). Sera should be tested undiluted or at 1:2 dilution, progressing in two- or four-fold dilutions, depending on the accuracy required. Titrations should extend to a dilution of 1:1024 in order to avoid "falsely negative" tests attributable to a prozone reaction. Two serum specimens taken at least a week apart should be compared, except in cases of ocular disease, when one specimen is sufficient. Although day-to-day reproducibility is high (47), specimens should be compared in a single day's test.

3. *Serological diagnosis.* In the acute disease, serological diagnosis by means of the dye test or IFAT is based on the demonstration of a four- to eight-fold antibody rise in two to three weeks, reaching a titer of over 1:1000 (Table 2). In the immunosuppressed patient, the antibody response may be slow and not diagnostic and difficult to distinguish from low, stable antibody titers or a remote infection. In such patients, finding of IgM antibody by use of the IFAT indicates newly elaborated antibody and active toxoplasmosis. An additional problem arises from the frequency with which these patients receive blood transfusions; and, since *Toxoplasma* antibodies are present in one-fourth to one-half of the adult population, a patient may receive a quantity of antibody-containing blood resulting in a titer suggesting an early active infection. Because chronic, latent toxoplasmosis is common in the United States, any positive laboratory findings

must be related specifically to the accompanying disease or must be classifiable in a syndrome, such as retinochoroiditis, the relation of which to toxoplasmosis has received statistical validation. Relapse of chronic toxoplasmosis encephalitis is not likely to be accompanied by a significant rise in antibody titer; isolation of the organisms and biopsy of the affected areas is helpful in such patients.

Four serological tests are commonly used. The Sabin and Feldman dye test is the standard reference test (42a, 43, 45). The indirect fluorescent antibody test measures apparently the same antibody as the dye test (35). A positive titer usually appears in the first two weeks after acute infection, with titers rising to levels between 1:1000 and 1:10,000 and remaining at this level for a year or more. Thereafter, titers decline, but in many instances antibody remains for decades, possibly for a lifetime. The interpretation of serological findings is illustrated in Table 2. The indirect hemagglutination test of Jacobs and Lunde (48) shows titers which generally are parallel to those of the dye test. However, they appear about a week later. This test avoids the need for organisms or a fluorescent microscope, but the significance of low titers is controversial. The complement-fixation test, for which several antigens have been prepared (49), shows antibody titers rising about a month after infection or later, with antibodies persisting for five to seven years only, when soluble antigen is used; a negative test does not exclude toxoplasmosis.

4. *Isolation of* Toxoplasma. Blood, sputum, cerebrospinal fluid, brain, liver, muscle, or other tissues, after maceration and suspension in saline, may be inoculated directly into the peritoneal cavity of laboratory mice or hamsters. Isolation in cell culture can be attempted; however, in general, mice and hamsters are more sensitive indicators of infection. *Toxoplasma* in tissues or body fluids usually is stable at 4–10°C, but the inoculation should be performed as soon as possible to avoid undue deterioration of the organisms. Blood should be centrifuged, and the buffy coat is injected into animals; the presence of antibody in the serum or plasma will impair the sensitivity of the isolation procedure.

The amount of tissue to be inoculated can be reduced by digestion (50) by using saline which contains 0.7–1% hydrochloric acid and 0.4–0.5% pepsin (1:10,000), maintaining this suspension for 1.5 hr at 37°C under agitation. Coarse particles are removed by passage through gauze or a tea strainer. The filtrate is centrifuged, and the sediment is washed by resuspension in saline and recentrifugation. The sediment finally is suspended in approximately twice its volume of saline; portions of up to 1 ml are injected intraperitoneally, and portions of up to 0.5 ml are injected subcutaneously into mice or hamsters.

After intraperitoneal inoculation, one can proceed in either of two ways.

a. Peritoneal fluid or suspensions of spleen and lung are subinoculated at four- to six-day intervals and before immunity is effective, in order to obtain successively higher inocula and to increase the likelihood of finding organisms in the peritoneal fluid or on microscopic examination. Any peritoneal fluid obtained is examined for the presence of *Toxoplasma* by staining impression films with Wright's or Giemsa stain (Fig. 4) or with fluorescent antibody. From the animals that die, imprints of organs or sections are made.

b. Animals inoculated by any route are kept for three to four weeks, after which time they are bled from the retroorbital sinus and tested for antibody. The finding of antibody in the inoculated animals and its absence in controls would indicate that *Toxoplasma* is present in the inoculum. Cysts can be found in the brains of such mice (Fig. 5).

Demonstration of parasites in the fluid or tissues of inoculated animals, or the finding of antibody, is evidence that the tissue

Figure 4. Crescentic *Toxoplasma* tachyzoites from the peritoneum of a mouse inoculated four days earlier with infected tissue. These are typical of an acute infection. (Giemsa, × 585) Inset, the organisms as they appear on a thicker imprint.

Figure 5. *Toxoplasma* bradyzoites in a cyst from the brain of a mouse inoculated two months earlier with infected tissue. Cysts are typical of a chronic infection. (Giemsa, × 585)

Figure 6. *Leishmania mexicana* organisms from a chiclero's ulcer were propagated subcutaneously in hamsters. Each organism contains a nucleus and a smaller kinetoplast. (Giemsa, × 585)

Figure 7. *Histoplasma capsulatum*, originally from an immunosuppressed patient. The round-to-ovoid organisms with eccentric nuclei are seen both in a macrophage and free; from the spleen of a hamster. (Giemsa, × 585)

Toxoplasmosis and Pneumocystosis

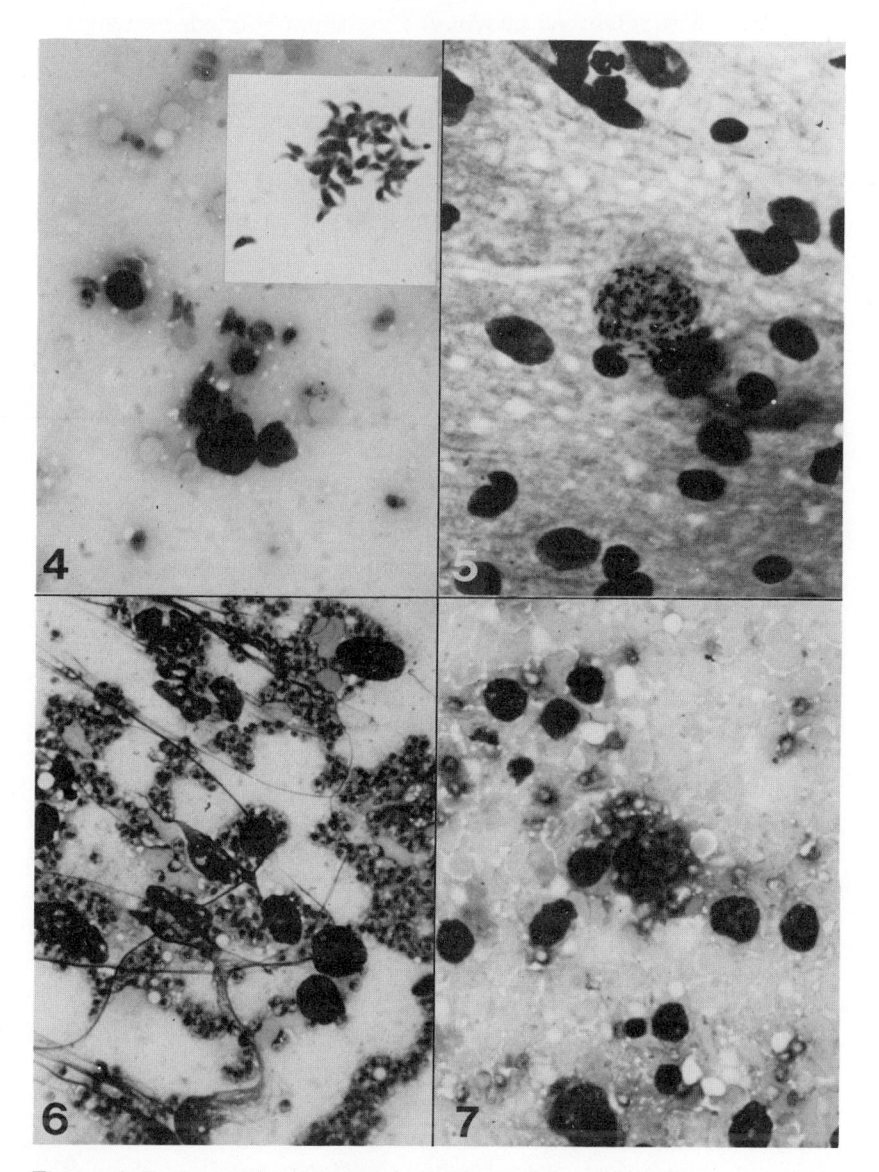

Figures 4–7. Comparison of small organisms on tissue imprints.

inoculated was infected, provided that uninoculated control animals are negative. Although mouse and hamster colonies generally are free from spontaneous toxoplasmosis, laboratory rabbits and guinea pigs have been found on some occasions to be infected (51). One should be cognizant of a common animal parasite, *Encephalitozoon*, which is sometimes mistaken for *Toxoplasma*, and which on repeated passage may give rise to ascites in the third and fourth weeks in mice. On peritoneal imprints, it is ovoid or, sometimes, refractile, and never crescentic; and, in sections, it stains with Goodpasture's carbol-fuchsin method, which leaves *Toxoplasma* unstained. The latter is stained by Giemsa and hematoxylin, which demonstrates *Encephalitozoon* poorly (51, 52). There is no cross-reaction serologically.

5. *Biopsies.* Lymph node biopsies are taken often, and the characteristic histological picture is one of epithelioid reticular cell hyperplasia involving germinal follicles and medullary cords, while necrosis and fibrosis are absent (53, 54). *Toxoplasma* cysts usually are rare and are found only by searching a large number of serial sections. The finding of *Toxoplasma* cysts can be aided by the periodic acid-Schiff stain, whereas tachyzoites of *Toxoplasma* are identified easily with hematoxylin and eosin. Brain biopsy is useful in diagnosing the case of an obscure encephalitis. The diagnosis of toxoplasmosis should be based on finding groups and cysts with accompanying lesions; the finding of *Toxoplasma* cysts without lesions only suggests infection.

6. *Peripheral blood.* Anemia, leukocytosis, or leukopenia may show in peripheral blood. Occasionally, atypical lymphocytes are seen, as have been described also in infectious mononucleosis, cytomegalovirus infection, and hepatitis. The heterophile test is negative.

7. *Cerebrospinal fluid.* The protein may be increased and there may be pleocytosis. *Toxoplasma* have been reported on occasion on microscopic examination of stained smears (55).

8. *Cat feces.* Since it has been proven that the infective form of *Toxoplasma* in cat feces is an isosporan oocyst measuring 10 × 12 μ (1, 56), there has been interest in detecting this oocyst to determine the infectivity of cats. Cat feces are floated in 40% sucrose, w/v, with a specific gravity of 1.15, and a drop of the top layer is examined under 100- and 400-× magnification. Care must

be exercised to differentiate the small *Toxoplasma* oocyst from the larger oocysts of *Isospora felis* (about 40 X 30 µ) and *Isospora rivolta* (about 25 X 20 µ). The two isosporas are seen readily at 100 X, where *Toxoplasma* is not recognized easily; however, at 400 X, *Toxoplasma* oocysts can be compared with about two diameters of human red blood cells (2). On the day of fecal shedding, the oocysts may show a single sporoblast, and they successively develop two sporoblasts, two sporocysts, and eight sporozoites. Sporulation is accomplished readily in 2% sulfuric acid or 2% potassium dichromate. A simplified method for flotation, sporulation, and animal inoculation has been described (57).

Mice are given injections of candidate sporulated oocysts after removal of the acid or the dichromate (57), and they can be tested serologically for the development of *Toxoplasma* antibody after three weeks. The two large isosporas do not give rise to the development of *Toxoplasma* antibody in mice. *Toxoplasma* oocysts are shed in cat feces usually for a period of about 10 days, after which the cats develop immunity; on the other hand, *I. felis* and *I. rivolta* are shed for long periods of time, and reinfection is accomplished easily.

9. *Morphological identification of* Toxoplasma. Tachyzoites are recognized on smears stained with Wright's or Giemsa as crescentic (toxon: bow, arc) bodies, 4–6 µ long and 2–3 µ wide, with a paracentral nucleus (Fig. 4). In sections, they are demonstrated easily by hematoxylin as groups of generally intracellular organisms of uniform size. They sometimes appear spherical, since only the nuclei are stained well (Fig. 9). On true lateral view, their elongate appearance can be discerned with Giemsa or other cytoplasmic stains. Proliferative tachyzoites usually give rise to destruction of individual cells, with accompanying inflammation. The term "pseudocyst" has lost all usefulness, since it has been used sometimes for groups of tachyzoites and at other times to designate cysts.

10. *Cysts.* These usually are intact and not accompanied by inflammation. They vary in size from 20 to over 200 µ. They are found in "normal" individuals as well as in patients with clinical toxoplasmosis. Only by identifying cyst-associated lesions and tachyzoites can one relate *Toxoplasma* to the disease observed. The intracystic bradyzoites store glycogen. Staining with periodic

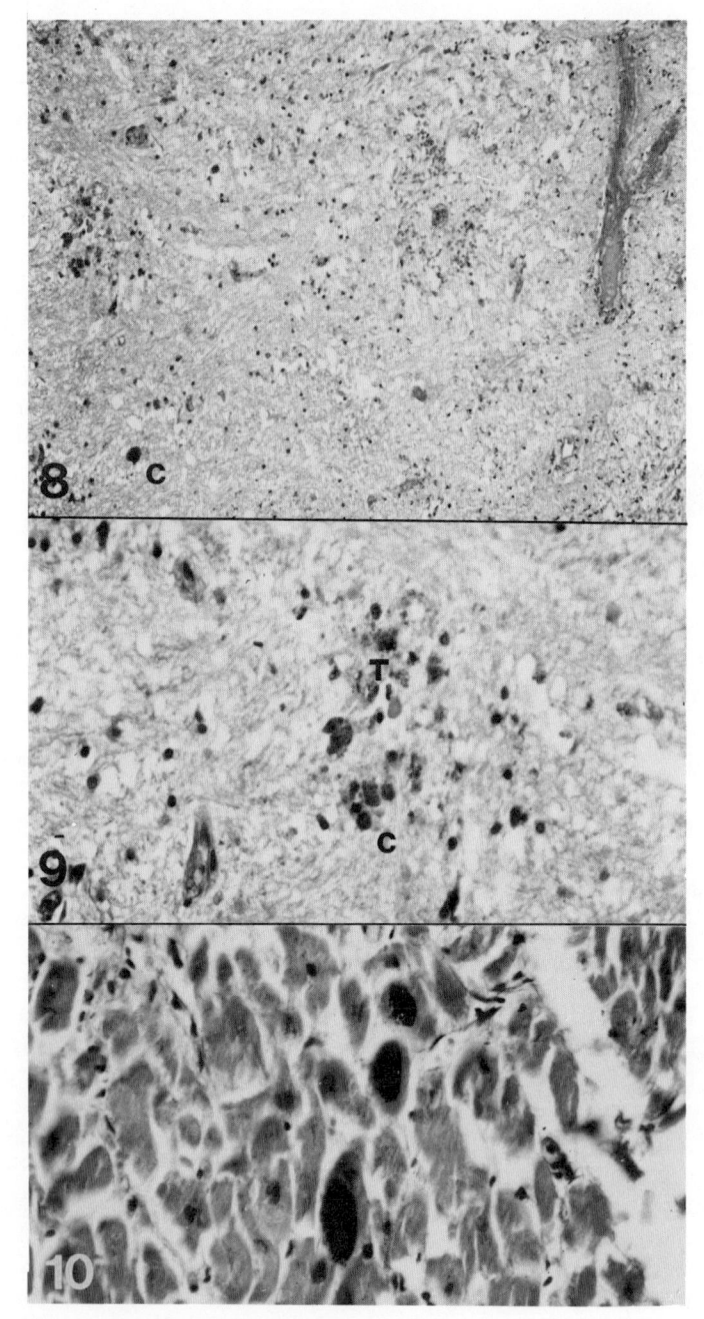

Figures 8–10. Chronic and relapsing toxoplasmosis as shown in tissue sections.

acid-Schiff, followed by hematoxylin, aids in recognition of cysts (Fig. 10). Bradyzoites measure about 7 × 2 μ. The cyst wall can be stained distinctively with the periodic acid-Schiff method (not prevented by diastase) and with silver, as used in Wilder's and Gordon-Sweet's reticulum techniques, and in Bodian's, and in some impregnations for glia. Cysts are spherical in the brain and elongate in muscle fibers (Figs. 9, 10). As cyst rupture gives rise to tissue necrosis from the associated hypersensitivity, and the liberated bradyzoites usually are destroyed, lesions may be seen without accompanying *Toxoplasma*.

11. *Oocysts.* These measure about 10 × 12 μ and are of isosporan type, containing two sporocysts, each with four sporozoites (Fig. 1). The stages in the cat gut resemble those of other coccidia, but can be differentiated from *I. felis* and *I. rivolta* of cats (58). Oocysts as well as tachyzoites accompanying the stages in the cat gut are identified best by their infectivity to mice, as described for the examination of cat feces (above).

The small size and simple organization of *Toxoplasma* present difficulties in distinguishing it from *Sarcocystis* and *Encephalitozoon (Nosema)*, also found in humans, from *Besnoitia*, found in animals, and from oval yeasts, occasionally found as contaminants. Specially stained sections and/or fluorescent and electron microscopy may aid differentiation. In fresh preparations, elongate, motile bradyzoites released from crushed cysts are characteristic of *Toxoplasma, Sarcocystis,* and *Besnoitia*. Tissue forms of *Trypanosoma cruzi* and *Leishmania* (Fig. 6) are distinguished by a kinetoplast and a parabasal body which *Toxoplasma* lacks. Great

---

Figure 8. Toxoplasmic encephalitis from a patient with Hodgkin's disease treated with cortisone, nitrogen mustard, and radiation. The border of a large area of tissue necrosis is shown (lower center and right), with groups and cysts of *Toxoplasma* at the periphery. (Hematoxylin and eosin, × 105)

Figure 9. Transitional area from border of necrosis (left center of Fig. 8), showing free tachyzoites and groups (T), as well as cysts (C) of *Toxoplasma*. (Hematoxylin and eosin, × 265) (Material courtesy of Dr. Javier Arias-Stella)

Figure 10. Three elongate *Toxoplasma* cysts in myocardium of a patient with an approximate 75-day history of toxoplasmosis. The bradyzoites in the cyst stain intensely with the periodic acid-Schiff technique. Use of this staining method facilitates searching for cysts under the scanning and low-power objective. (PAS hematoxylin, × 265) (Material courtesy of Dr. E. H. Kass)

caution is advised when any identification is made on the basis of fresh, nonpermanent preparations, since pollen grains and fungal spores have given rise to misidentifications in the past (59). A number of small organisms found in humans are compared in Figures 6 and 7, and those in animals have been treated elsewhere (6, 52).

E. Treatment

The multiplication of tachyzoites can be inhibited by sulfadiazine and pyrimethamine (Daraprim). Treatment is aimed at symptoms of disease and is continued until they abate and immunity becomes effective. Occasionally, chemotherapy is used prophylactically in sero-positive individuals, for example, to protect the fetus of a woman who acquires *Toxoplasma* antibody during pregnancy, or to prevent relapse in a patient treated with pharmacological doses of corticosteroids and cytostatic agents. However, in general, antibody does not indicate disease or the need for treatment.

The usual treatment dose is 0.5 g of sulfadiazine and 25 mg of pyrimethamine, four times per day. Since it takes a few days until an adequate tissue level of pyrimethamine is reached, 25 mg may be given three times daily for the first three days of treatment (60). These drugs act synergistically in sequential steps of folinic acid synthesis. They are effective against proliferating tachyzoites and bradyzoites but not against resting cysts (Table 3).

Side-effects of the drugs include thrombocytopenia and leukopenia, which should be checked for twice weekly, anorexia, and stomatitis. These can be counteracted by folinic acid (leucovorin calcium), the inhibited product, which can be incorporated into the biosynthetic pathway by man but not by the parasite. Hence, one can combat the side-effects of the drugs with leucovorin without impairing their chemotherapeutic effects; yeast further augments this effect (61) (Figs. 19 and 20).

The possible teratogenic effects of the antimicrobic combination are well recognized and mimic those of methotrexate (62, 63). For the management of toxoplasmosis in pregnancy, the newborn, and retinochoroiditis, a more detailed publication should be consulted (7).

Table 3. Chemotherapy of toxoplasmosis and pneumocystosis

Daily drug dose	First three days of treatment	Fourth day onward
Adults		
Pyrimethamine	75 mg	25 mg
Sulfadiazine[a]	500 mg 4 times daily	500 mg 4 times daily
Antagonists[b]		
Folinic acid (leucovorin)		2–10 mg
Baker's yeast		5–10 g
Children		
Pyrimethamine[c]	2 mg/kg	1 mg/kg
Sulfadiazine	25 mg/kg 4 times daily	25 mg/kg 4 times daily
Antagonists[d]		
Folinic acid (leucovorin)	1 mg	1 mg
Baker's yeast	100 mg	100 mg

[a] Sulfamerazine, sulfamethazine, sulfalene, and sulfadoxine may be substituted.

[b] If platelet counts are below 100,000 per mm^3, or prophylactically if twice weekly platelet counts are not feasible. Antagonists are given concomitantly with treatment.

[c] An intravenous form of pyrimethamine may become available, facilitating administration to the newborn (Burroughs Wellcome Co.).

[d] Antagonists may be administered prophylactically and simultaneously with the treatment to avoid the need for frequent bloodletting.

Certain other drugs have shown slight-to-moderate antitoxoplasmic activity in animals or humans, but are not recommended now. Lincomycin and analogs have shown a promising effect in mice (64).

Corticosteroids are used sometimes to control the symptoms of hypersensitivity in patients with uveitis caused by *Toxoplasma* and other agents. If there is a delay between cyst rupture and the appearance of hypercorticism and if immunity is at a high level, such treatment may be beneficial. However, cyst rupture in a patient already hypercorticoid may not permit immunity to kill all the liberated bradyzoites, and an actively progressive lesion may result. When corticoids are employed to treat a neoplasm or to support an organ transplant, relapse of toxoplasmosis is also a possibility. For this reason, in patients with *Toxoplasma* antibody, the antimicrobic sulfadiazine and pyrimethamine should be administered whenever the corticoids are used in high doses for prolonged periods, either for the depression of delayed hypersensitivity, against tumors, or to inhibit transplant rejection, since cellular immunity also may be impaired. Contrary to the often-cited interpretation of Shewell and Long (65), I consider humans to be highly corticoid sensitive. The cortisone dose of 50 mg per kg of body weight per day, which was used by these authors (65) to classify laboratory animals as either sensitive or resistant, would be equivalent to 3.5 g of cortisone for a 70-kg adult, or about 140 replacement doses for an Addisonian patient. This is an almost astronomical dose for humans, in whom usually 10–40 replacement doses are used to achieve pharmacological effects, and in whom 15 replacement doses have been shown to be immunosuppressive even in humans not compromised by underlying disease (66).

Cytostatic agents such as cyclophosphamide, antilymphocyte serum, and, to a lesser degree, aminopterin, chlorambucil, and total-body irradiation, are immunodepressive in experimental toxoplasmosis and probably in man (67–69). The antimicrobic effect of sulfadiazine and pyrimethamine is direct and need not be increased in the compromised host. However, the antimicrobic effect should be extended somewhat beyond the period of drug-induced immunosuppression to permit host immunity to recover. Since none of the available drugs will kill *Toxoplasma*, we must depend on a reasonably intact immune system to keep chronic, latent toxoplasmosis from becoming a disease.

F. Prevention

Toxoplasma can be acquired by the ingestion of oocysts and cysts and, occasionally, by transfer of tachyzoites. The principal situations to be scrutinized are contacts with cats and soil and handling or ingestion of raw or undercooked meat.

1. *Oocysts.* These are shed in cat feces and deposited in soil, litter pans, or elsewhere. These oocysts sporulate usually in one to five days at temperatures of over 70°F and with access to oxygen, and then are infectious. Winter temperatures with intermittent freezing delay sporulation but do not kill the oocysts (70a). Humans can become infected from soil contaminated by cat feces, which become unrecognizable after two weeks underground. Oocysts may remain viable in soil for weeks and months. Inadequately cleaned litter pans in which cats defecate are another possible source of infection. And, of course, so are the cats themselves, because when a million oocysts are shed for several days, it is possible to get a few in the fur. Hands should be washed after contact with cats and potentially contaminated soil, especially before eating. Infection of cats can be prevented by feeding only canned, cooked, or dry food and by restraining cats from hunting. Details on the shedding of oocysts by cats and the viability of oocysts have been presented (2).

2. *Cysts.* These are present in the meat of sheep, pigs, and cattle. Bradyzoites may enter humans through cuts or may be inoculated inadvertently when a person rubs his eyes or puts his fingers into the mouth. Some people eat raw meat as a delicacy, or as "health food," and the practice of eating rare meat is widespread. Adequate heating of meat to over 65°C (150°F) throughout is essential to avoid the ingestion of viable *Toxoplasma*. Freezing kills many organisms, but often is not sufficient to eradicate infection.

A rare mode of transmission is the transplacental one, in which a woman who becomes infected during or just before pregnancy transfers the tachyzoites to her infant in utero. As the intrauterine and neonatal infections are likely to be especially damaging, precautions about cats, soil, and meat apply to pregnant women in particular. Statistical considerations on the frequency of intrauterine transmission have been presented (70).

III. Pneumocystosis

Pneumocystis is an extracellular protozoan or fungus (71). It has been described as growing in the pulmonary alveoli of humans, rats (*Pneumocystis carinii*), rabbits, dogs, pigs, and other animals. Although transmission from animals to man has been suspected, there is no positive evidence of such spread, and some observations concerning species specificity have been presented (66). The cycle, as seen by electron microscopy in the alveoli of rats, consists of trophozoites, precysts, and cysts. The trophozoites measure 1–2 μ, with round or oval bodies and a smooth cell membrane, and larger, up to 5 μ. They are irregular parasites which undergo binary fission, with tubular extensions or filopodia. The precyst is a transitional stage, and the cysts are 4–6 μ in diameter, with three-layered membrane walls containing up to eight intracystic organisms (71). The cycle in humans appears to be similar (72). Crescentic, collapsed cysts devoid of interior organisms have also been described.

Although we may not know the entire cycle, that which is known suggests transmission of the cyst stages by direct contact, such as by kissing and by fomites. Our fragmentary knowledge of the infection in man has been supplemented by study of the infection in rats. In most colonies, and even in many so-called "specific pathogen-free" strains of rats, every animal appears to be infected, although subclinically. This latent infection develops into disease after a four- to six-week period of hypercorticism or the administration of cyclophosphamide (66). Prior to this time, it is difficult to make a diagnosis. In man, the incubation period is also long; however, available evidence from nursery infections and hospital epidemics indicates that the chronic carrier state is rare. For example, *Pneumocystis* disease developed in 10 out of 73 immunosuppressed transplant patients at Colorado General Hospital, but in none of 34 patients at the Denver Veteran's Hospital ($p < 0.03$). The hospitals are located within a block of each other and all patients were treated by the same surgical and medical teams (73).

Although it grows extracellularly, the organism has not yet been cultivated on artificial media. Its growth requisites are unknown.

As mentioned earlier, *Pneumocystis* grows quite slowly, irrespective of whether immunosuppressive treatment is given to an immune adult rat or a young rat recently infected. It takes about six weeks or longer to produce pulmonary fillings and death from *Pneumocystis*.

The numerous, tubular, filopodial projections which extend from the trophozoites and, to a lesser degree, from the cysts, attach to the cytoplasmic processes of alveolar pneumocytes and so anchor the parasites to the alveolar walls. This provides a plausible explanation for the deficient expectoration of the parasites and for the fact that alveoli may be filled with masses of *Pneumocystis* and the respiratory bronchus may be empty (Figs. 13 and 14). Few organisms are present ordinarily in sputum. However, I have seen disengagement and death of organisms in an atelectatic lobe of a rat lung, whereas, in the aereated lobes, the *Pneumocystis* were proliferating. In the immunosuppressed hypercorticoid rat with pneumocystosis, there is a minimal phagocytosis of living organisms. However, phagocytosis becomes active when corticosteroids are withdrawn, or when the infection is treated with sulfadiazine and pyrimethamine, or with pentamidine, even though the hypercorticism is maintained. This indicates that the immunological deficiency applies only to how the viable organisms are disposed of.

A. Infection versus Disease

Most *Pneumocystis* infections in man probably are asymptomatic and only a few give rise to disease. Pneumocystosis is the disease state resulting from alveolar filling with *Pneumocystis*, leading to progressive dyspnea with oxygen desaturation of the blood and thus suggesting an alveolar-capillary block. The disease states can be classified by their underlying pathogenic causes and other characteristics:

1. Interstitial plasma-cell pneumonia, usually in premature, institutionalized, and nutritionally deficient children;
2. Interstitial plasma-cell and mononuclear pneumonia in infants with congenital rubella;

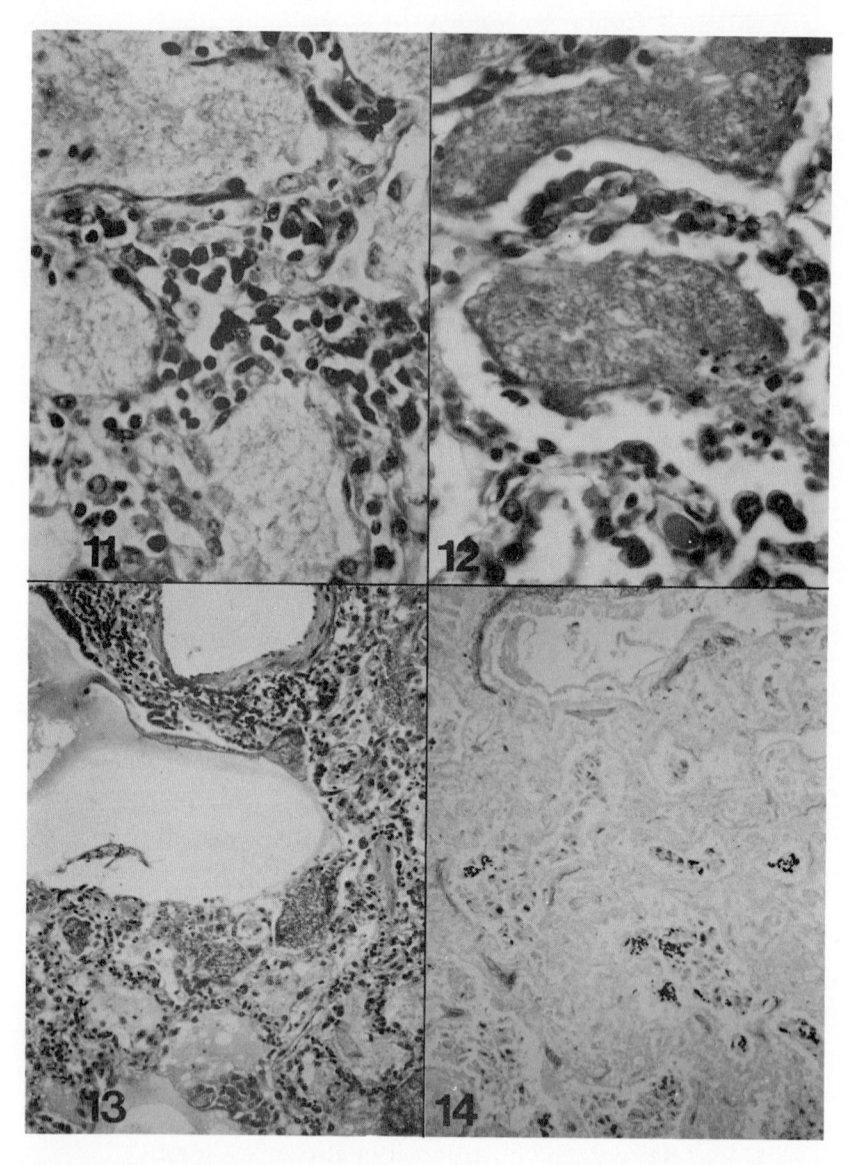

Figures 11–14. Pneumocystosis; comparison of staining methods for sections.

3. Alveolar filling, in children with hypo- or dysgammaglobulinemia, cellular and combined immuno-deficiency;
4. Familial pneumocystosis;
5. Alveolar filling, in recipients of organ transplants or in patients with nonneoplastic disease treated with high doses of immunosuppressive agents;
6. Alveolar filling, in patients with lymphoreticular neoplasms or leukemias treated with corticosteroids and cytostatic agents;
7. Alveolar filling—unknown predisposition;
8. Congenital pneumocystosis;
9. Extrapulmonary pneumocystosis;
10. Subclinical *Pneumocystis* infection.

A subclinical *Pneumocystis* infection is found occasionally at autopsy because of one of the above causes, and it is postulated also to occur as an acute infection and as a chronic carrier state. Furthermore, it is postulated that *Pneumocystis* is a normal saprophyte of man, giving rise to disease only exceptionally in immunodeficient hosts. As mentioned, infection is probably by contact

---

Figure 11. Interstitial plasma-cell pneumonia, accompanying alveolar filling with *Pneumocystis*. The plasma cells and lymphocytes are present almost entirely interstitially, and the "foamy" zoogloeal masses in the alveoli are associated only rarely with inflammatory cells. In sections, Giemsa stains *Pneumocystis* faintly. (Giemsa, × 365) (Slide Courtesy of Dr. Otto Jirovec)

Figures 12–13. Alveolar filling with *Pneumocystis* in a patient with malignant lymphoma, treated with corticosteroids. There is little interstitial infiltration; however, a few macrophages are commonly associated with the organisms.

Figure 12. With this hematoxylin and eosin stain, the nuclei and the foamy proteinaceous material are well demonstrated. (× 365)

Figure 13. In this slide stained with periodic acid-Schiff technique, the "foamy" alveolar masses (center) are well differentiated from edema fluid (bottom), even at × 240. The masses of organisms stick to the alveoli and are not discharged into the respiratory bronchiole (left and center). See also Fig. 15.

Figure 14. *Pneumocystis* in a patient with acute lymphocytic leukemia. Section is impregnated according to Grocott's methenamine silver method, which demonstrates cysts of *Pneumocystis* in several alveoli even at low magnification (× 95). Again, the bronchus (top) is free of organisms.

with respiratory secretions, judging from the nursing home epidemics (73, 74), and from infection studies in rats (66, 75).

B. Interstitial Plasma-Cell Pneumonia

This syndrome was common at about the end of World War II in institutions in several European countries in which premature children, foundlings, or orphans were nursed. This situation has been found more recently in Canada (76), Iran (77), Korea (78), and Spain (79). These infants were three to five months old and generally malnourished, especially with regard to protein, probably accounting for their inability to develop an effective immunity. In some of these infants, the slow weight gain was the reason for their prolonged hospitalization, and together with others who were orphans, institutionalization provided ample opportunity for infection by contact. Nutritional supplementation caused a reduction of incidence and severity of illness (80), although there was evidence of continuing subclinical infection.

Clinical symptoms are failure to gain weight, dyspnea, tachypnea, cough, cyanosis, and often fever. Radiographically, there is a uniform density, sometimes more marked in the hilar areas, and occasionally, atelectasis. Serologically, the plasma IgM levels were increased, but IgA and IgG levels were low. Complement-fixation tests have given variable results.

At postmortem examination, the interstitial plasma-cell infiltrate is prominent (Fig. 11). The organisms are present in the alveoli, often mixed with fibrin deposits, and with notably deficient intraalveolar cellular reaction. The presence of antibody, coating *Pneumocystis*, has been shown, as has a relative deficiency in complement deposits (81). This presence suggested to these authors that the immunodeficiency was in the expressor arm of the immune response, in a deficiency of complement rather than of antibody. However, Dutz (80) and collaborators, who found depressed plasma levels of IgA and IgG, attribute the immunodeficiency to these findings.

C. Interstitial Plasma-Cell and Mononuclear Pneumonia in Infants with Congenital Rubella

Although I know of only one published case (82) and one studied by myself (Kansas University Medical Center, case 5400), the pathogenesis of this category appears distinct. However, in neither of these cases were serum electrophoretic patterns available. Moderate numbers of plasma cells are represented in the mixed lymphocytic and mononuclear exudate which infiltrates the alveolar walls, causing marked thickening. Both children were born at or near term weighing 2500 g, and although both failed to gain weight, the infants were not as malnourished as those of the previous group. Our patient had a lenticular opacity and biventricular cardiac hypertrophy and ferrocalcinosis of the brain. The thymus weighed only 6 g. In the published case, rubella was isolated from heart, lungs, and bone. Both children still had a patent ductus arteriosus at three and four months, respectively; and the period from onset of symptoms of fever and pneumonia until death was 10 days.

D. Pneumocystosis of Children with Hypogammaglobulinemia and Dysgammaglobulinemia, Cellular and Combined Immunodeficiency

These are sporadic cases, usually becoming apparent clinically by cough, dyspnea, and repeated pulmonary infection in the first few months of life. Some of the infants were diagnosed as agammaglobulinemic (83) or as hypogammaglobulinemic with absence of plasma cells (84), as thymic alymphoplasic (Swiss type of agammaglobulinemia), as histiocytic (72), or as hypogammaglobulinemic of unspecified type. With refinement in diagnosis of primary immunodeficiency diseases, pneumocystosis may be found limited to only certain categories, as indicated by Burke and Good (83a).

Physical examination indicates difficult breathing, cyanosis, tachypnea, and sometimes evidence of other infection. Radiological findings include diffuse pulmonary infiltrates, occasionally with atelectasis and pulmonary and subcutaneous emphysema.

Laboratory findings showed low or absent gammaglobulin and, when studied, decrease or absence of IgA, IgM, and/or IgG.

Histologically, there is alveolar filling with *Pneumocystis;* plasma cells are absent, and lymphocytes or small mononuclear cells usually are present together with enlarged pneumocytes. Cytomegalovirus infection also may be present (85).

E. Familial Pneumocystosis

Clinically, this is a variant of the hypogammaglobulinemic group, with the apparent genetic factor's providing only an additional means of classification. In some instances, only IgA and IgM are decreased or absent; in others, IgG also is decreased or absent. Five sibling pairs have been reviewed, and one has been added recently (86). Additional reviews have been published by Becroft and Costello (87) and by Barnett et al. (88), and an interesting variant, with *Pneumocystis* in one sibling and progressive vaccinia in the other, has been published by Allibone, Goldie, and Marmion (89).

Clinical, radiological, and postmortem findings are similar to those in the previous group.

A familial occurrence in husband and wife, who died, and a daughter, who recovered, also has been reported (90). In June, the daughter developed breathing difficulty, fluctuating fever, malaise, and dry cough, with diffuse pulmonary densities on X-ray. Apparently, she recovered in August. The mother developed respiratory symptoms early in August and died in September. The father had been treated with corticosteroids and methotrexate for acute lymphatic leukemia; he developed respiratory symptoms at the end of August and died in September.

On postmortem examination, the father's lungs showed extensive involvement with *Pneumocystis*, accompanied by plasma cells; the bone marrow appeared normal, without evidence of leukemia. The mother's lungs showed slight pneumocystosis with plasma cells. No specific diagnosis was attempted in the daughter. One may wonder whether she represents the exceptional immunocompetent patient in whom the disease became manifest temporarily after a large inoculum.

F. Pneumocystosis Associated with Hypercorticism for Treatment of Nonneoplastic Disease

This group is of special interest, inasmuch as the disease is entirely treatment-related and therefore to be avoided. Also, this pathogenesis is investigated most easily in humans because there is no underlying immunodeficiency. The largest groups studied include 11 patients with renal transplants, reported by Rifkind et al. (73), three patients with renal or cardiac transplants and three with systemic lupus erythematosus, reported by Gentry, Ruskin, and Remington (91), and eight transplant patients who were mentioned from among 75 receiving pentamidine from Western, Perera, and Schultz (92).

Symptoms began with shortness of breath and nonproductive cough; although fever was common, it was "low-grade," probably in part because of hypercorticism. When illness progressed, there appeared tachypnea, cyanosis, and an increase of fever. Respiratory distress became marked. There were generally only a few moist rales and rhonchi, and there was diminution of breath sounds. Chest films demonstrated bilateral infiltrates, beginning in the hili and spreading to involve the entire lung field. There was no pleural reaction or hilar lymph node enlargement (73).

Prednisone was given to all these transplant patients, usually in doses of 40 mg per day or greater. Such pharmacological doses can be compared to 5.0 mg per day, which is the replacement dose for a patient with Addison's disease. The patients who died with *Pneumocystis* pneumonia received such doses of prednisone for a median duration of 113 days, as compared with an average duration of 49 days for all 51 fatal cases (comprising deaths after renal transplants from many causes) and 57 days from the total group of 107 transplant patients. *Pneumocystis* pneumonia occurred 69–599 days after transplantation and lasted 8–66 days before death of the patient. All of these patients also were treated with 75–200 mg of azathioprine per day (73).

Three patients with lupus erythematosus were treated with about 60 mg of prednisone for three, five, and seven years, accompanied either by nitrogen mustard for one month, or cyclophosphamide for one month and two years, respectively (91, 93).

Cytomegalovirus infection accompanied *Pneumocystis* pneumonia most frequently. It was present in 7 out of 10 *Pneumocystis* patients in Rifkind's series (73), compared to 53% in the total transplanted group. In addition, it was present in four out of six patients of Gentry's series (91).

The immunity-depressing dose of corticosteroids is of interest when one wishes to determine the risk levels in patients who are not otherwise immunosuppressed. Estimation of this dose level is aided by a series of patients studied by Kossell (94) and by Muller (95). *Pneumocystis* pneumonia appeared in children after an incubation period of two to three months when 3 mg of prednisone per kg of body weight were given orally. On the basis of 5 mg as a replacement dose for a 70-kg adult, the 3 mg per kg would seem to equal 40 such doses. In children, however, only the intramuscular administration can be related to the adult dose (96). The cortisol secretion rate in normal infants, children, and adults has been determined to be 12 ± 2 mg per m^2 per day (97). In children, by applying the surface area correction, the oral dose of prednisone appears to correspond to 10–20 replacement doses. In Rifkind's series (73), the dose was variable during the treatment of renal transplant rejection, and averaged 48 mg per day at the onset of pneumonia, or approximately 10 replacement doses. In view of the long incubation period until alveolar filling becomes symptomatic, the prior corticoid dose is also important. In general, it was higher, especially in those patients who developed pneumonia relatively soon after transplantation (median, 132 days; mean, 200 days).

Appearance of pneumonia is influenced also by the rapid reduction of the corticoid dose. Following transplantation, patients often receive 40 replacement doses (200 mg of prednisone) for one or two weeks, and this is tapered as indicated by renal function. In several such patients, a "transplantation pneumonia" appeared when the prednisone dose was lowered to 1 mg per kg of body weight per day, or about 14 replacement doses (98). This suggests that the clinical symptoms of pneumocystosis were masked by the higher corticoid dose, and when the corticoid dose was lowered and the inflammation reappeared, the inflammatory exudate was added to the *Pneumocystis* filling of the alveoli, increasing the alveolar-capillary block. Although most of the patients recovered and although both *Pneumocystis* and cytomegalovirus were found, in only one patient who died (98), this interpretation receives support by the observation of Kossell (94), who also observed that patients became sick, not at the time of the maximal dose, but when the dose was reduced.

In the rat model of pneumocystosis, 50 mg of cortisone acetate were given weekly to 200-mg rats, amounting to 35 mg per kg of body weight per day (66). Since rats secrete corticosterone, and there is no corticoid requirement if additional salt is given, it is not possible to compute the cortisone equivalent, but this dose appears to be at least 100 times the antiinflammatory equivalent of the corticosterone secreted.

For the development of clinical pneumocystosis, an exogenous source of infection appears to be important, as are the corticoid species, the dose (best expressed in replacement equivalents for a patient with Addisonian disease), the duration of hypercorticism, and the speed of tapering. As mentioned earlier, Rifkind et al. (73) noted a significant difference in the occurrence of *Pneumocystis* pneumonia, depending on the hospital in which the patients were cared for. Vivell (99) traced the epidemic to certain carriers. Although we have at present no means to identify these presumed sources of infection, it should be reemphasized that in human *Pneumocystis* infection, the carrier state appears to be rare, and that the observation from rats where the carrier state is the rule should not be applied to man (66). The statement that the carrier state in children might be as high as 40% (100) probably applied to an orphanage-foundling home population in Shiraz, Iran; Dutz (80) refers to the carrier state as 20%.

G. Pneumocystosis in Patients with Lymphoreticular Neoplasms or Leukemias Treated with Corticosteroids and Cytostatic Agents

This grouping represents the largest in the U. S. at present. In the pentamidine study (92), it accounted for 43 out of 75 patients; in the 1972 study by Gentry et al. (91), it accounted for 16 out of 24. This group accounted for 33 out of 40 patients with diffuse interstitial pneumonia, about 40% of which was due to *Pneumocystis* (101). In addition, several multi-case reports of

Pneumocystis associated with lymphoreticular disease have appeared (102–105).

Although a few instances of *Pneumocystis* have been reported from untreated patients with lymphoreticular neoplasms or leukemia (106) and during leukemia in remission (90), it appears that the antitumor treatment accounts for the majority of the cases. Corticosteroid agents were used in 14 out of 16 of Gentry's cases (91), in 11 out of 12 of Esterly's (101), and in all of the leukemia and Hodgkin's treatment protocols (103, 107). In the few patients not receiving corticosteroids, cyclophosphamide, which in rats causes relapse of *Pneumocystis* by itself, or chlorambucil, which potentiates corticosteroids, was given. Because several drugs often are employed and the patient already may be immunosuppressed by primary illness, the *Pneumocystis* pneumonia is often more severe in this patient group. In addition, the frequency of bacterial, fungal, and viral infections adds to the seriousness of the respiratory disease condition.

Signs and symptoms consist of fever, a dry cough, progressive dyspnea, and hyperpnea, with bronchial or bronchovesicular breath sounds and minimal rales and rhonchi. The roentgenogram showed diffuse or patchy interstitial pneumonia.

Histologically, the accumulation of *Pneumocystis* is associated more frequently with hyaline membranes, prominence of alveolar septal cells, and luminal macrophages. Frequently, it is associated with fibroblastic proliferation with organizing pneumonia, and, occasionally, it is associated with frank pulmonary fibrosis (108) (Figs 12–14).

For practical purposes, the infection should be regarded also as exogenously acquired and iatrogenous, in the sense that treatment of the underlying disease predisposes the patient to develop pneumocystosis. The clinical problem is how to adjust treatment so that the patient does not suffer more from infection than from the underlying malignancy.

H. Pneumocystosis without Known Predisposing Conditions

There are relatively few patients in this category. A patient was described by McMillan (109) as a Japanese woman, aged 60, with fatal inclusion disease pneumonia, characterized by breathing difficulty for seven weeks and accompanied by pneumocystosis. Another example, a 49-year-old Negro with cough lasting three months and who died after 20 days, had a plasma cellular pneumonia infiltrate accompanying *Pneumocystis* and hyaline membranes (110).

I. Congenital Pneumocystosis

Four such probable instances have been described: one by Pavlika (111) in a stillborn baby and another by Post et al. (77) in a baby that died seven days after delivery (case 6), and two in newborns with respiratory insufficiency who died after seven days, described by Abioye (112) and Bazaz et al. (112a). However, a patient who was reported by Montoya (113) and of whom I had the opportunity to examine the sections, could not be confirmed.

If not based on error or mix-up, the identification of apparent transplacental transmission of *Pneumocystis* is surprising.

J. Disseminated Pneumocystosis

Extrapulmonary pneumocystosis is another rarity; however, it is less subject to misinterpretation or error than is congenital pneumocystosis. Zandanell (114) reported isolated organisms in extrapulmonary locations. At least three reports of extensive accumulations of *Pneumocystis* exist. Jarnum et al. (115) observed a 54-year-old man with extensive weakness for one year and marked albumin turnover with a serum albumin level of only 0.2 g per 100 ml. *Pneumocystis* was diagnosed at lobectomy, and the patient died five months later, with *Pneumocystis* accumulation in liver, spleen, lymph node, and bone marrow. Barnett et al. (88) reported three patients with lymph node involvement, including one with splenic *Pneumocystis* accumulation in a 16-month-old baby with diminished IgG and IgA and increased levels of IgM. Awen and Baltzan (116) described generalized dissemination to lungs, liver, pancreas, kidney homograft, and hematopoietic bone marrow in a 54-year-old renal transplant recipient. He had been treated with prednisone equivalent in amounts of 80—400 mg per day for one week, 60—80 mg for the second week, 40—60 mg until the fourth week, and 20 mg by the end of the sixth week, accompanied by 150 mg of azathioprine per day. The prednisone equivalent was increased to 40 mg per day on the 86th day and was decreased to 20 mg per day on the 100th day. The patient became febrile and hypoxic on the 118th day and died on the 120th day. There was intravascular invasion by *Pneumocystis*, with the extrapulmonary dissemination mentioned above. The identity of the organism was supported by electron micrographs and methenamine silver staining. LeGolvan and Heidelberger described disseminated, chronic pneumocystosis with granulomas and necrosis in an immunoglobulin-deficient 4-year-old boy (116a).

K. Laboratory Diagnosis

1. *Serological tests.* Complement-fixing antigens have been prepared from the lungs of children with plasma-cell pneumonia and have been used generally in qualitative tests (99). Antibodies were found sporadically in the first week of illness, and more regularly in the second and third weeks, and also in some patient contacts (117). Dutz (80) states that the test becomes positive six to eight weeks after the disease. These tests were considered specific for infection, not only for disease, and if so, they appear to lack some sensitivity. Vivell (99) detected antibody in sera from North American patients, but Goetz (118) did not, and believed that there might be antigenic differences between European and North American strains of *Pneumocystis*. Rifkind et al. (73), using two types of antigens, found the complement-fixation test unsuccessful in demonstrating antibodies, and speculated that in the immunosuppressed patient, no antibody was developed. Since a majority of patients with *Pneumocystis* disease in this country are immunosuppressed, other tests have been investigated.

2. *Fluorescent-antibody tests.* These tests have been devised to search for antibody in the sera of patients and to identify orga-

nisms or antibody precipitates in the lungs. Norman and Kagan (119) reviewed previous findings and described the preparation of an antigen composed of isolated *Pneumocystis* organisms which are fixed on slides, dried, frozen, and used for an indirect fluorescent-antibody test. Antibody was found in only 44% of confirmed infections, in 14% of patient contacts, and in none of 50 healthy, young adults. The positive titers were not high and did not exceed 1:40 or 1:80 in the majority of cases. The authors state that controls from immunosuppressed patients without indication of *Pneumocystis* are needed. The test appears to be specific; the low sensitivity may relate to either the patients' immunosuppressed state or a deficiency in the test.

3. *Demonstration of* Pneumocystis. This has been attempted from the sputum, open lung biopsy, needle biopsy of the lung, and endobronchial brushing. *Sputum examination* was perhaps most successful in the hands of Le Tan-Vihn, Vu Trien-Dong, and Solonar (120), who devised an aspirator for obtaining expectorated material from the larynx and staining it with Gram-Weigert stain. These preparations were searched carefully, and the patient was not regarded as negative until 15 negative tests had been obtained. The success of this method apparently lies in the painstaking effort exerted by these experienced workers. In routine testing, or when tests are performed only from time to time, this method is rarely successful (Fig. 16). However, staining with methenamine silver or with the method of Chalvardjian and Grawe (121) does facilitate recognition of the organisms if they are present (Figs. 14 and 15).

An *open lung biopsy* is preferred by some for best control of surgical biopsy procedures, although it carries with it a greater morbidity [see, for example, Smith and Gaspar (122)]. The material obtained can be used for impression films to be stained with either silver or Giesma methods (Fig. 17) or for permanent sections.

Needle aspiration has been used by many with relatively few complications; see, for example, DeVita et al. (123). The material obtained may be used for either impression films or sections.

Endobronchial brush biopsy has been used successfully to obtain alveolar material for diagnosis (124). *Pneumocystis* was identified by means of 11 brushings in 10 patients, and it was missed in

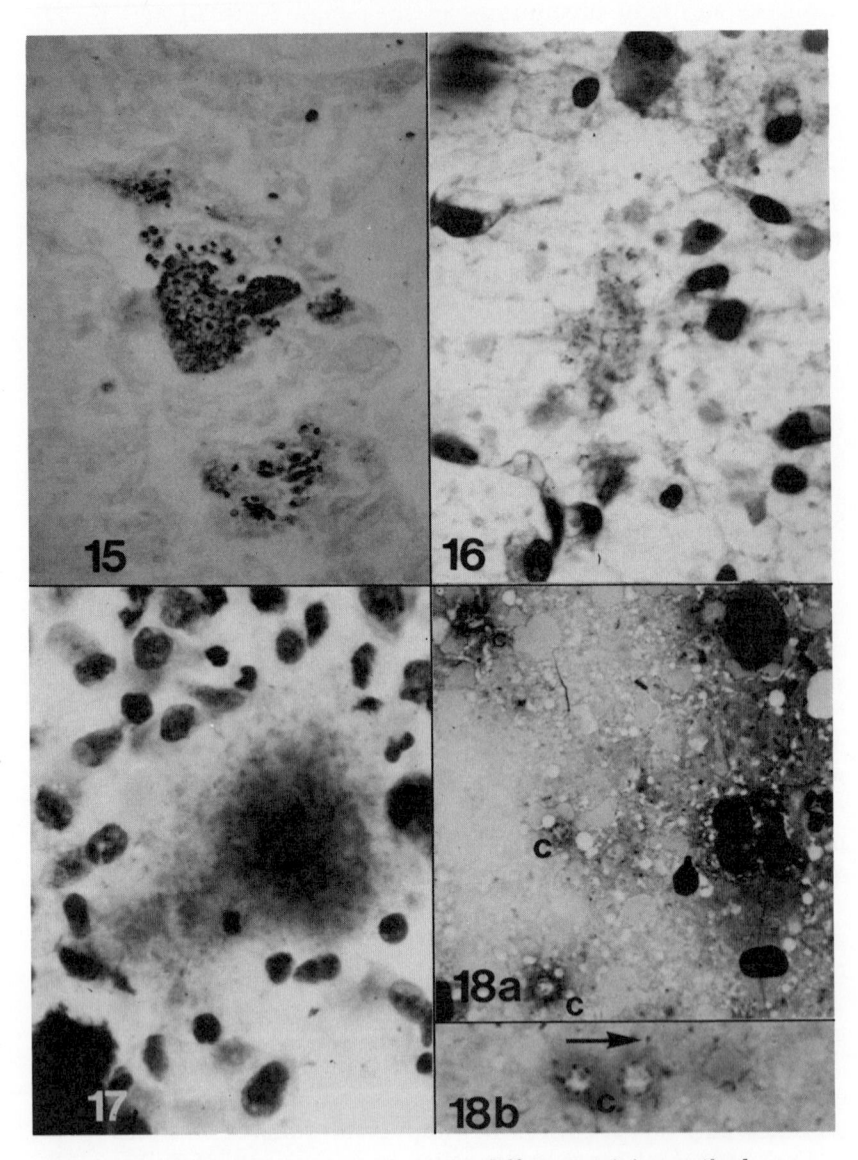

Figures 15–18. *Pneumocystis* as shown by different staining methods.

two patients diagnosed at autopsy. Another three patients may have been missed, if one interprets a slow response to treatment as indicating *Pneumocystis* infection.

The difficulty of using sputum and endobronchial brush examination results from the fact that the organisms stick to the alveolar wall and only a few are expectorated. It is possible that inhalation of mucolytic agents such as acetylcysteine may make more of the organisms available for diagnostic tests.

4. *Animal inoculation and cultures.* These diagnostic procedures have been unsuccessful. Since mice, rats, and rabbits have been found spontaneously infected with what is apparently their own species of *Pneumocystis*, experimental attempts at transmission are beset by difficulties (66, 125) (Fig. 18).

5. *Stains for* Pneumocystis. One of the methenamine silver methods is most useful in identifying the organisms (Fig. 14). A rapid staining technique has been described by Smith and Hughes (126), employing a dry impression film, dimethylsulfoxide, and the solutions employed in the standard method of Grocott (127). This method is described in many books on technique and is widely used for fungi. To avoid confusing *Pneumocystis* with fungi, a Giemsa preparation should be included to search for the eight-nucleated cysts (Figs. 17 and 18). The method of Chalvardjian and Grawe (121), employing toluidine blue, can be used successfully instead of the silver method (Fig. 15).

Figure 15. *Pneumocystis* stained in section by method of Chalvardjian and Grawe (121), permitting their recognition under low magnification. The lung parenchyma is almost unstained. (× 585) (from same patient as in Figs. 12 and 13)

Figure 16. *Pneumocystis* in lung imprint. No organisms were found in the sputum smears taken from this patient. Fixed and stained with Papanicolau's method. (× 585)

Figure 17. *Pneumocystis* group in lung imprint of a child with plasma-cell pneumonia, as shown in Fig. 11. The cohesiveness of the organisms is well demonstrated. Dry smear. (Giemsa, × 585)

Figure 18. *Pneumocystis* in lung impression of a rat that was treated with corticosteroids for six weeks. Several eight-nucleated cysts (C) are visible, as well as the nuclei of individual trophozoites (arrow). Dry smear. [Giemsa, × 585 (A); × 1100 (B)]

The organisms also may be stained with fluorescein-labelled antiserum prepared in rabbits against *Pneumocystis* of human origin (128). Antiserum against human complement or against human globulin (81) stains some of the protein precipitates accompanying and coating the organisms. It should be noted that the silver stain impregnates generally only the cyst walls, and that the trophozoites or the eight organisms within the cysts must be demonstrated with hematoxylin, Gram-Weigert, or a trichrome stain on sections and with Giemsa on dried, alcohol-fixed impression films. The periodic acid-Schiff method stains the entire zooglial mass, including trophozoites and cysts.

Table 4. Comparison of chemotherapeutic agents against pneumocystosis

	Sulfadiazine + Daraprim[a]	Pentamidine isethionate[b]
Manner of administration	Orally for 14–28 days (intravenous available)	Intramuscularly for 12–14 days; permission for intravenous administration granted on an individual basis
Recommended dose	Sulfadiazine: 1 g 4 times daily; pyrimethamine: 25 mg once or twice daily	4 mg/kg/day (150 mg/m^2 of body surface)
Static action	Effective	Effective
Lethal action	Partial	Partial
Recurrence observed if immunosuppression continued	Yes	Yes
Mode of action	Interference with dihydrofolate synthesis	Unknown

Table 4, continued

Toxicity	Folinic deficiency, with thrombocytopenia and leukopenia principally (5–10% when treated for ocular toxoplasmosis with similar doses for one to two months)	Renal, with azotemia, also hypoglycemia, hepatic dysfunction, pain at injection site and others in 69/164 patients (42%), with a total of 130 adverse reactions observed in 164 patients
Management of toxicity	Administration of leucovorin, the inhibited product, which humans can utilize, but which *Pneumocystis* cannot	No specific antagonist known
Prophylaxis	Practical (oral medication)	Impractical

[a] Based on dosages used by Kirby et al. (129), Rifkind et al. (73), and personal experience with the use of this drug combination in treatment of presumed ocular toxoplasmosis in similar doses for one to two months [Frenkel et al. (133); Frenkel and Hitchings (61)].

[b] Based largely on Western et al. (92).

L. Treatment

There are two different kinds of treatment available, sulfonamide plus pyrimethamine (Daraprim) as against toxoplasmosis, and pentamidine. The sulfadiazine-pyrimethamine combination was shown to be effective in rats at a time when no other drug was available for treatment in the U. S. (66). It was tried in humans by Rifkind et al. (73), who achieved pulmonary clearing of *Pneumocystis* in their patient, LD-47, which had been diagnosed from tracheal aspirates; he died with *Aspergillus* pneumonia. Additional patients successfully treated with the drug combination survived

(129). Pentamidine first was used for the treatment of *Pneumocystis* by Ivady and Paldy (130), and their experience was summarized in 1967 (131). The drug had been used widely in Europe and elsewhere, but had not been introduced for clinical use in the U. S. However, several enterprising physicians were able to obtain pentamidine and showed its effectiveness in the U. S. [for example, Robbins et al. (132) and Patterson et al. (84)]. In 1967, a Parasitic Diseases Drug Service was established by the Center for Disease Control, Atlanta, Ga., which filed a Notice of Claimed Investigational Exemption for pentamidine isethionate with the Food and Drug Administration. The Parasitic Diseases Drug Service of the Center for Disease Control has been the sole distributor of pentamidine in the U. S. (92).

Inasmuch as both drug regimens are similarly effective against *Pneumocystis* infections of rats and humans and the main differences lie in drug action, side-effects, and their management, these

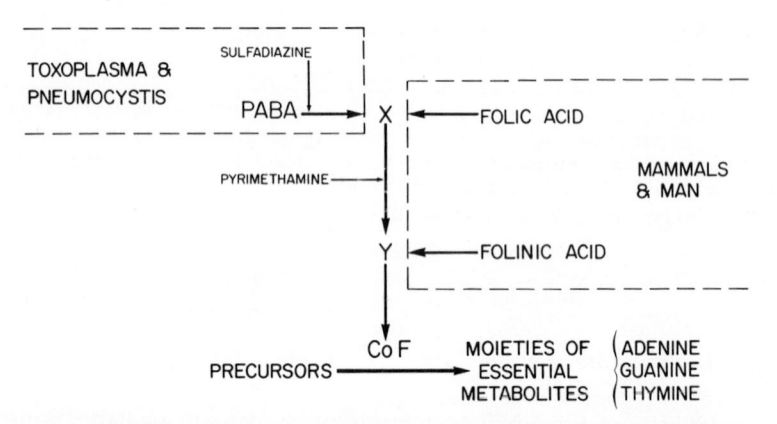

Figure 19. Biosynthetic pathway from paraaminobenzoic acid to coenzyme F, via folic (X) and folinic (Y) acids. The sequential sites of inhibition by sulfadiazine and pyrimethamine (Daraprim) explain the synergistic effect of this drug combination. The enclosure at left indicates that the biosynthesis in *Toxoplasma* and *Pneumocystis* necessarily begins with paraaminobenzoic acid or a close analog. Mammals and man can utilize folinic acid (leucovorin) as indicated by the enclosure at right. Hence, leucovorin can be used to counteract the toxic effects of sulfadiazine and pyrimethamine without impairing their chemotherapeutic effectiveness.

are compared in Table 4. Essentially, the side-effects are uncommon with the sulfadiazine-pyrimethamine combination, and those that do occur can be managed by providing the inhibited vitamin, folinic acid (leucovorin), either orally or intramuscularly (Table 3). It has been shown with toxoplasmosis in mice and humans, and with pneumocystosis in rats and humans, that the administration of this antagonist does not interfere with the chemotherapeutic action (61, 129, 133) (Figs. 29 and 20).

Unfortunately, a comparative study has not yet been organized. Although termed "investigational," pentamidine is "sent automatically on the verbal assurance that *P. carinii* had been documented histologically, or that results of appropriate diagnostic studies were pending" (92). In view of its availability, pentamidine is accepted readily. Because many physicians are not familiar with the availability of another treatment method with similar effectiveness and significantly less toxicity, the sulfadiazine-pyrimethamine combination has not been given a comparable trial.

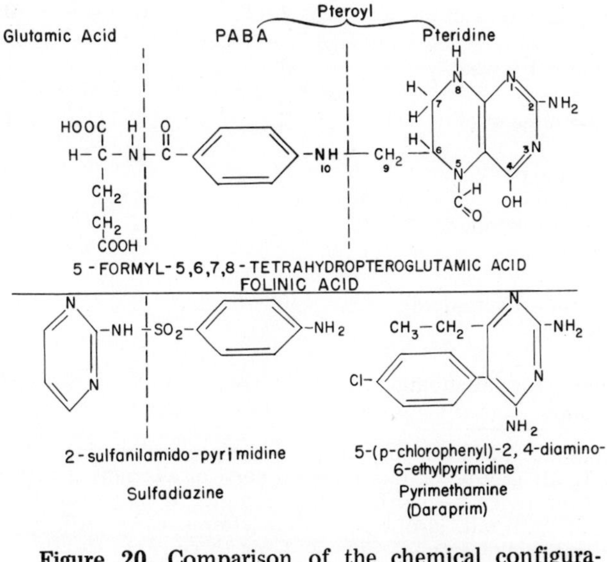

Figure 20. Comparison of the chemical configurations of the vitamin folinic acid with the inhibitory drugs sulfadiazine and pyrimethamine, to emphasize their structural similarities. (By permission of Antibiotics and Chemotherapy; from Ref. 61).

Initial enthusiasm is common after the introduction of most drugs, and the side-effects often are recognized slowly (134). The variety and frequency of such side-effects, listed by Western et al. (92), is notable (Table 4). In addition, interstitial pulmonary fibrosis has been reported both from humans and from 4 out of 15 rats treated with pentamidine (66, 108). In the rat model, the fibrosis apparently was associated with especially rapid killing of

Table 5. Effects of sulfadoxine alone, and in combination with pyrimethamine, on the prevention of pneumocystosis in rats hypercorticoid for 100 days[a]

Drug	No. of Rats Negative	No. of Rats Positive	*Pneumocystis* rating (mean)
None	0	17	2.8[b]
Sulfadoxine daily	6	1	0.07
Sulfadoxine alternate days	7	0	0.0
Sulfadoxine twice weekly	0	8	1.6
Sulfadoxine once weekly	0	6	1.7
Pyrimethamine daily	6	1	0.07
Pyrimethamine + sulfadoxine alternate days	4	2	0.5
Pyrimethamine + sulfadoxine twice weekly	0	6	1.1
Pyrimethamine + sulfadoxine once weekly	0	7	2.6

[a] Sulfadoxine, 200 mg per 100 g of food; pyrimethamine, 10 mg per 100 g of food. All groups of rats received cortisol alternating with cortisone acetate, given twice weekly in 25-mg amounts to 200-g rats for immunosuppression. All rats also received chlortetracycline HCl, 100 mg% in drinking water, and amphotericin B, 1 mg three times weekly, subcutaneously.

[b] 0, none; 1/2, rare organism detected; 1, few organisms present in few alveoli; 2, few organisms in many alveoli; 3, about half of alveoli filled with moderate number of organisms; 4, more than half of lung involved with pneumocystosis.

Pneumocystis by pentamidine, whereas the destruction of the organisms during sulfadiazine-pyrimethamine treatment was by phagocytosis. In humans, the pulmonary fibrosis has been observed also without pentamidine treatment (135).

Recurrent pneumocystosis has been seen in humans after pentamidine treatment by Hughes and Johnson (136) and others, and there is evidence from rats that neither pentamidine nor the sulfadiazine-pyrimethamine mixture eradicates the infection completely to prevent recurrence. The delay until the appearance of clinical pneumocystosis after sulfadiazine-pyrimethamine prophylaxis is longer than the delay after pentamidine prophylaxis in immunosuppressed rats, probably because of the longer tissue storage of pyrimethamine, in comparison to pentamidine (133).

Prophylaxis of epidemic infantile pneumocystosis has been carried out recently with a 20:1 combination of sulfadoxine and pyrimethamine (Fansidar; Roche Laboratories, Inc., Nutley, N. J.), giving 40 mg per kg of body weight every seven or 14 days (137). Sulfadoxine is a long-acting sulfonamide which has been used for malaria prophylaxis by weekly or biweekly administration (138). This drug combination also has been tested in immunosuppressed rats, in which it was effective prophylactically (Table 5). Since the half-life of sulfadoxine in mice and probably in rats is about 36 hr, compared to 200 hr in humans, only the daily and alternate daily administration were effective.

Prophylaxis must be used continuously or intermittently during the period of hypercorticism to prevent recurrence. There is no need to reduce hypercorticism or immunosuppression that is therapeutic for the primary disease process, because both treatment regimens were active concurrently.

M. Prevention

Infection cannot be prevented easily in humans, since carriers are not readily identified at present. Any isolation methods restricting respiratory and fomite contamination should be helpful. Once the disease becomes epidemic in an institution (73, 103), the contact between newly admitted patients and those admitted some time previously should be avoided to prevent intrainstitutional spread.

Serological testing of all family members, nursing, and medical personnel in contact with immunosuppressed patients might provide information about possible carriers to be futher investigated epidemiologically.

A prophylactic weekly or biweekly dose of sulfadoxine-pyrimethamine could be employed to inhibit the development of subclinical infection into clinically significant pneumocystosis. Inasmuch as this combination is not yet licensed in the U. S., four daily doses of 0.5 g of sulfadiazine and a weekly dose of 25—50 mg of pyrimethamine could be substituted.

Acknowledgment

I am grateful to Drs. S. Jarnum and A. S. Ohlsen for making available for study the slides of their patient, described in Section III-J of this chapter.

Literature Cited

1. Frenkel, J. K., J. P. Dubey, and N. L. Miller. *Toxoplasma gondii:* fecal stages identified as coccidian oocysts. Science 167: 893, 1970.
2. Frenkel, J. K., and J. P. Dubey. Toxoplasmosis and its prevention in cats and man. J. Infect. Dis. 126: 664, 1972.
3. Frenkel, J. K. Toxoplasmosis: Parasite life cycle, pathology, and immunology. *In* D. M. Hammond and P. L. Long (eds.), The Coccidia: *Eimeria, Isospora, Toxoplasma,* and Related Genera, p. 343. University Park Press, Baltimore, 1973.
4. Alford, C. A., J. W. Foft, W. J. Blankenship, G. Cassady, and J. W. Benton. Subclinical central nervous system disease of neonates: A prospective study of infants born with increased levels of IgM. J. Pediat. 75(6, Pt. 2): 1167, 1969.
5. Couvreur, J. Prospective study of acquired toxoplasmosis in pregnant women with a special reference to the outcome of the foetus. *In* D. Hentsch (ed.), Toxoplasmosis, p. 119. Hans Huber, Bern, 1971.
6. Frenkel, J. K. Toxoplasmosis. *In* R. Marcial-Rojas (ed.), Pathology of Protozoal and Helminthic Diseases, p. 254. Williams & Wilkins, Baltimore, 1971.
7. Frenkel, J. K. Toxoplasmosis. Mechanisms of infection, laboratory diagnosis and management. Curr. Topics Pathol. 54: 28, 1971.

8. Saxon, S. A., W. Knight, D. W. Reynolds, S. Stagno, and C. A. Alford. Intellectual deficits in children born with subclinical congenital toxoplasmosis. J. Pediat. 82: 792, 1973.
9. Pinkerton, H., and R. G. Henderson. Adult toxoplasmosis. A previously unrecognized disease entity simulating the typhus-spotted fever group. JAMA 116: 807, 1941.
10. Ludlam, G. B., and C. P. Beattie. Pulmonary toxoplasmosis? Lancet 2: 1136, 1963.
11. Kass, E. H., S. B. Andrus, R. D. Adams, F. C. Turner, and H. A. Feldman. Toxoplasmosis in the human adult. Arch. Intern. Med. 89: 759, 1952.
12. Sexton, R. C., D. E. Eyles, and R. E. Dillman. Adult toxoplasmosis. Amer. J. Med. 14: 366, 1953.
13. Vischer, T. L., C. Bernheim, and E. Engelbrecht. Two cases of hepatitis due to *Toxoplasma gondii*. Lancet 2: 919, 1967.
14. Manschot, W. A., and C. B. F. Daamen. Connatal ocular toxoplasmosis. Arch. Ophthalmol. 74: 48, 1965.
15. Wising, P. Akut adult toxoplasmos med lymphadenopathi och chorioretinit. Nord. Med. 47: 563, 1952.
16. Brown, J., and L. Jacobs. Adult toxoplasmosis: Report of a case due to laboratory infection. Ann. Intern. Med. 44: 565, 1956.
17. Lunde, M. N., A. H. Gelderman, S. L. Hayes, and C. L. Vogel. Serologic diagnosis of active toxoplasmosis complicating malignant diseases. Cancer 25: 637, 1970.
18. Siegel, S. E., M. N. Lunde, A. H. Gelderman, R. H. Halterman, J. A. Brown, A. S. Levine, and R. G. Graw. Transmission of toxoplasmosis by leukocyte transfusion. Blood 37: 388, 1971.
19. Wertlake, P. T., and T. S. Winter. Fatal *Toxoplasma* myocarditis in an adult patient with acute lymphocytic leukemia. New Engl. J. Med. 237: 438, 1965.
20. Frenkel, J. K. Pathogenesis of toxoplasmosis with a consideration of cyst rupture in *Besnoitia* infection. Surv. Ophthalmol. 6(6, Pt. 2): 799, 1961.
21. Frenkel, J. K. Ocular lesions in hamsters with chronic *Toxoplasma* and *Besnoitia* infections. Amer. J. Ophthalmol. 39: 203, 1955.
22. Wilder, H. C. *Toxoplasma* chorioretinitis in adults. Arch. Ophthalmol. 48: 127, 1952.
23. Zimmerman, L. E. Ocular pathology of toxoplasmosis. Surv. Ophthalmol. 6(6, Pt. 2): 832, 1961.
24. Hoeprich, P. D. Toxoplasmosis. Clinical notes. Med. Sci. 15: 89, 1964.
25. Hooper, A. D. Acquired toxoplasmosis. Arch. Pathol. 64: 1, 1957.
26. Prick, J. J. G., and J. A. M. Prick-Hoefnagels. Étude clinique et anatomo-

pathologique de la toxoplasmose chez l'homme. Folia Psychiat. Neurol. Neurochir. Neerl. 53: 352, 1950.
27. Sabin, A. B. Toxoplasmic encephalitis in children. JAMA 116: 801, 1941.
28. Bobowski, S. J., and W. G. Reed. Toxoplasmosis in an adult, presenting as a space-occupying cerebral lesion. Arch. Pathol. 65: 460, 1958.
29. Koeze, T. H., and G. H. Klingon. Acquired toxoplasmosis. Arch. Neurol. 11: 191, 1964.
30. Hemsath, F. A., and H. Pinkerton. Disseminated cytomegalic inclusion disease and disseminated toxoplasmosis in an adult with myeloid metaplasia. Amer. J. Clin. Pathol. 26: 36, 1956.
31. Vietzke, W. M., A. H. Gelderman, P. M. Grimley, and M. P. Valsamis. Toxoplasmosis complicating malignancy. Cancer 21: 816, 1968.
32. Frenkel, J. K., J. Arias-Stella, and B. Nelson. Clinical and experimental aspects of immunodepression and toxoplasmic encephalitis. (In preparation)
33. Cheever, A. W., M. P. Valsamis, and A. S. Rabson. Necrotizing toxoplasmic encephalitis and herpetic pneumonia complicating treated Hodgkin's disease. New Engl. J. Med. 272: 26, 1965.
34. Ghatak, N. R., T. P. Poon, and H. M. Zimmerman. Toxoplasmosis of the central nervous system in the adult. Arch. Pathol. 89: 337, 1970.
35. Walton, B. C., B. M. Benchoff, and W. H. Brooks. Comparison of the indirect fluorescent antibody test and methylene blue dye test for detection of antibodies to *Toxoplasma gondii*. Amer. J. Trop. Med. Hyg. 15: 149, 1966.
36. Takumi, K., I. Takebayashi, H. Takeuchi, H. Ikeda, and N. Toshioka. The use of lyophilized parasites in indirect fluorescent antibody technique for detection of *Toxoplasma* antibody. Jap. J. Microbiol. 10: 189, 1966.
37. Suggs, M. T., K. W. Walls, and I. G. Kagan. Comparative antigenic study of *Besnoitia jellisoni*, *B. panamensis* and five *Toxoplasma gondii* isolates. J. Immunol. 101: 166, 1968.
38. Goldman, M. Fluorescent Antibody Methods. Academic Press, New York, 1968. 303 p.
39. Remington, J. S. The present status of the IgM fluorescent antibody technique in the diagnosis of congenital toxoplasmosis. J. Pediat. 75(6, Pt. 2): 1116, 1969.
40. Halling, L. W. Problems in establishing diagnosis of toxoplasmic lymphadenitis. Amer. J. Clin. Pathol. 47: 370, 1967.
41. Carver, R. K., and M. Goldman. Staining *Toxoplasma gondii* with fluorescein-labeled antibody. Amer. J. Clin. Pathol. 32: 159, 1959.
42. Desmonts, G. Sur la technique de l'epreuve de lyse des toxoplasmes. Sem. Hôp. Paris 31: 1, 1955.

42a. Sabin, A. B., and H. A. Feldman. Dyes as microchemical indicators of a new immunity phenomenon affecting a protozoon parasite (Toxoplasma). Science 108:660, 1948.
43. Frenkel, J. K., and L. Jacobs. Ocular toxoplasmosis: Pathogenesis, diagnosis and treatment. Arch. Ophthalmol. 59: 260, 1958.
44. Stewart, G. L., and H. A. Feldman. Use of tissue culture cultivated *Toxoplasma* in the dye test and for storage. Proc. Soc. Exp. Biol. Med. 118: 542, 1965.
45. Wallace, G. D. Sabin-Feldman dye test for toxoplasmosis. Amer. J. Trop. Med. Hyg. 18: 395, 1969.
45a. Desmonts, G. Some remarks about the Sabine-Feldman test and other serological methods used in the diagnosis of toxoplasmosis. *In* D. Hentsch (ed.), Toxoplasmosis, p. 91. Hans Huber, Bern, 1971.
46. Feldman, H. A., and G. A. Lamb. A micromodification of the Toxoplasma dye test. J. Parasitol. 52: 415, 1966.
47. Sulzer, A., and E. C. Hall. Indirect fluorescent antibody tests for parasitic diseases. IV. Statistical study of variation in the indirect fluorescent antibody (IFA) test for toxoplasmosis. Amer. J. Epidemiol. 86: 401, 1967.
48. Jacobs, L., and M. Lunde. A hemagglutination test for toxoplasmosis. J. Parasitol. 43: 308, 1957.
49. Fulton, J. D., and F. Fulton. Complement-fixation tests in toxoplasmosis with purified antigen. Nature 205: 776, 1965.
50. Jacobs, L., J. S. Remington, and M. L. Melton. The resistance of the encysted form of *Toxoplasma gondii*. J. Parasitol. 46: 11, 1960.
51. Perrin, T. L. *Toxoplasma* and *Encephalitozoon* in spontaneous and in experimental infections of animals. A comparative study. Arch. Pathol. 36: 568, 1943.
52. Frenkel, J. K. Protozoal diseases of laboratory animals. *In* R. Marcial-Rojas (ed.), Pathology of Protozoal and Helminthic Diseases, p. 318. Williams & Wilkins, Baltimore, 1971.
53. Saxen, E., and L. Saxen. The histological diagnosis of glandular toxoplasmosis. Lab. Invest. 8: 386, 1959.
54. Tenhunen, A. Glandular toxoplasmosis. Occurrence of the disease in Finland. Acta Pathol. Microbiol. Scand. 172(Suppl.): 9, 1964.
55. Robinson, P. A case of toxoplasmosis. With recovery. Ann. Paediat. 168: 134, 1947.
56. Dubey, J. P., N. L. Miller, and J. K. Frenkel. The *Toxoplasma gondii* oocyst from cat feces. J. Exp. Med. 132: 636, 1970.
57. Dubey, J. P., G. V. Swan, and J. K. Frenkel. A simplified method for isolation of *Toxoplasma gondii* from the feces of cats. J. Parasitol. 58: 1005, 1972.
58. Dubey, J. P., and J. K. Frenkel. Extra-intestinal stages of *Isopora felis*

and *I. rivolta* (protozoa: Eimeriidae) in cats. J. Protozool. 19: 89, 1972.
59. Langer, H. Die Bedeutung der latenten mutterlichen *Toxoplasma*-Infektion fur die Gestation. *In* H. Kirchhoff and H. Kraubig (eds.), Toxoplasmose, p. 123. Georg Thieme Verlag, Stuttgart, 1966.
60. Kaufman, H. E., and L. A. Caldwell. Pharmacological studies of pyrimethamine (Daraprim) in man. Arch. Ophthalmol. 61: 885, 1959.
61. Frenkel, J. K., and G. H. Hitchings. Relative reversal by vitamins (−aminobenzoic, folic, and folinic acids) of the effects of sulfadiazine and pyrimethamine on *Toxoplasma* mouse and man. Antibiotics Chemother. 7: 630, 1957.
62. Nelson, M. M. Mammalian fetal development and antimetabolites. *In* Antimetabolites and Cancer, p. 107. American Association for the Advancement of Science, Washington, D.C. 1955.
63. Krahe, M. Untersuchungen uber die teratogene Wirkung von Medikamenten zur Behandlung der Toxoplasmose wahrend der Schwangerschaft. Arch. Gynekol. 202: 104, 1965.
64. McMaster, P. R. B., K. G. Powers, J. F. Finerty, and M. N. Lunde. The effect of two chlorinated Lincomycin analogues against acute toxoplasmosis in mice. Amer. J. Trop. Med. Hyg. 22: 14, 1973.
65. Shewell, J., and D. A. Long. A species difference with regard to the effect of cortisone acetate on body weight, γ-globulin and circulating antitoxin levels. J. Hyg. 54: 452, 1956.
66. Frenkel, J. K., J. T. Good, and J. A. Schultz. Latent *Pneumocystis* infection of rats, relapse, and chemotherapy. Lab. Invest. 15: 1559, 1966.
67. Wilson, H. R., and J. K. Frenkel. Immunosuppressive agents in intracellular infection: Besnoitiosis in hamsters. Infect. Immun. 3: 756, 1971.
68. Frenkel, J. K., and H. R. Wilson. Effects of radiation on specific cellular immunities: Besnoitiosis and a herpes virus infection of hamsters. J. Infect. Dis. 125: 216, 1972.
69. Strannegard, O., and E. Lycke. Effect of antithymocyte serum on experimental toxoplasmosis in mice. Infect. Immun. 5: 769, 1972.
70. Frenkel, J. K. *Toxoplasma* in and around us. BioScience 23:343, 1973.
70a. Frenkel, J. K., and J. P. Dubey. Effects of freezing on the viability of Toxoplasma oocysts. J. Parasitol. 59: 587, 1973.
71. Vavra, J., and K. Kucera. *Pneumocystis carinii* Delanoe, its ultrastructure and ultrastructural affinities. J. Protozool. 17: 463, 1970.
72. Campbell, W. G. Ultrastructure of *Pneumocystis* in human lung. Life cycle in human pneumocystosis. Arch. Pathol. 93: 312, 1972.
73. Rifkind, D., T. Faris, and R. B. Hill. *Pneumocystis carinii* pneumonia: Studies on the diagnosis and treatment. Ann. Intern. Med. 65: 943, 1966.

74. Kucera, K. Exact correlation in epidemics of *Pneumocystis* pneumonia. Folia Parasitol. 13: 343, 1966.
75. Hendley, J. O., and T. H. Weller, Activation and transmission in rats of infection with *Pneumocystis*. Proc. Soc. Exp. Biol. Med. 137: 1401, 1971.
76. Berdnikoff, G. Fourteen personal cases of *Pneumocystis carinii* pneumonia. Can. Med. Assoc. J. 80: 1, 1959.
77. Post, C., W. Dutz, and I. Nasarian. Endemic *Pneumocystis carinii* pneumonia in South Iran. Arch. Dis. Child. 39: 35, 1964.
78. Hyun, B. H., F. Varga, and L. J. Thalheimer. *Pneumocystis carinii* pneumonitis occurring in an adopted Korean infant. JAMA 195: 784, 1966.
79. Moragas, A., and M.-T. Vidal. *Pneumocystis carinii* pneumonia. First autopsy series in Spain. Helv. Paediat. Acta 26: 71, 1971.
80. Dutz, W. *Pneumocystis carinii* pneumonia. Pathol. Ann. 5: 309, 1970.
81. Brzosko, W. J., K. Madalinski, K. Krawczynski, and A. Nowoslawski. Immunohistochemistry in studies on the pathogenesis of *Pneumocystis* pneumonia in infants. Ann. N. Y. Acad. Sci. 177: 156, 1971.
82. Lingeman, C. H., D. M. Schulz, and J. W. Lukemeyer. *Pneumocystis carinii* pneumonia in congenital rubella. Amer. J. Dis. Child. 113: 585, 1967.
83. Burke, B. A., J. L. Krovetz, and R. A. Good. Occurrence of *Pneumocystis carinii* pneumonia in children with agammaglobulinemia. Pediatrics 28: 196, 1961.
83a. Burke, B. A., and R. A. Good. Pneumocystis carinii infection. Medicine 52: 23, 1973.
84. Patterson, J. H., I. L. Lindsey, E. S. Edwards, and W. D. Logan. *Pneumocystis carinii* pneumonia and altered host resistance: Treatment of one patient with pentamidine isethionate. Pediatrics 38: 388, 1966.
85. Kramer, R. I., V. C. Cirone, and H. Moore. Interstitial pneumonia due to *Pneumocystis carinii*, cytomegalic inclusion disease and hypogammaglobulinemia occurring simultaneously in an infant. Pediatrics 29: 816, 1962.
86. Gentry, L. O., and J. S. Remington. *Pneumocystis carinii* pneumonia in siblings. J. Pediat. 76: 769, 1970.
87. Becroft, D. M., and J. M. Costello. *Pneumocystis carinii* pneumonia in siblings: Diagnosis by lung aspiration. N. Z. Med. J. 64: 273, 1965.
88. Barnett, R. N., J. G. Hull, V. Vortel, and J. Schwarz. *Pneumocystis carinii* in lymph nodes and spleen. Arch. Pathol. 88: 175, 1969.
89. Allibone, E. C., W. Goldie, and B. P. Marmion. *Pneumocystis carinii* pneumonia and progressive vaccinia in siblings. Arch. Dis. Child. 39: 26, 1964.
90. Watanabe, J. M., H. Chinchinian, C. Weitz, and S. K. McIlvanie. *Pneumocystis carinii* pneumonia in a family. JAMA 193: 685, 1965.

91. Gentry, L. O., J. Ruskin, and J. S. Remington. *Pneumocystis carinii* pneumonia. Problems in diagnosis and therapy in 24 cases. Calif. Med. 116: 6, 1972.
92. Western, K. A., D. R. Perera, and M. G. Schultz. Pentamidine isethionate in the treatment of *Pneumocystis carinii* pneumonia. Ann. Intern. Med. 73: 695, 1970.
93. Ruskin, J., and J. S. Remington. The compromised host and infection. I. *Pneumocystis carinii* pneumonia. JAMA 202: 1070, 1967.
94. Kossell, A. Interstitielle plasmazellulare Pneumonie beim alteren Kind als Folge langdauernder Corticosteroidbehandlung. Dt. Med. Wschr. 87: 1133, 1962.
95. Muller, G. Interstitielle plasmacellulare Pneumonie nach Corticosteroidbehandlung. Frankf. Z. Pathol. 70: 657, 1960.
96. Wilkins. L., R. M. Blizzard, and C. J. Migeon. The Diagnosis and Treatment of Endocrine Disorders in Childhood and Adolescence. 3rd Ed. Charles C Thomas, Springfield, Ill., 1965. 619 p.
97. Kenny, F. M., C. Preeyasombat, and C. J. Migeon. Cortisol production rate. II. Normal infants, children and adults. Pediatrics 37: 34, 1966.
98. Rifkind, D., T. E. Starzl, T. L. Marchioro, W. R. Waddell, D. T. Rowlands, and R. B. Hill. Transplantation pneumonia. JAMA 189: 808, 1964.
99. Vivell, O. Die Serologie der interstitiellen Pneumonie. Mschr. Kinderheilk. 108: 146, 1960.
100. Post, C. A., W. F. Dutz, A. T. Fakouhi, E. I. Kohout, and S. Ball-Fritschi. Prophylaxis and therapy of epidemic infantile *Pneumocystis carinii* pneumonia. *In* Fifth International Congress of Infectious Diseases. Vol. IV, p. 169. Verlag der Wiener Medizinischen Akademie, Vienna. 1970.
101. Goodell, B., J. B. Jacobs, R. D. Powell, and V. T. DeVita. *Pneumocystis carinii:* The spectrum of diffuse interstitial pneumonia in patients with neoplastic diseases. Ann. Intern. Med. 72: 337, 1970.
102. Esterly, J. A., and N. E. Warner. *Pneumocystis carinii* pneumonia. Arch. Pathol. 80: 433, 1965.
103. Perera, D. R., K. A. Western, H. D. Johnson, W. W. Johnson, M. G. Schultz, and P. V. Akers. *Pneumocystis carinii* pneumonia in a hospital for children. JAMA 214: 1074, 1970.
104. Luna, M. A., G. P. Bodey, A. M. Goldman, and B. Lichtiger. *Pneumocystis carinii* pneumonia in cancer patients. Texas Rep. Biol. Med. 30(Suppl.): 41, 1972.
105. Rosen, P., D. Armstrong, and C. Ramos. *Pneumocystis carinii* pneumonia. A clinicopathologic study of twenty patients with neoplastic diseases. Amer. J. Med. 53: 428, 1972.

106. Jirovec, O., and J. Vanek. Zur Morphologie der *Pneumocystis carinii* und zur Pathogenese der *Pneumocystis*-Pneumonie. Zentbl. Allg. Pathol. Pathol. Anat. 92: 424, 1954.
107. Johnson, H. D., and W. W. Johnson. *Pneumocystis carinii* pneumonia in children with cancer. JAMA 214: 1067, 1970.
108. Whitcomb, M. E., M. I. Schwarz, M. A. Charles, and P. H. Larson. Interstitial fibrosis after *Pneumocystis carinii* pneumonia. Ann. Intern. Med. 73: 761, 1970.
109. McMillan, G. C. Fatal inclusion-disease pneumonitis in an adult. Amer. J. Pathol. 23: 995, 1947.
110. Hennigar, G. R., K. Vinijchaikul, A. L. Roque, and H. A. Lyons. *Pneumocystis carinii* pneumonia in an adult. Amer. J. Clin. Pathol. 35: 353, 1961.
111. Pavlika, F. The first observation of congenital pneumocystic pneumonia in a fully developed stillborn child. Ann. Paediat. 198: 177, 1962.
112. Abioye, A. A. Interstitial plasma cell pneumonia (*Pneumocystis carinii*) in Ibadan: Report of a case. W. Afr. Med. J. 16: 130, 1967.
112a. Bazaz, G. R., O. L. Manfredi, R. G. Howard, and A. A. Claps. *Pneumocystis carinii* pneumonia in three full-term siblings. J. Pediat. 76: 767, 1970.
113. Montoya, V. M. Patologia, y bacteriologia en mortinatos y muertos neonatales. Anot. Pediát. 4: 753, 1962.
114. Zandanell, E. Pneumozystisbefund ausserhalb der Lunge bei interstitieller plasmazellularer Pneumonie der Sauglinge und Fruhgeburten. Zentbl. Allg. Pathol. Pathol. Anat. 92: 74, 1954.
115. Jarnum, S., E. F. Rasmussen, A. S. Ohlsen, and A. W. S. Sorensen. Generalized *Pneumocystis carinii* infection with severe idiopathic hypoproteinemia. Ann. Intern. Med. 68: 138, 1968.
116. Awen, C. F., and M. A. Baltzan. Systemic dissemination of *Pneumocystis carinii* pneumonia. Can. Med. Assoc. J. 104: 809, 1971.
116a. LeGolvan, D. P., and K. P. Heidelberger. Disseminated, granulomatous *Pneumocystis carinii* pneumonia. Arch. Pathol. 95: 344, 1973.
117. Goetz, O. Erfahrungen mit der Komplementbindungreaktion auf interstitielle plasmacellulare Pneumonie. Z. Kinderheilk. 82: 209, 1959.
118. Goetz, O. Serologische Befunde interstitieller Pneumonien aus den Vereinigten Staaten. Arch. Kinderheilk. 170: 60, 1964.
119. Norman, L., and I. G. Kagan. A preliminary report of an indirect fluorescent antibody test for detecting antibodies to cysts of *Pneumocystis carinii* in human sera. Amer. J. Clin. Pathol. 58: 170, 1972.
120. Le Tan-Vinh, C., A. M. Vu-Trieu-Dong, and W. Solonar. Diagnostic in vivo de la pneumonie a *Pneumocystis*. Arch. Fr. Pédiat. 20: 773, 1963.
121. Chalvardjian, A. M., and L. A. Grawe. A new procedure for the identifi-

cation of *Pneumocystis carinii* cysts in tissue sections and smears. J. Clin. Pathol. 16: 383, 1963.
122. Smith, E., and I. Gaspar. 1. Pentamidine treatment of *Pneumocystis carinii* pneumonitis in adult with lymphatic leukemia. Amer. J. Med. 44: 626, 1968.
123. DeVita, V. T., M. Emmer, A. Levine, B. Jacobs, and C. Berard. *Pneumocystis carinii* pneumonia. Successful diagnosis and treatment of two patients with associated malignant processes. New Engl. J. Med. 280: 287, 1969.
124. Repsher, L. H., G. Schroter, and W. S. Hammond. Diagnosis of *Pneumocystis carinii* pneumonitis by means of endobronchial brush biopsy. New Engl. J. Med. 287: 340, 1972.
125. Sheldon, W. Experimental pulmonary *Pneumocystis carinii* infection in rabbits. J. Exp. Med. 110: 147, 1959.
126. Smith, J. W., and W. T. Hughes. Rapid staining technique for *Pneumocystis carinii*. J. Clin. Pathol. 25: 269, 1972.
127. Grocott, R. G. Stain for fungi in tissue sections and smears using Gomori's methenamine silver nitrate technic. Amer. J. Clin. Pathol. 25: 975, 1955.
128. Minielly, J. A., F. C. McDuffie, and K. E. Holley. Immunofluorescent identification of *Pneumocystis carinii*. Arch. Pathol. 90: 561, 1970.
128a. Lim, S. K., R. H. Jones, and W. C. Eveland. Fluorescent antibody studies on experimental pneumocystosis. Proc. Soc. Exp. Biol. Med. 136: 675, 1971.
129. Kirby, H. B., B. Kenamore, and J. C. Guckian. *Pneumocystis carinii* pneumonia treated with pyrimethamine and sulfadiazine. Ann. Intern. Med. 75: 505, 1971.
130. Ivady, G., and L. Paldy, Ein neues Behandlungsverfahren der interstitiellen plasmazelligen Pneumonie Fruhgeborener mit funfwertigem Stibium und aromatischen Diamidinen. Mschr. Kinderheilk. 106: 10, 1958.
131. Ivady, G., L. Paldy, M. Koltay, G. Toth, and Z. Kovacs. *Pneumocystis carinii* pneumonia. Lancet 1: 616, 1967.
132. Robbins, J. B., R. H. Miller, V. M. Arean, and H. A. Pearson. Successful treatment of *Pneumocystis carinii* in a patient with congenital hypogammaglobulinemia. New Engl. J. Med. 272: 708, 1965.
133. Frenkel, J. K., R. W. Weber, and M. N. Lunde. Acute toxoplasmosis. Effective treatment with pyrmethamine, sulfadiazine, leucovorin calcium and yeast. JAMA 173: 1471, 1960.
134. Western, K. A., and M. G. Schultz. Pentamidine nontoxicity. Ann. Intern. Med. 70: 234, 1969.
135. Nowak, J. Late pulmonary changes in the course of infection with *Pneumocystis carinii*. Acta Med. Pol. 7: 23, 1966.

136. Hughes, W. T., and W. W. Johnson. Recurrent *Pneumocystis carinii* pneumonia following apparent recovery. J. Pediat. 79: 755, 1971.
137. Post, C., T. Fakouhi, W. Dutz, B. Banarizadeh, and E. Kohout. Prophylaxis of epidemic infantile pneumocystosis with a 10:1 sulfadoxine and pyrimethamine combination. Curr. Ther. Res. 13: 273, 1971.
138. Laing, A. B. G. Antimalarial effects of sulphormethoxine, diaphenylsulphone and separate combinations of these with pyrimethamine: A review of preliminary investigations carried out in Tanzania. J. Trop. Med. Hyg. 71: 27, 1968.
139. Dubey, J. P., and J. K. Frenkel. Cyst-induced toxoplasmosis in cats. J. Protozool. 19: 155, 1972.

14

Cytomegalovirus, A Model for Herpesvirus Opportunism

John L. Randall and Stanley A. Plotkin

I. Clinical Manifestations of Herpes Agents

The human herpes viruses, varicella-zoster (VZ), herpes simplex I and II (HSV), cytomegalovirus (CMV), and Epstein-Barr virus (EBV) comprise a group of viral agents that commonly causes disease in opportunistic clinical situations. In the normal host, the clinical expressions of these agents are well known. VZ causes chickenpox during primary infection and the appearance of shingles in the older patient as an expression of recrudescence. HSV I and II in limited primary infection cause superficial ulcerations on the oral mucosa (type I) and on the genital mucosa (type II). Recurrent infections of herpes labialis (type I) and chronic cervical infection (type II) are well described. In its more serious form, CMV causes severe infection of the fetus and newborn infant, with resultant hepatitis, bone marrow suppression, and encephalitis, often with residual brain damage. Two other forms of primary limited disease have been suggested for CMV in older patients, in upper respiratory infection, with a resultant croup or pertussis syndrome, and, recently (1), in venereal infection. EBV, implicated as the cause of infectious mononucleosis (2), also causes many inapparent upper respiratory infections which may go unrecognized by the physician. It is often found in association with Burkitt's lymphoma, but its status as an etiological agent is uncertain.

Some infections caused by herpes group viruses are serious problems to the patients and to the clinician (Table 1). These infections may represent an extension of primary disease or of secondary or latent infection in the altered host. Depending on the degree of immune compromise, the extent of infection seen in altered hosts ranges from inapparent infection to severe disease. Both humoral and cell-mediated immunity are important in herpes group infection; however, specific deficiencies which allow extension of disease are not yet completely defined. Practical experience has delineated certain groups of patients undergoing specific types of therapy who are in danger of extension of herpes group disease. These include patients with burns or eczema (3–5), fetuses or premature infants (6–8), patients being treated with steroids (9, 10) or with some other immunosuppression (e.g., patients with Hodgkin's disease) (11, 12). When signs of infection develop in these clinical situations, the clinician, microbiologist, pathologist, and other members of the hospital support team must suspect and search for the presence of herpes agents. Furthermore, these patients should be protected from contact with those known to have active herpetic disease.

II. Epidemiology and Biology

The epidemiology and biology of the herpes agents tend to favor their expression as opportunists. They are ubiquitous, not only in the human species, but also in many phyla and species throughout the natural world. From the herpes-like phage of a marine *Pseudomonas* to the Marek's-virus of chickens or Lucké frog virus, they all become manifest under appropriate conditions in their respective hosts.

All herpes agents possess the potential for latency following primary infection and exist in a cell-associated state, most likely through the remainder of the life of the infected host. Moreover, herpes agents are inducible following latency. UV light, X-ray, and

Table 1. Clinical infection by herpesvirus

Agent	Normal host — Primary infection	Normal host — Recrudescent infection	Altered host or extension of primary or recurrent disease
HSV I	Oral ulcers Inapparent early infection	Lip ulcers	Neonatal hepatitis and encephalitis Encephalitis in adult Severe generalized skin eruption
HSV II	Genital ulcerations	Cervicitis (chronic) Skin ulceration (chronic)	Neonatal syndrome, hepatitis, encephalitis, systemic infection
VZ	Chickenpox Unapparent infection	Shingles	Severe pneumonia Generalized zoster Encephalitis Systemic infection
CMV	Inapparent neonatal infection Heterophile-negative infectious mononucleosis syndrome Croup, pertussis syndrome Postperfusion syndrome	Asymptomatic viruria	Intestinal pneumonia Hepatitis Encephalitis Hemolytic anemia Severe neonatal syndrome
EBV	Infectious mononucleosis	?	Encephalitis Hepatitis Severe infectious mononucleosis

probably chemical mutagens allow herpes viruses in their latent phases to initiate replicative cycles in the whole animal. Induction following latency makes the epidemiology of this group of agents more complicated. For example, patients undergoing radiation therapy for oncological disease have developed herpes zoster at the site of radiation. Another example is the high incidence of herpetic group infections in patients undergoing renal transplant. They may have received blood carrying CMV and EBV, and they are immunosuppressed, which tends to favor the extension of latent foci of infection. Furthermore, it has been suggested that the rejection process in these patients may stimulate replication of latent virus. Thus, at times, it is difficult to delineate clearly the origin of the infection. At all times, the potentiality for reactivation of latent infection exists.

III. Pathology, Classification, and Morphology

The pathology of the lesions caused by herpes agents in tissue culture and in the host demonstrates several general characteristics. These include cell-rounding, intranuclear inclusions, and giant cell formation, with ultimate lysis and destruction of the cell.

Sections of a lesion of chickenpox demonstrate cell-rounding and giant cell formation at the base of the lesion (see Figs. 1 and 2). Figure 3 demonstrates a similar pattern in tissue culture infected with CMV, with the addition of classical type A intranuclear inclusions.

Consideration of cell-virus relationships has led to the classification of the herpes agents into group A and group B. Herpes I and II (group A) demonstrate a more lytic type of infection in cell culture and fulminating disease in patients, while VZ, CMV and EBV (group B) are more cell associated and have a more insidious clinical presentation.

Electron microscopy of these agents has demonstrated a close resemblance to each other, with all containing 162 capsomers with several enveloping membranes, depending on the site and nature of the specimen. The virus cores contain DNA.

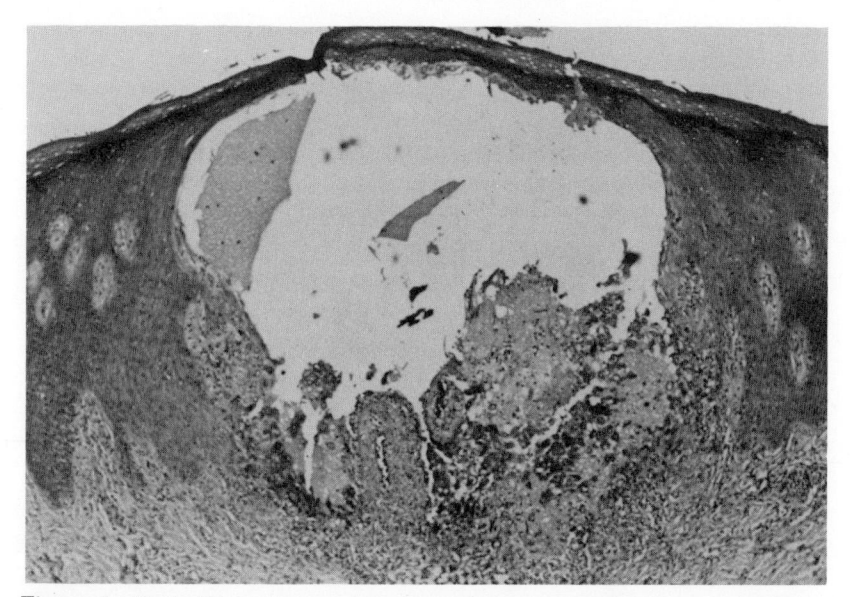

Figure 1. Varicella vesicle demonstrating cell rounding at the base of the lesion. (× 10)

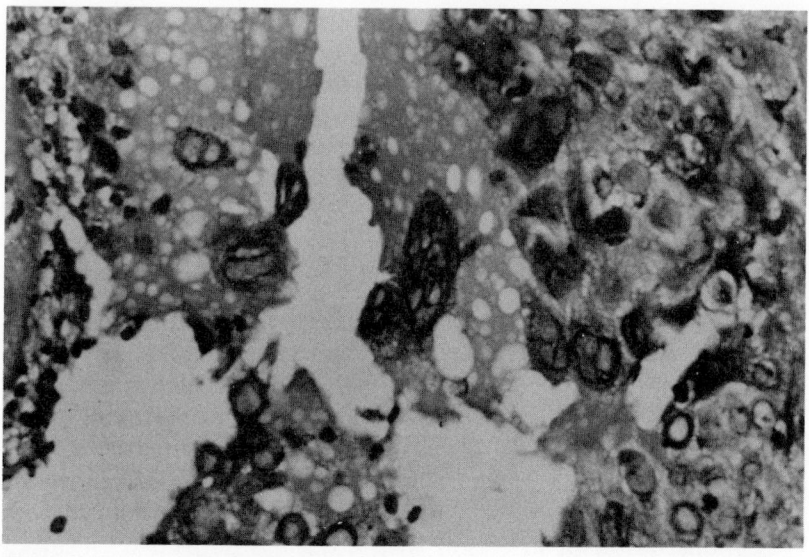

Figure 2. Giant cell formation at the base of the varicella vesicle. (× 40)

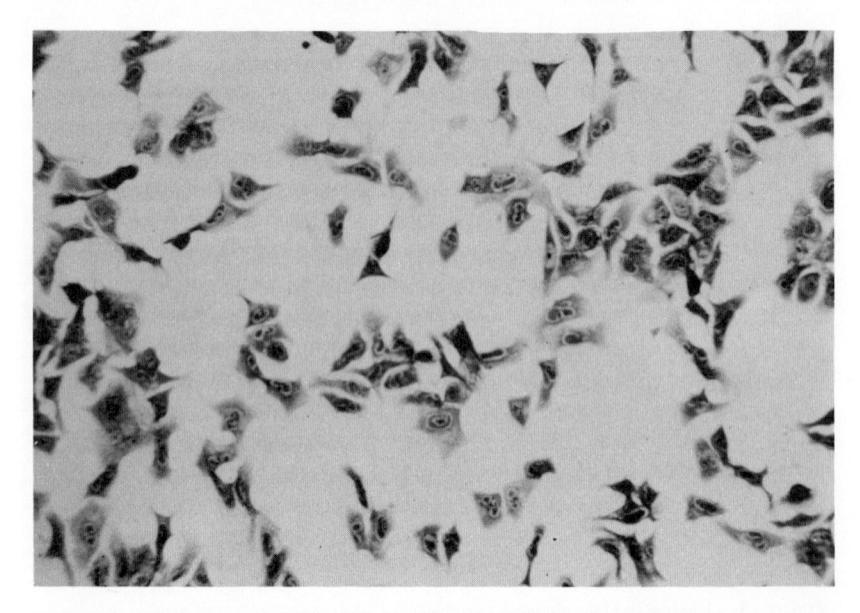

Figure 3. WI-38 human fibroblasts five days following infection with high-titer CMV. Demonstrating "type A" intranuclear inclusions. (× 40)

The continuing presence of herpes agents in the human population and their ability to express themselves in disease states as a result of primary and relapsing infection make a unique and complicated story. It is not within the scope of this presentation to describe each virus. Of all the members of the Herpes group, CMV tends to become manifest most readily in altered host situations and therefore it serves as a suitable example for discussion.

IV. Cytomegalovirus

During the 16 years following its original isolation, much information has been collected regarding the epidemiology, clinical expression, physical characteristics, and modes of replication of CMV.

Demonstration of infection with CMV has depended on several methods. Early studies called attention to the presence of inclusion bodies in cells at postmortem examination (13). Following the first isolation of the virus from the submaxillary gland of a dead infant (14) and the simultaneous isolation of the agent from explants of adenoidal tissue (15), the use of tissue culture gradually became a relatively easy method for the isolation and identification of the agent. The use of tissue culture is cumbersome, however, for large epidemiological studies, and most large-scale work has used the complement-fixation (CF) test. Complement-fixation testing has been performed, for the most part, by using strain AD169 as the antigen, although some studies have employed test strains indigenous to a particular area. Different strains of CMV may react variably when neutralization with heterologous antisera is performed (16). However, they appear to share complement-fixing antigens. It is not clear for how long a period levels of complement-fixing antibodies persist. In one study (17), two of 21 patients lost detectable CF titers over a three-year period. With these facts in mind, one can then look at the available serological data.

A. *Epidemiology*

Testing of human sera for the presence of complement-fixing antibodies to several standard strains has indicated two seroepidemiological patterns (Table 2) (18). In the United States and

Table 2. Prevalence of CMV (CF) antibody in several populations*

Location	5–9 years	45–49 years
Seattle	16%	67%
London	15%	51%
Puerto Rico	21%	52%
Japan	47%	54%
Easter Island	65%	81%

* From Ref. 18.

England, 15% of the population appears to have developed antibody to CMV by the age of 10. This pattern is also found in the Easter Islands (19) and Japan (20). By the time middle age is reached, one can expect complement-fixing antibodies in 50–70% of the American and English populations and in 85–95% of the Japanese and Easter Island populations. The rapidity with which a given population acquires antibody varies inversely with the socio-economic level and directly with population density. Those at the lower level in more densely populated areas acquire antibody more rapidly. How these antibodies are acquired is not known fully, but one may assume that a large percentage of the population experiences inapparent infection.

B. Infection of the Normal Host

The pattern of disease caused by CMV over the life span is as follows. The fetus is most clearly in jeopardy. Approximately 1% of infants born in the United States and England excrete CMV (21–23). The total morbidity associated with this infection is not yet clear; however, it is estimated by one author that at least 10% of those infected will have central nervous system damage (7). The syndrome of congenital CMV infection, described classically as a severely ill child with hepatosplenomegaly, intrauterine growth retardation, and intracranial calcifications (24) has now been shown to be an extreme manifestation of a broad spectrum of illness. Infection during pregnancy may result in abortion if the fetus is infected in an early period of gestation. Later infection may lead to generalized disease, but may also result in asymptomatic viruria.

Transmission of the virus to the fetus occurs for the most part by the transplacental route. However, one group of investigators (25) has described the appearance of CMV in two infants following intrauterine blood transfusion. In addition, studies in Pittsburgh indicate that virus can be isolated from approximately 5% of cervices of women in the third trimester of pregnancy. In the same study, Navajo women were found to have a 14% excretion rate (26). This represents another way in which large numbers of infants may thus be exposed to CMV during birth. Furthermore, Diosi et al. (27) have isolated the virus from breast milk in several cases, thus indicating an alternate route for acquisition of the virus. Following infections that are acquired either within the uterus or neonatally, infants shed virus in the urine for prolonged periods, despite the presence of high circulating neutralizing antibody.

Evidence exists to indicate the presence of early infection in 10–20% of children in the first year of life. The mode of transmission is not clear, however. In one study in Thailand, virus was isolated frequently from the respiratory tract of children with pertussis syndrome and respiratory diseases (27a). This observation was made in a tropical climate and in a low socioeconomic population, and it remains to be seen how frequently this form of disease occurs in other settings.

A group of young adult patients with symptoms resembling infectious mononucleosis but negative for heterophile antibody has been described. In a study from Finland (28), these patients did not have pharyngeal symptoms or evidence of lymphadenopathy. All were young adults, and all had typhoidal-type disease. All but one were seronegative for CMV at the time of the acute illness and later showed a serological conversion. Recently, we have seen an 11-year-old boy with similar symptoms: fever, hepatic involvement, and a hemolytic anemia. His heterophile antibody test was negative, but CMV was in his urine. The incidence of hemolytic anemia in CMV infection is unknown, but several cases have been reported (29, 30).

EBV appears to be the most important agents in the heterophile-positive cases of infectious mononucleosis syndrome. In a prospective study of 268 students at Yale University who were seronegative for EBV, 15% later developed a syndrome of infectious mononucleosis (31). Of 275 patients studied in Helsinki with clinical histories suggesting infectious mononucleosis, 60 were heterophile negative. Forty-four of these sera were checked for antibody to CMV and EBV. Of these, 19, or 7% of the total cases, showed significant rise in CF antibody to CMV and 8 demonstrated rise to EBV (28).

Recently, the potential for venereal transmission of CMV has been suggested by epidemiological data and by the isolation of the virus from seminal fluid and cervical secretions in patients attending venereal disease clinics (1).

C. Altered Host Infection

The fact that patients who show seroconversion to CMV and who excrete virus may not show active disease has been confusing, particularly in the case of the compromised host. The situation is further complicated by other agents that are often present, such as *Pneumocystis* and *Toxoplasma*. CMV may not be a pathogen at all times, despite the laboratory evidence for infection.

Three major patient groups are at risk from CMV infection:

1. Patients receiving large amounts of blood
2. Patients receiving renal transplants
3. Patients having oncological disease and receiving immunosuppressive therapy

It is difficult to subdivide these groups, inasmuch as most patients who have serious illness and who are receiving immunosuppressive therapy and those receiving transplants require large numbers of transfusions. However, by examining only the group of patients who have received large amounts of blood, one can gain a general idea of the results of exposure to CMV.

Table 3. Incidence of CMV antibody rise (CF) in patients receiving multiple blood transfusions

Study	No. of patients	No of patients with rise	%
Prince et al., 1971 (36)	72	15	21
Henle et al., 1970 (62)	72	17	23
Stevens et al., 1970 (63)	41	13	32
Perham et al., 1971 (64)	55	21	38
Paloheimo et al., 1968 (65)	63	19	30

In various studies (Table 3), from 20 to 40% of patients who received blood in large quantities or who were on extra corporeal circulation showed seroconversion to CMV. Within three to 12 weeks following transfusions, 10–15% of these patients developed a postperfusion syndrome consisting of fever, hepatosplenomegaly, and lymphocytosis.

Attempts to screen donors of blood for the presence of CMV have given variable results, which may be related to the techniques employed. Some laboratories have been able to isolate virus from donor blood (32), and others have not (33). In one study, Lang (34) observed a carrier rate of approximately 6%.

Several mechanisms of infection have been suggested to explain the occurrence of seroconversion or titer rise in this patient population, for example:

1. Direct transmission of the virus from the blood of the donor to the patient
2. Reactivation of the infection in the recipient by a mixed lymphocyte reaction

In a small study using lymphocyte-depleted blood for transfusions, the incidence of CMV infection was diminished, in comparison with a control population (35). It has been suggested that the use of fresh blood tends to increase the incidence of infection. However, Prince et al. (36) have demonstrated an increase in seroconversion which was directly related to the number of transfusions received, irrespective of the age of the blood. In one study, CMV was recovered from banked blood for as long as 28 days following its inoculation with a high-titer laboratory strain (37).

Little evidence exists to date to support the hypothesis of reactivation by a mixed lymphocyte reaction. Nor, to our knowledge, has lymphocyte stimulation been known to reactivate the virus in vitro.

The situation in patients undergoing immunosuppression for renal transplant is more complicated. In patients receiving renal transplants, the incidence of CMV seroconversion or of significant titer rise by CF method is quite high, approaching 80% in various studies. Yet, as stated previously, the incidence of clinically recognizable disease is much lower (38–40).

Table 4. CMV (CF) antibody in renal transplant patients

Study	No. of patients studied	No. of patients with rise	%
Craighead, 1967 (40)	50	43	86
Nagington, 1971 (38)	41	30	73

Patients undergoing renal transplant have shown evidence of either acquired infection or reactivation. In one study, Craighead, Hanshaw, and Carpenter (40) demonstrated that patients with serological evidence of CMV prior to renal transplant had titer rises in 22 of 24 cases (91%), while only 8 of 17 (47%) with titers negative for CMV before surgery demonstrated significant titer rise. These data strongly suggest a combination of reactivation and primary infection. The hypothesis that mixed lymphocyte reaction activates the virus from its latent state as part of the rejection process has been suggested. An additional consideration in explaining the high rate of seroconversion or titer rise in this population is the possibility of nosocomial infection (34). Patients who are undergoing immunosuppressive therapy and who have CMV infection may have prolonged excretion of virus in the urine similar to that occurring in the neonatal form of the disease, and therefore constitute a potential source of cross-infection in the hospital.

Several studies of children with leukemia and other forms of neoplastic disease who were undergoing immunosuppressive therapy have not indicated a higher rate of infection (41–43). The potential for other opportunistic pathogens to cause combined disease with CMV in leukemic children is stressed by Armstrong et al. (41) and deserves careful attention. Recently, Henson and co-workers (44) demonstrated an excretion rate of 27% when repeated cultures of throat and urine were obtained. Furthermore, in this study, five of seven children receiving marrow transplants were positive for virus, similar to the prevalence found in cases of renal transplantation.

The combination of immunosuppressive therapy and exposure to large blood volumes tends to provide fertile soil for CMV infection. In those patients who do show clinical symptoms, the pattern ranges from disseminated disease resembling the neonatal syndrome to the more confined expressions of either infiltrative pulmonary disease, hepatic dysfunction, or, in rare instances, hemolytic anemia. Autopsy findings in these patients also range from disseminated disease to normal findings, with virus isolation as the only sign of its presence.

D. Diagnosis

Diagnosis of CMV has depended on several methods. The presence of the virus has been suggested by evidence of intranuclear inclusions either at autopsy or in biopsy specimen. CMV may be present, however, in the absence of inclusions (45), and other viruses, particularly of the herpes group, may show similar inclusions. Cytological examination of the urine has not proved reliable (46). The presence of complement-fixing antibody to CMV indicates previous exposure; however, its absence does not eliminate the possibility that the patient has been exposed to the virus in the past or that recent exposure to a different antigenic strain had occurred (47). Attempts to define the antigenic makeup by neutralization and by precipitin reaction are now under way (48, 49). The use of indirect hemagglutination also has been studied (50, 51). A platelet-aggregation test for CMV antibody has been described as more sensitive than CF, but its appearance seemed to parallel that of CF antibody in the patients studied (52). Indirect hemagglutination has the advantage of measuring both IgG and IgM fractions of the serum and may prove to be more sensitive.

The development of fluorescent techniques has provided a method to distinguish IgM antibody from IgG. This distinction has proven to be quite valuable in diagnosis of neonatal disease, in which the demonstration of specific IgM for CMV is evidence of a fetal reaction, inasmuch as only maternal IgG will cross the placenta. The value of this test in the diagnosis of adult infection, however, is not as clear (53). CMV IgM antibody has been shown to develop in patients who had had IgG antibody previously (38). Thus, an IgM response does not seem necessarily to indicate only primary infection, inasmuch as it may occur in reinfection or relapse. Recently, CMV antigen used in the test has been shown to react with macroglobulin generated by other herpes group virus infections (54). The specificity of the test is therefore less than had been anticipated.

E. Cell-Virus Relationships

More understanding of the expression of CMV and its relationship to the host may be gained by observing the activity of the virus in various cell lines. In our laboratory, three separate phenomena have been observed.

Following infection with high-titer CMV in WI-38 human fibroblasts, early rounding of the cells occurs, followed in four to five days by the appearance of cell-free virus in the tissue culture fluid as a result of lytic infection. These cells continue to shed virus for a period of up to approximately six weeks and then gradually die off (55).

Following similar infection of VA4 cells (SV40 transformed fibroblasts), little change is noted in cell morphology; but if these cells are tested for the presence of virus, persistent shedding is noted as with WI-38. If the VA4 cells then are passaged, they appear normal, although shedding of virus at low titer persists. Such virus shedding has been continuous over a six-month period.

In addition, in our laboratory, Dr. Fioretti has observed early rounding and cytopathic effect following infection of guinea pig embryo cells with high-titer CMV (55a). After this early change, the cells return to normal within 48 hours. Attempts to recover virus from these cells have been unsuccessful. Thus, in tissue culture, CMV will cause chronic, lytic, or abortive infection.

F. Isolation

Attempts to isolate virus from patients require consideration of the different modes of cellular expression. Isolation of virus from the urine of patients is accomplished readily because the virus is in a cell-free state, similar to that following lytic infection of WI-38. Many patients tend to excrete virus in low titer for long periods of time after acute infection; and, if cultures inoculated with these specimens are managed carefully, one is rewarded with isolation. In some instances, isolation of virus from the blood of patients requires prolonged culturing of cells and use of cocultivation techniques, which are also useful in isolation of other cell-associated viruses. Several factors deserve mention with regard to culturing from the blood:

1. Anticoagulant: heparin versus citrate. While isolation of the virus is recorded in the presence of heparin, some evidence exists to show that herpes agents are inhibited by the presence of heparin (56).
2. Heat lability. CMV is unstable when frozen even at −60°C unless stabilizer is added. Clinical specimens from urine and throat swabs appear to preserve better after storage at 4°C (57).
3. Cell association. Viral agents that are cell associated can be rescued, in some cases, only after prolonged cultivation either by cocultivation with receptor cells (i.e., WI-38) or by explant technique. In the case of CMV blood cultures, it may be necessary to add fresh receptor cells several times before cultures can be called negative. Some cultures have been maintained for four to five months before the appearance of small foci of viral cytopathic effect. Explant culture and the culturing of whole cells seem to be preferable to the use of cells disrupted by sonication or mincing (58).

G. Pathogenesis

How is the host affected by CMV? Several possible pathogenic mechanisms exist.

1. Infection may lead to cell destruction and death, as evident in the fulminating neonatal syndrome, and is most likely present in other forms of the disease.
2. Tissue culture cells will respond to infection by slowing of growth and alteration in morphology. Further work on the effects of the latent viral state on cell growth and metabolism is needed.
3. Osborn, Blaskovec, and Walker (59) have demonstrated a period of immunoblockade during murine CMV infection. Whether or not this occurs in man is not clear, although Craighead (45) reports focal areas of superinfection in parts of lung associated with inclusion. Infection of key protective cells, such as the plasma cell, could lead to widespread effects on the host.
4. Occurrences of hemolytic anemia, cryoglobulins, rheumatoid

factor, and other abnormal proteins have been found in patients with the postperfusion syndrome. The possibility of immune mediated disease deserves exploration (60).

5. Finally, the herpes agents have been described as providing helper activity in several viral systems. Cells infected with CMV can be superinfected with other agents (61). CMV may make cells more susceptible to other agents that are more pathogenic.

The final description of host-virus relationships of members of the herpes group awaits answers to fundamental questions in virology and immunology. Only then can the problem of opportunism be understood and specific therapy be designed. Until then, awareness of the disease patterns and modes of transmission of these agents will help in their recognition as potential pathogens in the altered host.

Literature Cited

1. Lang, D. J., and J. F. Klummer. Demonstration of cytomegalovirus in semen. New Engl. J. Med. 287: 756, 1972.
2. Henle, G., W. Henle, and V. Diehl. Relation of Burkitt's tumor-associated herpes-type virus to infectious mononucleosis. Proc. Natl. Acad. Sci. U.S.A. 59: 94, 1968.
3. Nash, G., M. J. Asch, F. D. Foley, and B. A. Pruitt, Jr. Disseminated cytomegalic inclusion disease in a burned adult. JAMA 214: 587, 1970.
4. Foley, F. D., K. A. Greenwald, G. Nash, and B. A. Pruitt, Jr. Herpes virus infection in burned patients. New Engl. J. Med. 282: 652, 1970.
5. Rook, A., D. S. Wilkinson, and F. J. G. Ebling. Textbook of Dermatology. Vol. I, p. 773. F. A. Davis Co., Philadelphia, 1968.
6. Nahmias, A. J., E. A. Alford, and S. B. Korones. Infection of the newborn with herpes virus hominis. Adv. Pediat. 17: 185, 1970.
7. Hanshaw, J. B. Congenital cytomegalovirus infection: A fifteen year perspective. J. Infect. Dis. 123: 555, 1971.
8. Rinvik, R. Congenital varicella encephalomyelitis in surviving newborn. Amer. J. Dis. Child. 117: 231, 1969.
9. Finkel, K. C. Mortality from varicella in children receiving adrenocortico steroids and adrenocorticotropin. Pediatrics 28: 436, 1961.
10. Chiba, S., S. Ikeda, Y. Agatsuma, F. Nakao, and Y. Saheki. Active infection with cytomegalovirus and herpes-group virus in children receiving corticosteroid therapy. Tohoku J. Exp. Med. 106: 265, 1972.

11. Sokal, J. E., and D. Firat. Varicella-zoster infection in Hodgkin's disease. Amer. J. Med. 39: 452, 1965.
12. Keidan, S. E., and D. Mainwaring. Association of herpes-zoster with leukemia and lymphoma in children. Clin. Pediat. 4: 13, 1965.
13. Farber, S., and S. B. Wolbach. Intranuclear and cytoplasmic inclusions (protozoan-like bodies) in the salivary glands and other organs of infants. Amer. J. Pathol. 8: 123, 1932.
14. Smith, M. G. Propagation in tissue culture of a cytopathogenic virus from human salivary gland virus disease (SGV). Proc. Soc. Exp. Biol. Med. 92: 424, 1956.
15. Rowe, W. P., J. W. Hartley, S. Waterman, H. C. Turner, and R. J. Huebner. Cytopathic agent resembling human salivary gland virus recovered from tissue culture of human adenoids. Proc. Soc. Exp. Biol. Med. 92: 418, 1956.
16. Anderson, H. K. Serological differentiation of human cytomegalovirus strains using rabbit hyperimmune sera. Arch. Ges. Virusforsch. 33: 187, 1971.
17. Starr, J. G., D. Calafiore, and H. L. Casey. Experience with a human cytomegalovirus compliment fixing antigen. Amer. J. Epidemiol. 86: 507, 1967.
18. Wentworth, B., and E. R. Alexander. Seroepidemiology of infections due to members of the herpes-virus group. Amer. J. Epidemiol. 94: 496, 1971.
19. Haldane, E. V., J. A. Embil, and A. D. Wall. A serological study of cytomegalovirus infection in the population of Easter Island. Bull. W.H.O. 40: 969, 1969.
20. Numazaki, Y., N. Yano, T. Morizuka, S. Takai, and N. Ishida. Primary infection with human cytomegalovirus: Virus isolation from healthy infants and pregnant women. Amer. J. Epidemiol. 91: 410, 1969.
21. Stern, H. Isolation of cytomegalovirus and clinical manifestations of infection at different ages. Brit. Med. J. 1: 665, 1968.
22. Birnbaum, G., J. Lynch, A. M. Margileth, W. M. Lonergan, and J. L. Sever. Cytomegalovirus infections in newborn infants. J. Pediat. 75: 789, 1969.
23. Starr, J. G., R. D. Bart, and E. Gold. Inapparent congenital cytomegalovirus infection: Clinical and epidemiological characteristics in early infancy. New Engl. J. Med. 282: 1075, 1970.
24. Weller, T. H., J. C. Macauley, J. M. Craig, and P. Wirth. Isolation of intranuclear producing agents from infants with illness resembling cytomegalic inclusion disease. Proc. Soc. Exp. Biol. Med. 94: 4, 1957.
25. King-Lewis, P. A., and S. Gardner. Congenital cytomegalic inclusion disease following intrauterine transfusion. Brit. Med. J. 2: 603, 1969.

26. Montgomery, R., L. Youngblood, and D. N. Medearis, Jr. Recovery of cytomegalovirus from the cervix in pregnancy. Pediatrics 49: 524, 1972.
27. Diosi, P., L. Babusceac, O. Nevinglovschi, and G. Kun-Stoicu. Cytomegalovirus infection associated with pregnancy. Lancet ii: 1063, 1967.
27a. Olson, L. C., R. Ketusinha, P. Mansuwan, and R. Snitban. Respiratory tract excretion of cytomegalovirus in Thai children. J. Pediat. 77: 499, 1970.
28. Klemola, E., R. Von Essen, G. Henle, and W. Henle. Infectious-mononucleosis-like disease with negative heterophile agglutination test. Clinical features in relation to Epstein-Barr virus and cytomegalovirus antibodies. J. Infect. Dis. 121: 608, 1970.
29. Zuelzer, W., R. Mastrangelo, C. Stulberg, M. D. Poulik, R. H. Page, and R. I. Thompson. Autoimmune hemolytic anemia: Natural history and viral-immunologic interactions in childhood. Amer. J. Med. 49: 80, 1970.
30. Coombs, R. R. H. Cytomegalic inclusion-body disease associated with acquired autoimmune haemolytic anaemia. Brit. Med. J. 2: 743, 1968.
31. Evans, A. S., J. C. Niederman, and R. W. McCollum. Seroepidemiologic studies of infectious mononucleosis with EB virus. New Engl. J. Med. 279: 1121, 1968.
32. Diosi, P., E. Moldovan, and N. Tomescu. Latent cytomegalovirus infection in blood donors. Brit. Med. J. 4: 660, 1969.
33. Mirkovic, R., J. Werch, M. A. South, and M. Benyesh-Melnick. Incidence of cytomegaloviremia in blood-bank donors and in infants with congenital cytomegalic inclusion disease. Infect. Immun. 3: 45, 1971.
34. Lang, D. J. Cytomegalovirus infections in organ transplantation and post transfusion. Arch. Ges. Virusforsch. 37: 365, 1972.
35. Lang, D. J., P. A. Ebert, B. M. Rodgers, H. P. Boggess, and R. S. Rixse. Reduction of postperfusion cytomegalovirus infections after the use of leukocyte-depleted blood. J. Clin. Invest. 51: 53a, 1972.
36. Prince, A. M., W. Szmuness, S. J. Millian, and D. S. David. A serologic study of cytomegalovirus infections associated with blood transfusions. New Engl. J. Med. 284: 1125, 1971.
37. Armstrong, D., M. Ely, and L. Steger. Post-transfusion cytomegaloviremia and persistence of cytomegalovirus in the blood. Infect. Immun. 3: 159, 1971.
38. Nagington, J. Cytomegalovirus antibody production in renal transplant patients. J. Hyg. Camb. 69: 645, 1971.
39. Rifkind, D., N. Goodman, and R. B. Hill. The clinical significance of cytomegalovirus infection in renal transplant recipients. Ann. Intern. Med. 66: 1116, 1967.
40. Craighead, J. E., J. B. Hanshaw, and C. B. Carpenter. Cytomegalovirus infection after renal allotransplantation. JAMA 201: 725, 1967.

41. Armstrong, D., M. Haghbin, S. L. Balakrishnan, and M. L. Murphy. Asymptomatic cytomegalovirus infection in children with leukemia. Amer. J. Dis. Child. 122: 404, 1971.
42. Sutton, R. N. P., C. W. Darby, and S. M. Gumpel. Cytomegalovirus infection in childhood leukemia. Brit. J. Haematol. 20: 437, 1971.
43. Caul, E. O., V. A. Dickinson, A. P. Roome, M. G. Mott, and P. A. Stevenson. Cytomegalovirus infections in leukemic children. Internatl. J. Cancer 10: 213, 1972.
44. Henson, D., S. E. Siegal, D. A. Fuccillo, E. Matthew, and A. S. Levine. Cytomegalovirus infections during acute childhood leukemia. J. Infect. Dis. 126: 469, 1972.
45. Craighead, J. E. Pulmonary cytomegalovirus infection in the adult. Amer. J. Pathol. 63: 487, 1971.
46. Weller, T. H., and J. B. Hanshaw. Virologic and clinical observations on cytomegalic inclusion disease. New Engl. J. Med. 266: 1233, 1962.
47. Weller, T. H. Cytomegaloviruses: The difficult years. J. Infect. Dis. 122: 532, 1970.
48. Waner, J. L., and T. H. Weller. Serological and cultural studies bearing on the persistent nature of cytomegaloviral infections in man. In M. Pollard (ed.), Perspectives in Virology. Vol. VIII, p. 211, Academic Press, New York, 1973.
49. Furakawa, T., F. Jensen, A. Fioretti, and S. A. Plotkin. Precipitin antibody in human cytomegalovirus infection. Abstracts of Annual Meeting of the American Society for Microbiology, Atlantic City, p. 246, 1972.
50. Huraux, J. M., P. Guillermin, and F. Bricout. Indirect haemagglutination of human cytomegalovirus. Rev. Eur. Étud. Clin. Biol. 16: 616, 1971.
51. Fuccillo, D. A., F. L. Moder, L. W. Catalano, M. M. Vincent, and J. L. Sever. Micro indirect hemagglutination test for cytomegalovirus. Appl. Microbiol. 21: 104, 1971.
52. Penttinen, K., L. Kääriäinen, and G. Myllylä. Cytomegalovirus antibody assay by platelet aggregation. Archiv. Virusforsch. 29: 189, 1970.
53. Hanshaw, J. B., H. J. Steinfeld, and C. J. White. Fluorescent-antibody test for cytomegalovirus macroglobulin. New Engl. J. Med. 279: 566, 1968.
54. Hanshaw, J. B., J. C. Niederman, and L. N. Chessin. Cytomegalovirus macroglobulin in cell-associated herpes virus infections. J. Infect. Dis. 125: 304, 1972.
55. Furukawa, T., and S. A. Plotkin. Some characteristics of high titer cytomegalovirus from WI-38 human diploid cells. Fed. Proc. 31: 810, 1972.
55a. Fioretti, A., J. Furukowa, D. Santoli, and S. Plotkin. Nonproductive

infection of guinea pig cells with human cytomegalovirus. J. Virol. 11: 998, 1973.
56. Vaheri, A. Heparin and related polyionic substances as virus inhibitors. Acta Pathol. Microbiol. Scand. 171(Suppl): 98, 1964.
57. Lennette, E. H., and N. J. Schmidt (eds.). Diagnostic Procedures for Viral and Rickettsial Infections. 4th Ed. American Public Health Association, New York, 1969. p. 715.
58. Shope, T. E., J. Klein-Robbenhaar, and G. Miller. Fatal encephalitis due to herpes virus hominis: Use of intact brain cells for isolation of virus. J. Infect. Dis. 125: 542, 1972.
59. Osborn, J. E., A. A. Blazkovec, and D. L. Walker. Immunosuppression during acute murine cytomegalovirus infection. J. Immunol. 100: 835, 1968.
60. Kantor, G. L., L. S. Goldberg, B. L. Johnson, M. M. Dereehin, and E. V. Barnett. Immunologic abnormalities induced by post perfusion cytomegalovirus infection. Ann. Intern. Med. 73: 553, 1970.
61. Seto, D. S., and D. H. Carver. Interaction between cytomegalovirus and Newcastle disease virus as mediated by intrinsic interference. J. Virol. 4: 12, 1969.
62. Henle, W., G. Henle, M. Scriba, C. R. Joyner, F. S. Harrison, R. von Essen, J. Paloheimo, and E. Klemola. Antibody responses to the Epstein-Barr virus and cytomegaloviruses after open-heart and other surgery. New Engl. J. Med. 282: 1068, 1970.
63. Stevens, D. P., L. F. Barker, A. S. Ketcham, and H. M. Meyer, Jr. Asymptomatic cytomegalovirus infection following blood transfusion in tumor surgery. JAMA 211: 1341, 1970.
64. Perham, T. G. M., E. O. Caul, P. J. Conway, and M. G. Mott. Cytomegalovirus infection in blood donors—a prospective study. Brit. J. Haematol. 20: 307, 1971.
65. Paloheimo, J. A., R. von Essen, E. Klemola, L. Kääriäinen, and P. Siltanen. Subclinical cytomegalovirus infections and cytomegalovirus mononucleosis after open heart surgery. Amer. J. Cardiol. 22: 624, 1968.

15

Control of Opportunistic Infections in Hospitals— A Position Paper

N. Joel Ehrenkranz, George W. Counts,
J. Leilani Kicklighter,
and Phineas J. Hyams

I. Introduction

Opportunistic infections are those which occur because of decreased host resistance to microbial invasion, rather than increased microbial virulence. Hence, a quantitative relation between susceptibility and disease caused by opportunistic microflora can be inferred. The minimal disease-producing number of such microorganisms presumably decreases as host susceptibility increases. Healthy subjects, by contrast, should be able to withstand exposure to similar or even larger numbers of microorganisms by the same route with no ill effect. In the context of this discussion, microorganisms generally associated with nosocomial infections will be considered as opportunistic invaders. Among the important ingredients in the epidemiology of these infections are certain people, certain inanimate objects, and the indiscriminate use of antimicrobial agents.

Supported by the Florida Regional Medical Program Project No. 46.

The people involved with opportunistic infections are of two groups: those more likely to acquire infection because of intrinsic change in resistance, called "susceptibles," and those who are particularly efficient in dissemination, called "spreaders." Among the latter are persons with overt infections and those who are seemingly healthy. Both types are found in hospitals, as patients and as employees. Those with overt infection are the easier to identify. One index of opportunistic infection, and therefore of microbial spread, may be derived from systematic observations of certain highly susceptible patients whose increased risk to infection is readily apparent. Such individuals may serve as "sentinels" in the epidemiological sense and may lead to detection of healthy and sick spreaders as well as of other sources of infection.

Inanimate objects not only permit survival and person-to-person transfer of opportunistic microflora, but may serve also as numerical amplifiers of the microbial population. Since minimal substrate, such as distilled water, saline, and Ringer's solution can support growth of bacteria responsible for nosocomial infection (1), environmental studies are important. However, indiscriminate studies of microbial distribution in the hospital environment are herculean tasks which may be totally unrewarding in terms of infection control. Thus, microbial surveillance of the environment should be carried out in a way that is calculated to yield information relevant to human infection.

Antimicrobial therapy renders patients susceptible to new infection with opportunistic microbes. Moreover, antibiotic usage influences patterns of drug susceptibility of nosocomial microflora by selecting resistant microorganisms for survival (2). Although it has long been clear that excessive usage results in new infections with resistant microorganisms, programs of antibiotic limitations clearly are beset with difficulty. Effective methods for restriction of antibiotics in the usual hospital setting remain to be demonstrated, but such limitations are not likely to result from simple administrative fiat.

Thus, control of opportunistic infections in hospitals should be accomplished by surveillance of specific people and fomites and by discouragement of unrestricted antimicrobial therapy. Sound epidemiological principles, guided by selectivity and discretion, are necessary for success, and much yet remains to be learned.

II. Organization of the Infection Control Service

In our view, hospital infection control requires the professional approach of a skilled group, consisting of a full-time infection control nurse or nurses, a trained physician-epidemiologist, and a competent microbiologist, organized into a single administrative unit, the Infection Control Service. Adequate facilities for in-depth diagnostic and epidemiological microbiology are essential. Clerical support and equipment should be available for recording, calculating, and storing data and for rapid recall of infection rates.

This concept of a professional group for hospital infection control extends from the original programs of nurse epidemiology (3, 4) and physician involvement in hospital infection epidemiology (5). In our experience, an infection control nurse is not effective without the regular consultation and support of a clinician-epidemiologist. Similarly, a microbiologist is at a distinct disadvantage by himself. Parenthetically, nurses, physicians, and microbiologists knowledgable in infection control and hospital epidemiology have not been easy for us to find, and, of necessity, we have developed our own training programs.

Before outlining details of our approach to control of opportunistic infection, it is appropriate to set forth three basic propositions which we feel are implicit in the successful functioning of the program.

1. An enlighted hospital administration is an absolute necessity. The Infection Control Service must have adequate funds, space, equipment, and personnel, and regular meetings with administration. Ideally, the physician-epidemiologist should be the hospital administrator responsible for infection control. In order to avoid a conflict of interest, he should not be chairman of the hospital infection committee. A review of the standards set forth by the Joint Commission on Hospital Accreditation, relating to hospital infection and antibiotic control, may be useful for administration and the hospital staff for purposes of orientation:

Standard IV*

Responsibility for the control of infection within the hospital, and for the evaluation of the infection potential of the related environment, shall be vested in a multidisciplinary committee of the medical staff. Responsibility for this function should be given to a committee made up of representatives of the medical staff, the administration, the microbiology laboratory, and the nursing service.

[T]he committee should meet on a regular basis ... [and] review data obtained since the previous meeting. Such review may include: reports of hospital-associated infections that include identification of patients requiring isolation; reports of tests conducted on sterilization devices; and reports of bacteriological studies of personnel, of patients, or of environment.

Standard IV*

The [Hospital Infection] Committee should do at least the following:
• Develop written standards for hospital sanitation and medical asepsis. These standards should include a definition of infection for the purpose of surveillance, as well as specific indications of the need for the procedures to be used in isolation.
• Develop, evaluate and revise on a continuing basis the procedures and techniques for meeting established sanitation and asepsis standards.
• Develop a practical system for reporting, evaluating and keeping records of infections among patients and personnel in order to provide an indication of the endemic level of all nosocomial infections, to trace the sources of infection and to identify epidemic or potential epidemic situations.
• Review periodically the use of antibiotics as they relate to patient care within the hospital.

2. The expertise, advice, and on-the-scene help of the Hospital Infections Section of the Center for Disease Control, U. S. Public Health Service, Atlanta, Ga., are freely available for both prevention and investigation of infection problems. Their criteria for hospital-associated infection and tabulation forms are especially valuable and will provide for uniformity in analyses (6).
3. The recording of microbial cultures of people or things and/ or the tabulation of rates of infection do not equal infection control. However, monthly data on rates of infection, pre-

---

* Accreditation Manual for Hospitals, Environmental Services, Standard IV, p. 9. Joint Commission of Accreditation of Hospitals, Chicago, 1970.

pared by the Infection Control Service in a consistent way, do permit intelligent analyses if certain components are included (Table 1).

III. Responsibilities of the Infection Control Service

A. Clinical and Epidemiological Responsibilities

Hospital-associated infection should be identified and classified according to anatomical site and causative organisms, and recorded by geographical area, professional service, and involved procedure or equipment.

Table 1. Components of hospital infection surveillance report

I. Presentation of monthly statistics of nosocomial infections
   A. Calculated by:
      1. Anatomical site
      2. Ward
      3. Service
      4. Infecting microorganisms
   B. Discussion of changes in rates includes:
      1. Possible clusters
      2. Sampling variations
      3. Changes in surveillance technique
      4. Changes in patient population
      5. Secular trends
      6. Effective control measures
   C. For clusters of nosocomial infection: implications, proposed further investigations and possible means of control
   D. Discussion of selected nosocomial infections

II. Results of prevalence walk: observation of infections and comments on reporting disparities

III. Employee health problems: analysis of occurrence of hepatitis, tuberculosis tuberculin converters; programs for influenza, rubella immunizations, and other preventive measures.

IV. Autopsy review: relation of nosocomial infections to patient deaths

V. Surveillance of antibiotic usage.

A continuing program of in-house patient surveillance is vital. We feel that this is best accomplished by the Service's identification and prospective observation of specific high-risk patients—the above-mentioned "sentinels"—to determine their rates of acquisition of infection. In addition, regular reports from various patient areas are solicited. Educational activities concerning the criteria of hospital infection, means of reporting, and hospital policy with regard to prevention of infection are carried out in small groups for various nursing units and physician groups. Much useful information is gained from reports by floor nurses and physicians; however, interpretation may be difficult unless the Infection Control Service compares these reports with its own regular observations (7). Thus, the prevalence of infections should be determined weekly by the Service in a bed-to-bed survey on one or more nursing units. Reported discrepancies then are discussed with the personnel of the units.

Retrospective evaluation alone, particularly that done from hospital records after patient discharge, is of limited value in identifying current problems in time for control. However, when taken together with observations of current infection, systematic retrospective evaluations are useful. For example, we review all autopsies monthly for the possible presence of opportunistic infection and make a judgment of its role in the patient's demise.

In addition to patients, employees risk acquiring and spreading infection. Such conditions as diarrhea or skin infections, or more virulent infections such as tuberculosis* and hepatitis,* may be hazardous to patients and employees alike. An effective employee health program is an integral part of infection control. Infections in employees should be recorded by the hospital employee health office and evaluated by members of the Infection Control Program to determine their possible relation to patient infection.

B. Microbiological Responsibilities

Precise microbiology is an obvious prerequisite for intelligent investigations of outbreaks, and is necessary for determining

---

* These are not opportunistic infections, but rather are nosocomial infections.

sources of opportunistic infection and individuals colonized with opportunistic microorganisms, as well as identifying those who are clinically involved. These investigations often necessitate quantitative as well as qualitative studies, and the logistics can be formidable. The microbiologist needs laboratory resources with the capacity to undertake the increased work load of epidemic investigation and must be aware of his limitations in this regard, so that he can obtain help when necessary.

In addition to the investigation of outbreaks, relevant environmental surveillance is an appropriate responsibility of the microbiologist. For example, inhalation therapy equipment used by selected susceptible patients should be regularly evaluated during use to determine the level of contamination and the relation between that contamination and patient infection (8, 9). Random checks on the sterility of so-called sterile equipment and on the efficacy of sterilization equipment also need to be carried out.

Human microbial surveillance may be of value, but this needs further definition. Quantitative studies of *Pseudomonas* skin colonization may help to determine when therapy of the highly susceptible burn patient should be instituted (10); similarly, quantitative studies of *Staphylococcus aureus* colonization may indicate when simple carriers become dangerous spreaders (11). However, routine, qualitative skin, nasopharyngeal, or stool cultures of patients or personnel taken in the absence of clinical or epidemiological leads not only are useless but frankly are wasteful of limited resources. Similarly, routine cultures of floors, silverware, air conditioners, etc., are unnecessary for infection control, although they may indicate the general level of cleanliness. Microbiological studies which are not interpreted or are uninterpretable are to be avoided.

It is important to perform antibiotic sensitivity studies in a reliable and reproducible manner. Regular in-house publication of recent opportunistic pathogens and their antibiotic sensitivity patterns can greatly influence and aid selection of appropriate antibiotic therapy by physicians in that hospital.

C. Advice to Administration

The Infection Control Service should advise the hospital administration on a number of matters. Physical facilities play an important role in control of opportunistic infection. For example, the availability and placement of sinks, design of traffic flow, function of ventilation systems, and types of housekeeping equipment are all considerations pertinent to infection control. The need for "life island" isolation, rooms with air locks, laminar air flow, and ultraviolet lights for protection against nosocomial infection are important considerations. These structures occasionally may be necessary to prevent spread or acquisition of infection; however, administrative decisions concerning their installation should include the judgments of the Infection Control Service. Continuous evaluation to determine the efficacy of these structures once they are installed is necessary to avoid false security (12, 13).

Administrative aspects of patient placement are also under the purview of the Infection Control Service. To prevent opportunistic infections, bed assignments for patients admitted to the hospital must be made with knowledge of the patient's susceptibility to infection and his ability to disseminate it. Such bed assignments and the institution of appropriate isolation techniques require an objective evaluation of the patient's ability to spread or acquire infection. This evaluation should supercede both the attending physician's opinion about placement of his patient and the patient's desires, not withstanding his financial status. Strict criteria can be supplied by the Service. Since nonprofit hospitals now share legal responsibility for physician's errors (14), cooperation of all parties concerned can be obtained if bed assignments are made diplomatically and impartially.

The assignment of type and number of employees in some patient areas often can be critical in infection control. For example, harried or undertrained personnel may not carry out simple handwashing as a necessary precaution prior to contact with each patient. Personnel with mild diarrhea or inconspicuous furunculosis may continue to work so as not to "let the team down." "Floating" of personnel from one floor of the hospital to another, especially on the 11 P.M. to 7 A.M. shift, can be a pernicious practice contributing to spread of infection. For example, if the employee "floats" between infected gynecological patients, normal obstetrical patients, and the newborn nursery, the stage will be set for spread of infection to infants or mothers.

Policies, procedures, and purchase of equipment which bear on infection should be evaluated by the Infection Control Service. New products must be investigated with a search for unbiased evidence of effectiveness.

D. Prevention

Intelligent intervention, based on clinical and microbiological studies, is the goal of the Infection Control Service. The weekly prevalence walk of infection is extremely useful in this regard. One may detect overcrowding of patients or the mingling of susceptibles and spreaders in a multibed room and may arrange for redistribution. One may observe faulty techniques of patient isolation, unsterile techniques in changing surgical dressings, and prolonged placement of therapeutic foreign bodies such as intravascular or intraurethral catheters, and may correct the errors on the spot. One can seek potential and actual sources of microbial contamination and eliminate them before infections occur. One may find that the disparity between announced policy and actual practice often is considerable. An inquiry into a head nurse's reasons for being unable to implement infection control policy may reveal a variety of difficulties which the Infection Control Service can help to remedy. Interference between a physician and his patient obviously must be avoided. Administrative abuses in the name of infection control cannot be permitted. Only those practices which are known to influence infections are in the legitimate realm of the Infection Control Service.

To maintain the good will of the professional staff, physicians and nurses alike, the Infection Control Service must investigate carefully and sympathetically the circumstances of departure from fixed policy, but ultimately must act with total fairness. To this end, it may be useful for the physician-epidemiologist serving one or more community hospitals to be based in a university hospital and not to be economically dependent upon a practice in the former.

E. Limitation of Antibiotic Usage

For the past 25 years, it has been known that successful antibiotic therapy of infections may be followed by superinfection with opportunistic microorganisms (15). Antibacterial agents have several distinct effects which promote opportunistic infections. These include:

1. Colonization of the host with new organisms as a result of therapy's decreasing the variety and numbers of his usual body microflora. For example, the toe web studies of Taplin (16) have demonstrated a shift from Gram-positive to Gram-negative microflora on skin as a result of assiduous application of antibacterial soap (17). Others have shown similar results with systemic antibiotic treatment (18, 19). Colonization with opportunistic microflora on skin, respiratory, or enteric epithelium permits their subsequent invasion of the host or person-to-person dissemination.
2. One-way population pressures as a result of antibiotic exposure result in selection and concentration of antibiotic-resistant microorganisms in the hospital environment. These microorganisms may grow in fomites containing minimal support media and then may invade the susceptible host via respiratory therapy equipment, along various therapeutic foreign bodies in common use, or after first colonizing his mucous membranes. Bacteria such as *Klebsiella* which have a particularly high frequency of resistance transfer factors may have a biological advantage in this regard (20), along with other organisms, such as *Pseudomonas* and *Serratia* species, which are naturally resistant to many antibiotics.
3. Tetracycline treatment enhances an individual's environmental dissemination, autoinfection, and person-to-person spread of tetracycline-resistant *S. aureus* and tetracycline-resistant pneumococci (21, 22). Thus, the seemingly profligate usage of tetracyclines in hospitals (23) merits further examination. Indeed, in view of the availability of other equally effective antibiotics, one may well ask whether there are many indications for tetracycline therapy in hospitalized patients.

None of this is particularly new, yet virtually nothing has been achieved in the efforts to curb excessive usage of antibiotics in hospitals. Scheckler and Bennett (23) have reported that more than 30% of 5286 patients in seven community hospitals were receiving antibiotics at the time of survey, i.e., between 1967 and 1969; in less than half of those being treated was evidence of infection apparent in the record. Hence, we share the view of Finland (2) that some limitations of unrestricted antibiotic usage in hospitals are indicated. This view must be taken as an admission of our failure as educators.

There are a number of ways to curtail excessive antibiotic therapy in hospitals. These include:

1. Withholding selected antibiotics for use in specifically defined, life-threatening infections. The drugs are to be made available when certain clinical or clinical plus microbiological conditions have been met. Members of the Infection Control Service who are not involved with the patient's care are to see that the conditions are met before the antibiotic is released.
2. Limiting broad-spectrum antibiotic therapy or its equivalent, including penicillin in dosage of greater than 3 million units per day, to five days of usage. More extended therapy requires an explanatory note in the record by the physician. Such notes are reviewed by physicians who are not involved with the patient's care, and inappropriate usage is brought to the physician's attention.
3. Analyzing antibiotic usage in a utilization committee by reviewing records for evidence of infection at the time at which antibiotic therapy was begun, and for selection, dose, and duration of therapy. The findings are evaluated according to predetermined accepted criteria of good antibiotic usage. Repeated inappropriate usage on the part of a physician carries a predetermined penalty.
4. Voluntarily restricting certain antibiotics on the basis of in-house antibiotic sensitivity studies of selected infections and analyses of distribution of opportunistic infections in the hospital. Physicians not complying with the advice not to use certain drugs will be reminded to do so in a monthly therapy review conference.

Whether any or all of these alternatives, or various combinations of them, will, in fact, decrease excessive antibiotic usage without concurrently diminishing appropriate therapy remains to be demonstrated. We are exploring this possibility now.

Along these lines, it may be appropriate for the microbiologist to record but not to report patterns of sensitivity to chloramphenicol for aerobic bacteria and perhaps to other selected antibiotics in an effort to limit their use. Such information would be available only upon the physician's request.

IV. Summary

The goals of a hospital Infection Control Service are to seek small clusters of opportunistic infections by time, place, and microorganism; to identify sources of infection, both animate and inanimate, early enough to permit corrective measures before serious consequences occur; to institute preventive measures on a broad front, involving the cooperation of professional and administrative personnel; and to conduct these activities in a manner consistent with the best possible patient care.

Literature Cited

1. Favero, M. S., L. A. Carson, W. W. Bond, and N. J. Petersen. *Pseudomonas aeruginosa:* Growth in distilled water from hospitals. Science 173: 836, 1971.
2. Finland, M. Changing patterns of susceptibility of common bacterial pathogens to antimicrobial agents. Ann. Intern. Med. 76: 1009, 1972.
3. Davis, N. C. The infection control sister. Her role in a large hospital. Lancet ii: 1321, 1963.
4. Gardner, A. M. N., M. Stamp, J. A. Bowgen, and B. Moore. The infection control sister. A new member of the control of infection team in general hospitals. Lancet ii: 710, 1962.
5. Langmuir, A. D. Significance of epidemiology in medical schools. J. Med. Educ. 39: 39, 1964.
6. Outline for Surveillance and Control of Nosocomial Infection. U. S. Department of Health, Education and Welfare, Center for Disease Con-

trol, Epidemiology Program, Bacterial Diseases Branch, Hospital Infections Section, Atlanta, Ga., 1970.
7. Eickhoff, T. C., P. S. Brachman, J. V. Bennett, and J. Brown. Surveillance of nosocomial infections in community hospitals. I. Surveillance methods, effectiveness and initial results. J. Infect. Dis. 120: 305, 1969.
8. Reinarz, J. A., A. K. Pierce, B. B. Mays, and J. P. Sanford. The potential role of inhalation therapy equipment in nosocomial pulmonary infection. J. Clin. Invest. 44: 831, 1965.
9. Sanders, C. V., J. P. Luby, W. G. Johanson, J. A. Barnett, and J. P. Sanford. *Serratia marcescens* infections from inhalation therapy medications: Nosocomial outbreak. Ann. Intern. Med. 73: 15, 1970.
10. Brentano, L., C. A. Moyer, D. L. Gravens, and W. W. Monafo. Bacteriology of large human burns treated with silver nitrate. Arch. Surg. 93: 456, 1966.
11. White, A. Increased infection rates in heavy nasal carriers of coagulase-positive staphylococci. *In* J. C. Sylvester (ed.), Antimicrobial Agents and Chemotherapy, p. 667. American Society for Microbiology, Ann Arbor, 1963.
12. Burke, J. F. A bacteria controlled nursing unit and individual patient isolation facility. *In* Proceedings of the International Conference on Nosocomial Infections. Center for Disease Control, p. 216. American Hospital Association, Chicago, 1970.
13. Lidwell, O. M. Hospital uses of unidirectional ("laminar") air flow. *In* Proceedings of the International Conference on Nosocomial Infection. Center for Disease Control, p. 207. American Hospital Association, Chicago, 1970.
14. Springer, E. W. Medical staff law and the hospital. New Engl. J. Med. 285: 952, 1971.
15. Weinstein, L. The spontaneous occurrence of new bacterial infections during the course of treatment with streptomycin or penicillin. Amer. J. Med. Sci. 214: 56, 1947.
16. Taplin, D. The use of antibiotics in dermatology. *In* W. Montagna, R. B. Stoughton, and E. J. VanScott (eds.), Pharmacology and the Skin. Vol. 12, p. 315. Appleton-Century-Crofts, New York, 1972.
17. Ehrenkranz, N. J., D. Taplin, and P. Butt. Antibiotic-resistant bacteria on the nose and skin, colonization and cross-infection. *In* G. L. Hobby (ed.), Antimicrobial Agents and Chemotherapy, p. 255. American Society for Microbiology, Ann Arbor, 1966.
18. Smith, D. T. The disturbance of the normal bacterial ecology by the administration of antibiotics with the development of new clinical syndromes. Ann. Intern. Med. 37: 1135, 1952.
19. Sprunt, K., and W. Redman. Evidence suggesting importance of role of

interbacterial inhibition in maintaining balance of normal flora. Ann. Intern. Med. 68: 579, 1968.
20. Pollack, M., P. Charache, R. E. Nieman, M. P. Jett, J. A. Reinhardt, and P. H. Hardy, Jr. Factors influencing colonisation and antibiotic-resistance patterns of gram-negative bacteria in hospital patients. Lancet ii: 668, 1972.
21. Ehrenkranz, N. J. Person-to-person transmission of *Staphylococcus aureus*. Quantitative characterization of nasal carriers spreading infection. New Engl. J. Med. 271: 225, 1964.
22. Turner, G. C. Tetracycline-resistant pneumococci in a general hospital. Lancet ii: 1292, 1963.
23. Scheckler, W. E., and J. V. Bennett. Antibiotic usage in seven community hospitals. JAMA 213: 264, 1970.

Index

Absidia, 156, 163, 166, 168
  lichtheimi, 169
  ramosa, 169
Actinomadura, 186, 187, 190–191, 196
  dassonvillei, 191, 194, 198
  madurae, 186, 191, 198
  pelletierii, 186, 191, 198
Actinomyces, 121, 199
  israeli, 94
Addiction
  to drugs, and yeast infection, 139
  to heroin, and superinfection, 14, 15
Adrenal hormones, 8
Aeromonas, 2, 65, 66, 77–78
  hydrophila, 69, 77
  punctata, 77
Agar dilution method, for testing susceptibility of opportunistic pathogens, 120–121, 123
Amphotericin B, use of. *See also* Antibiotic therapy
  in treatment of cryptococcosis, 148
  in treatment of mucormycosis, 169
Ampicillin. *See also* Antibiotic therapy
  ineffectiveness of, 77
  resistance to, 69, 70, 73, 75, 78
  sensitivity to, 82
  susceptibility to, 73, 75, 125

Anaerobic bacteria
  culture and identification of, 87–103
  incubation of, 87
  in opportunistic infections, 65–82
  sensitivity to antibiotic therapy, 69, 70, 105–109
  susceptibility to antibiotics, 105–116
  methods for testing, 109–115
  transport of, 90
Anaerobe laboratory, 88, 89
  methods used by, 90–92, 94–100
  susceptibility tests by, 106, 109–115
Animal bites, and infection of humans, 80
Antibiotic therapy
  and nosocomial infection, 282
  and superinfection, 3–8, 15, 290
  ineffectiveness of, 105–106, 125
  need for limitation of, 290–292
  sensitivity to
    by anaerobes, 69, 70
    by hemophili, 80
    by opportunistic pathogens, 287
  susceptibility to
    by anaerobes, 105–116
    by opportunistic pathogens, 119–126
    by yeasts, 130–131
Antimicrobial agents
  and Enterobacteriaceae, 70, 73, 77

Index

Antimicrobial agents—*Continued*
  efficacy of, 126
  therapy with, and nosocomial infection, 282
Antitumor agents, and superinfection, 9–10
Arachnia, 191
  propionica, 199
Arizona hinshawii, 70
Aspergillosis
  and leukemia, 2
  detected by immunodiffusion, 148
  in the compromised host, 169–174
  serodiagnosis of, 154–156
Aspergillus, 2, 3, 8, 10, 11, 16, 148, 156, 169–174, 245
  flavus, 156, 172
  fumigatus, 154–156, 171, 172, 174
  nidulans, 156, 172
  niger, 156, 172
  niveus, 172
  restrictus, 172
  sydowi, 172
  terreus, 156
  versicolor, 172
Asthma, and immunodiffusion techniques, 151
Australia antigen, detected by immunoelectroosmophoresis, 157

Bacitracin
  in cultures, 80
  ineffectiveness of, 80
Bacteremia
  and antibiotic therapy, 126
  and trauma, 20–21
  as superinfection, 1
Bacteriocin typing, 49
  applicability of, 56–60
  method of, 50–56
  use of, 50, 60–62

Bacterium typhi flavum, 75
Bacteroides, 94, 100, 102
  fragilis, 100, 108, 110
  melaninogenicus, 98, 100, 102
Besnoitia, 223
Besnoitiosis, 211
Birth control pills, and susceptibility to yeast infection, 138
Blastomyces, 12
  dermatitides, 12
Broth dilution method, for testing susceptibility of opportunistic pathogens, 120
Brucella, 110
Brucellaceae, identification of, 77
Burn wounds
  and herpes group disease, 262
  and infection, 20, 26, 31, 44
  and nosocomial infection, 287
  in the compromised host, 163, 167, 174

Candida, 2, 3, 7, 8, 9, 10, 14, 15, 16, 126, 136, 137, 144, 148, 150–153
  albicans, 9, 15, 129, 130, 132–133, 137–138, 139, 142–144, 150, 151, 152, 153, 154, 182
  parakrusei, 9
  parapsilosis, 131, 138–139, 144, 152
  pseudotropicalis, 134
  stellatoidea, 132, 142
  tropicalis, 131, 133, 137, 138–139, 144
Candidiasis, 1
  and antibiotic therapy, 7–8
  and leukemia, 2
  and needles and catheters, 8–9
  serodiagnosis of, 147, 150–154
Carbenicillin
  resistance to, 73, 75

Index

sensitivity to, 73
susceptibility to, 75
Catheters
  and nosocomial infection, 289
  and opportunistic infection, 44
  and superinfection, 8–9
Central nervous system, damaged by cytomegalovirus, 268
Cephalosporins
  effectiveness of, 106
  resistance to, 73
  sensitivity to, 75
  susceptibility to, 125
Cephalothin
  ineffectiveness of, 77
  resistance to, 70, 78, 82
  sensitivity to, 82
  susceptibility to, 75
Cetrimide, 22
Chickenpox
  caused by varicella-zoster, 261
  pathology of, 264
Chloramphenicol. *See also* Antibiotic therapy
  effectiveness of, 106
  resistance to, 73
  sensitivity to, 75, 78, 82
  use of
    in isolation of *Nocardia* species, 184, 185
    in isolation of yeasts, 130
Citrobacter
  Bethesda, 46
  diversus, 73–75
  freundii, 70, 73–75
Clindamycin. *See also* Antibiotic therapy
  effectiveness of, 106–108
Clostridium, 106
  perfringens, 94, 100, 110, 112
Coccidioides immitis, 3

Colistin
  resistance to, 78
  sensitivity to, 73, 75
Computers, use of
  in bacteriocin typing, 56
  in susceptibility tests, 123
Corynebacterium, 191–192, 198
Cross-infection
  and bacteriocin typing, 58–59
  and cytomegalovirus, 272
Cryptococcosis
  and listeriosis, 14
  and nocardiosis, 14
  and tuberculosis, 14
  association with impaired hosts, 139
  serodiagnosis of, 147, 148–150
Cryptococcus, 136, 144, 148
  albidus, 131, 137
  laurentii, 137
  neoformans, 3, 13, 130, 131, 136–137, 139–142, 148, 149
Cycloheximide. *See also* Antibiotic therapy
  use of, in isolation of *Nocardia* species, 184
Cyclophosphamide, treatment with, 235
Cystic fibrosis
  and antibody response, 40
  and susceptibility to infection, 42
Cysts, of *Toxoplasma*, 210–211, 225
Cytomegalovirus, 266
  and leukemia, 2
  and pneumocystosis, 234, 235–236
  and transplantation, 10, 270, 271–272
  clinical manifestations of, 261–262
  diagnosis of, 273
  epidemiology of, 267–268
  in the compromised host, 270–273
  in the normal host, 268–270

Index

Cytomegalovirus—*Continued*
  isolation of, 274–275
  pathogenesis of, 275–276
  pathology and morphology of, 264–266
  relationship to cell lines, 274

Dermatophilus, 188, 190
Diabetes
  and susceptibility to yeast infection, 139
  in the compromised host, 163, 164, 166, 167, 169
Diagnostic laboratory, 89
  methods used by, 92–102
Disc diffusion method
  for testing anaerobes, 111–113
  deficiency of, 113
  for testing opportunistic pathogens, 121–124
DNA, in herpes virus agents, 264

Eczema, and herpes group disease, 262
Edwardsiella tarda, 69
Encephalitis
  in the fetus and newborn infant, 261
  related to *Toxoplasma*, 211–212
Encephalitozoon, 220, 223
Endocarditis
  and antibiotic therapy, 126
  and superinfection, 14
  caused by yeast infection, 138
  in compromised hosts, 73, 172
  subacute bacterial, 38
Enterobacter, 26, 28–30, 32–34, 75
  aerogenes, 28, 29, 44
  agglomerans, 75

  cloacae, 28, 39–40, 46, 73
  hafniae, 28
  liquefaciens, 28
Enterobacteriaceae
  and antimicrobial agents, 70, 73, 77
  and cystic fibrosis, 42–43
  as opportunists, 66
  identification of, 26, 33, 34, 39, 75, 77
Epstein-Barr virus
  clinical manifestations of, 261–262
  pathology and morphology of, 264–266
Erwinia, 39, 46, 75
Erythromycin. *See also* Antibiotic therapy
  effectiveness of, 106
  sensitivity to, 82
Escherichia coli, 38, 42–43, 45, 77

Fungemia, caused by yeast infection, 139
Fusobacterium, 100

GasPak, for incubation of anaerobic bacteria, 87, 93, 94–100, 110–112
Gentamicin. *See also* Antibiotic therapy
  ineffectiveness of, 106
  sensitivity to, 73, 75, 78
  susceptibility to, 122
  use of, in isolation of yeasts, 130
Geotrichum candidum, 133
Germ tubes, use of, in identification of yeasts, 132–133, 142, 144
Glaucoma, related to *Toxoplasma*, 211

Index

Glove-box chamber, for isolation of anaerobic bacteria, 88, 91–92, 113, 114
Guizotia abyssinica, 137

Haemophilus, 65, 80
 influenzae, 66, 78–80
 parainfluenzae, 66, 78–80
Hansenula, 144
Hepatitis
 as nosocomial infection, 286
 in the fetus and newborn, 261
Herbicola-Lathyri, 75
Heroin addiction, and superinfection, 14, 15
Herpes simplex I and II
 clinical manifestations of, 261–262
 pathology and morphology of, 264–266
Herpes virus, human
 clinical manisfestations of, 261–262
 epidemiology and biology of, 262–264
 pathology, classification, and morphology of, 264–266
Hetacillin. *See* Antibiotic therapy
Histoplasma capsulatum, 3, 11, 13
Hodgkin's disease, and *Nocardia asteroides*, 178

Immune response
 in candidiasis, 153–154
 of leukemia patients, 43–44
 to opportunistic pathogens, 37–39, 41, 46
Immunodiffusion
 compared with immunoelectroosmophoresis, 157
 for serodiagnosis, 147, 150–151, 152, 154–156
Immunoelectroosmophoresis, for serodiagnosis, 147, 151, 157–158
Influenza, and superinfection, 13
Isospora, 204
 felis, 221, 223
 rivolta, 221, 223

Kanamycin
 ineffectiveness of, 106
 resistance to, 73
 sensitivity to, 75, 78, 82
 susceptibility to, 122
Klebsiella, 26, 28–34, 44, 290
 ozaenae, 26
 pneumoniae, 26, 28
 rhinoscleromatis, 26
Klebsiella-Aerobacter, 26
Klebsiella-Enterobacter, 20, 26, 30
Klebsiella-Enterobacter-Serratia, 32, 49, 54, 61–62
Kluyveromyces fragilis, 134

Leishmania, 223
Leucosporidium, 142
Leukemia
 acute, 2
 and cytomegalovirus infection, 272
 and immunodiffusion techniques, 151, 155–156
 and infections, 2, 10, 11, 14
 susceptibility to, 43–44
 and pneumocystosis, 234, 237–238
 and prolonged therapy, 2–3
 in the compromised host, 163, 165, 166, 169, 172, 174–175, 178, 179

299

Index

Levinea malonatica, 73
Lincomycin
  ineffectiveness of, 80
  resistance to, 82
Listeria, 82
  monocytogenes, 3, 65, 66, 82
Listeriosis
  and cryptococcosis, 14
  as typical opportunistic infection, 82
Lymphoma
  and superinfection, 3, 11
  Burkitt's, and Epstein-Barr virus, 262
  in the compromised host, 167, 172, 178, 179

Melioidosis
  identification of causative organism, 25
  in Vietnam veterans, 21, 25
Meningitis
  and cryptococcosis, 148
  caused by yeast infection, 139
Methicillin, ineffectiveness of, 80
Microbispora, 188
Micromonospora, 188
Mima-Herellea, 34
Minimal bactericidal concentration, and antibiotic susceptibility tests, 120
Minimal inhibitory concentrations, and antibiotic susceptibility tests, 110, 113–114, 120, 124–125
Mitomycin C, use of, in bacteriocin typing, 52, 60, 61
Mononucleosis, infectious
  and cytomegalovirus, 269
  and Epstein-Barr virus, 261, 269

Mucor, 2, 8, 10, 156, 163, 166, 168
  corymbifera, 169
  hiemalis, 169
  ramosissimus, 169
Mucoraceae, and the compromised host, 163
Mucormycosis (opportunistic phycomycosis)
  and leukemia, 2
  detected by immunodiffusion, 148
  in the compromised host, 163–169
  serodiagnosis of, 156
Mycobacterium, 190–192, 198
  fortuitum, 187
  tuberculosis, 3, 180

Neomycin, ineffectiveness of, 106
Neoplastic disease
  affected by *Nocardia asteroides*, 179
  and cytomegalovirus infection, 272
  and pneumocystosis, 237–238
  and superinfection, 182
Nitrofurantoin
  sensitivity to, 73, 78, 82
  susceptibility to, 75
Nocardia, 121, 177, 182–193, 196, 198
  asteroides, 3, 10, 177–180, 183, 184–185, 188, 195, 198
  brasiliensis, 177–179, 183, 194–195, 198
  caviae, 177–179, 194–195, 198
Nocardiosis, 177, 178
  and cryptococcosis, 14
  diagnosis of, 180
  systemic, cause of, 179
Nosema, 223
Nosocomial infection, 19, 281–292
  and antibiotic susceptibility tests, 120

Index

and cytomegalovirus, 272
  control of, 283–292

Opportunistic phycomycosis. *See* Mucormycosis
Oxacillin, ineffectiveness of, 80

Padlewskia, 73
Papovavirus, and transplantation, 11
Pasteurella
  haemolytica, 80
  multocida, 66, 80–82
  pneumotropica, 80
  ureae, 80
Penicillin. *See also* Antibiotic therapy
  as substrate, 25
  effectiveness of, 106, 108
  need for limitation of treatment with, 291
  resistance to, 108
  sensitivity to, 80, 82, 124, 125, 184
  use of, in isolation of *Nocardia* species, 184, 185, 193
Pentamidine, treatment with, 245–249
Peritonitis
  and antibody response, 41, 45
  and reduced resistance, 42
Phagocytosis, and antibiotic therapy, 6
Phenethicillin. *See* Antibiotic therapy
Pichia, 144
Pityrosporum, 130
Pneumocystis, 3, 10, 203, 228–232, 234–249, 270
  carinii, 2, 9, 10, 228, 247

Pneumocystosis, 203, 204
  definition of, 228–232
  diagnosis of, 240–244
  disease states of, 232–240
  prevention of, 249–250
  transplacental transmission of, 239
  treatment of, 245–249
Pneumonia
  and aspergillosis, 169–171
  and pneumocystosis, 232–233, 235–236, 237, 239
  and reduced resistance, 42
  and superinfection, 6, 11
Polymixins
  ineffectiveness of, 82, 106
  resistance to, 69, 73
  sensitivity to, 82
Prednisone, treatment with, 235, 236, 240
Pregnancy
  acquisition of pneumocystosis during, 239
  and cytomegalovirus infection, 268–269, 273
  and herpes group disease, 262
  and superinfection, 13
  infection by *Toxoplasma* during, 224
  susceptibility to yeast infection during, 138
Proteus, 20, 21, 22, 30–34, 49, 50, 51, 61, 68, 69
  mirabilis, 30, 61, 68
  rettgeri, 68
  vulgaris, 30, 68
Providencia, 20, 30–33, 69
  alcalifaciens, 31
  stuartii, 31
Pseudomonadaceae, 77
Pseudomonas, 2, 3, 10, 20, 21–26, 34, 49, 75, 262, 287, 290
  acidovorans, 21, 24

Index

Pseudomonas—Continued
  aeruginosa, 21–24, 42, 50, 51, 54, 58, 60, 122
  cepacia, 21
  fluorescens, 21, 22
  maltophila, 21, 22, 26
  multivorans, 21, 22
  pseudomallei, 21, 25
  putida, 21, 22
  stutzeri, 21, 22, 24, 25, 26
Pyrimethamine, treatment with, 245–249

Radiation therapy, and herpes virus infection, 264
Retinochoroiditis, related to *Toxoplasma*, 209, 210–211
Rhizopus, 156, 163, 164–168, 174
  arrhizus, 168
  microsporus, 169
  nigricans, 169
  oryzae, 156, 168
  rhizopodiformis, 169
Rhodotorula, 136
  rubra, 139
Roll tube method
  for isolation of anaerobic bacteria, 88
  inconvenience of, 91
Rubella, congenital, and pneumocystosis, 233

Saccharomyces, 134
  carlbergensis, 134
  cerevisiae, 134
  uvarum, 134
Salmonella, 38, 70–73
  cholerae-suis, 70
  enteritidis, 70
  bioser. Paratyphi A, 70
  bioser. Paratyphi C, 70
  ser. typhimurium, 73
  typhi, 70
Sarcocystis, 223
Serratia, 14, 28–30, 40–41, 46, 69, 290
  marcescens, 28, 30, 52, 58–60, 61–62
Shigella, 38, 54, 65
  sonnei, 51
Shingles, caused by varicella-zoster, 261
Sputum analysis, quantitative, uses of, 6–7
Staphylococcus, 3
  aureus, 14, 119, 124, 287, 290
Steroids. *See also* Antibiotic therapy; Antitumor agents
  and herpes group disease, 262
  and transplantation, 10
  cortical, therapy with
    in the compromised host, 163–164, 165, 166, 167, 169, 174, 179, 211, 224
    for pneumocystosis, 236, 237–238
    for toxoplasmosis, 225
Streptococcus
  mitis, 38
  pyogenes, 119
  viridans, 38
Streptomyces, 183, 186, 187, 188, 190–191, 194–195, 196, 199
  somaliensis, 186, 194
Streptomycin. *See also* Antibiotic therapy
  ineffectiveness of, 106
  resistance to, 73
  sensitivity to, 82
Sulfonamides
  effects of, in susceptibility tests, 122

Index

ineffectiveness of, 106
   treatment with, 245–249
Superinfection, 1, 16
   and adrenal hormones, 8
   and antibiotic therapy, 3–8
   and antitumor agents, 9–10
   and cytomegalovirus, 275
   and environment, 12–14
   and needles and catheters, 8–9
   and prolonged therapy, 2–3
   and transplantation, 10
   detected by use of hypertonic media, 14–15
   dual, 6–7, 14
   related to geography, 11–12
Swarming, as characteristic of *Proteus*, 30
Syphilis
   misdiagnosis of, 211
   treated by penicillin, 125

Tests
   assimilation, for identification of yeasts, 134–135
   complement-fixation, for diagnosis of toxoplasmosis, 217
   dye, for diagnosis of toxoplasmosis, 213–216, 217
   fermentation, for identification of yeasts, 135–136
   indirect fluorescent-antibody
     for antibody detection, 149, 152–153
     for diagnosis of toxoplasmosis, 212–213, 217
   slide-agglutination, for identification of yeasts, 137
   slide-latex agglutination, for detection of antigen, 147, 149, 152, 158

Tetracycline. *See also* Antibiotic therapy
   effectiveness of, 106, 108
   need for limitation of treatment with, 290
   resistance to, 73, 108
   sensitivity to, 75, 78, 82
Torulopsis, 144, 154
   glabrata, 129, 139, 154
Torulopsosis
   detected by immunodiffusion, 148
   diagnostic serology of, 154
Toxoplasma, 204–227, 270
   gondii, 3
Toxoplasmosis, 203, 204
   acquisition of, during pregnancy, 224, 227
   acute, 209–210
   in the compromised host, 209
   chronic, 210–212
   definition of, 204–209
   diagnosis of, 212–224
   prevention of, 226–227
   treatment of, 224–226
Transfusions, blood, and cytomegalovirus, 270–271
Transplantation
   and infections, 10–11, 14, 45, 46
     by cytomegalovirus, 270, 271–272
     by herpes virus, 264
   and pneumocystosis, 235–236
Transtracheal puncture, risk involved in, 7
Treponema pallidum, 119, 126
Trichosporon, 133, 136, 144
Trypanosoma cruzi, 223
Tuberculosis
   and cryptococcosis, 14
   as nosocomial infection, 286
   in the compromised host, 172, 178

Index

Tuberculosis—*Continued*
  misdiagnosis of, 211
  similarity to nocardiosis, 180

Vaginitis, 138, 139
Vancomycin, ineffectiveness of, 80
Varicella-zoster
  clinical manifestations of, 261–262
  pathology and morphology of, 264–266
Veillonella, 102
Venereal infection
  and cytomegalovirus, 269–270
  and Epstein-Barr virus, 261
Vibrio, 77
  alginolyticus, 77
  cholerae, 77
  parahaemolyticus, 77
Vincristine. *See* Antitumor agents

Xanthomonas, 75

Yeasts
  identification and ecology of, 129–144
  infection by
    and antibiotic therapy, 7–8
    and hyperalimentation, 9
Yersinia
  enterocolitica, 66, 69, 77
  pestis, 77
  pseudotuberculosis, 77